MECHANISMS OF
CELL-MEDIATED
CYTOTOXICITY II

ADVANCES IN EXPERIMENTAL MEDICINE AND BIOLOGY

Recent Volumes in this Series

MECHANISMS OF CELL-MEDIATED CYTOTOXICITY II

Edited by

Pierre Henkart

National Institutes of Health
Bethesda, Maryland

and

Eric Martz

University of Massachusetts
Amherst, Massachusetts

PLENUM PRESS • NEW YORK AND LONDON

Library of Congress Cataloging in Publication Data

International Workshop on Mechanisms in Cell-Mediated Cytotoxicity (2nd: 1984:
Annapolis, Md.)
    Mechanisms of cell-mediated cytotoxicity II.

    (Advances in experimental medicine and biology; v. 184)
    "Proceedings of the Second International Workshop on Mechanisms in Cell-Mediated
Cytotoxicity, held June 10–13, 1984, in Annapolis, Maryland"—T.p. verso.
    Includes bibliographies and index.
    1. Cell-mediated cytotoxicity—Congresses. I. Henkart, Pierre. II. Martz, Eric. III.
Title. IV. Title: Mechanisms of cell-mediated cytotoxicity 2. V. Series. [DNLM: 1.
Cytotoxicity, Immunologic—congresses. W1 AD559 v.184 / QW 568 I62 1984m]
QR185.5.I57   1985   615.9   85-6532
ISBN 978-1-4684-8328-4   ISBN 978-1-4684-8326-0 (eBook)
DOI 10.1007/978-1-4684-8326-0

Proceedings of the Second International Workshop on
Mechanisms in Cell-Mediated Cytotoxicity,
held June 10–13, 1984, in Annapolis, Maryland

©1985 Plenum Press, New York
Softcover reprint of the hardcover 1st edition 1985
A Division of Plenum Publishing Corporation
233 Spring Street, New York, N.Y. 10013

PREFACE

        This book is derived from contributions to the Second
International Workshop on Mechanisms in Cell-Mediated
Cytotoxicity, held in Annopolis, Maryland, June 10-13, 1984.
This workshop was organized by an international committee of
immunologists interested in lymphocyte cytotoxic mechanisms (G.
Berke, W.R. Clark, P. Golstein, M. Hanna, P. Henkart, R.
Herberman, H.R. MacDonald, E. Martz, and C. Nathan), who strove
to invite participants who have made major contributions to this
field. The Workshop was a follow-up to the highly successful
1981 Workshop, whose proceedings Workshop were published by
Plenum as Mechanisms in Cell-Mediated Cytotoxicity, edited by
W.R. Clark and P. Golstein. That volume has been much
appreciated by researchers and students since it contains
accounts of most of the current approaches to understanding
cytotoxic lymphocyte mechanisms all in one volume. The present
book may be viewed as a follow-up to the first one, and in our
opinion fairly summarizes the varying current viewpoints on
lymphocyte cytotoxic mechanism.
        It should be noted that the discussions have been
transcribed directly by us, and the participants have not had an
opportunity to edit their remarks. We have tried to maintain
some of the style of the actual discussion in these transcripts.
In some cases technical problems prevented usable transcriptions
from being made, and hence not all of the actual discussion at
the workshop is reproduced here.

                                        Pierre Henkart
                                        Eric Martz

ACKNOWLEDGMENTS

The following organizations have provided invaluable financial assistance to the Second International Workshop on Mechanisms in Cell-Mediated Cytotoxicity. Their generous support is gratefully acknowledged by the Organizing Committee.

NATIONAL CANCER INSTITUTE

E.I. DUPONT CO.

GENENTECH

HOFFMAN-LA ROCHE

MERCK, SHARP AND DOHME

PFIZER

SMITH, KLINE & FRENCH

CONTENTS

SECTION 1. NON-LYMPYHOCYTE MEDIATED CYTOTOXICITY

INTRODUCTION

From a broad biological perspective, the ability of one cell type to destroy another is widely distributed in nature, and fulfills several different purposes. A study of these diverse cytotoxic systems is fascinating in its own right, but goes far beyond the scope of the present volume. In this section Bhakdi and collaborators describe lytic agents from bacteria and serum which function by creating membrane pores. As will be seen in the next chapter, these may be relevant to effector molecules from cytolytic lymphocytes.

Michel Joseph and Jerrold Weiss describe the cytotoxic mechanisms of blood platelets and neutrophils which are directed against helminths and bacteria, respectively. In both these systems, effector cell granules contain the cytotoxic components which are exposed to the targets after an initial cell surface recognition. These systems thus bear some resemblence to the granule mechanisms for lymphocyte cytotoxicity discussed in the next section.

The last three contributions in this section describe aspects of macrophage cytotoxicity. The selective lysis of tumor cells by activated macrophages was described in Mechanisms of Cell-Mediated Cytotoxicity and has been the object of continued study. It appears that macrophages can kill various target cells via several different pathways depending on the circumstances. One such route of target cell damage is described by Granger, et al., and involves oxidative phosphorylation in target mitochondria. A secreted factor with protease activity as described by Adams, et al., appears to provide another independent pathway of tumor killing by activated macrophages. Finally, macrophages can utilize their Fc receptor to provide target cell recognition, as desrcibed by Johnson and collaborators. In these circumstances reactive oxygen metabolites have been suggested to play a role in target cell damage, as previously shown by Carl Nathan and collaborators.

FORMATION OF PROTEIN CHANNELS IN TARGET MEMBRANES

Sucharit Bhakdi and Jørgen Tranum-Jensen

Institute of Medical Microbiology, Univ. of Giessen
D-6300 Giessen, GFR
Anatomy Inst. C, The Panum Institute
Univ. of Copenhagen, DK-2200 Copenhagen N, Denmark

INTRODUCTION

Many membrane-damaging proteins act at a physical level by inserting themselves into the target lipid bilayer and generating hydrophilic transmembrane channels. The first clear documentation of this principle was made in the complement field, where it was found that self-association of the terminal five serum complement components into channel-forming C5b-9 protein complexes inserting into the target bilayer constituted the molecular principle underlying the phenomenon of immune cytolysis. Subsequently, the recognition emerged that membrane damage by channel formers occurred in a similar fashion in many other instances. The present discussion will focus on the cytolytic C5b-9 complement complex and on two prototypes of channel-forming bacterial exotoxins that we have been studying. Attention will be drawn to the numerous analogies now recognized to exist among these protein systems.

Certain features appear common to all channel-formers. The proteins are produced as water-soluble polypeptides, but they undergo an irreversible transition from a hydrophilic to an amphiphilic state after binding and insertion into the target bilayer. In their final, membrane-bound form, they thus assume properties characteristic of integral membrane proteins. This is possible because of exposure of lipid-binding, apolar surfaces on the molecules that firmly anchor them to the lipid matrix. Membrane insertion and channel formation is invariably the consequence of self-association (oligomerisation) of the protein monomers on and in the lipid bilayer. Lipids and proteins of the membrane targets, although sometimes involved in the initial binding of native toxin molecules to the cell surface, probably never themselves signifi-

3

cantly contribute to formation of the channel structures <u>per se</u>.

The initial binding of the channel-formers to the membrane surface requires specific "binder" or "acceptor" molecules in some cases but may require none in others. Examples for the former category of molecules are the C9 complement component, and the sulf-hydryl-activated bacterial exotoxins such as streptolysin-O. C9 binds to membrane-bound C5b-8 "precursor" terminal complexes, whereas the sulfhydryl-activated toxins bind to membrane choleste-rol. These proteins will not bind to membranes lacking the respective binder molecules. Examples for membrane insertion of proteins without the apparent requirement for specific binders are given in the case of precursor C5b6/C5b-7 complement complexes and sta-phylococcal α-toxin. These proteins bind to Protein-free liposomes and specific lipidic binders have also not been unequivocally identified. When specific binders are present, membrane attachment is generally very effective even at low protein molarity. In con-trast, binding of proteins directly to the bilayer in the absence of a high-affinity acceptor is generally of low efficacy. For this reason, the presence of relatively high concentrations of the latter category of channel-formers as opposed to the former is usually required to generate the channels and induce cytolysis.

The protein channels may constitute a homogeneous population of structures (e.g. staphylococcal α-toxin hexamers), or they may exhibit marked heterogeneity due to the presence of varying num-bers of monomeric subunits harbored in a given polymer. Examples for the latter are the channels formed by C9, which is the major channel-forming subunit of the C5b-9 complement complex, and by the sulfhydryl-activated toxins such as streptolysin-O. The pro-cess of oligomerisation directly leads to exposure of lipid-bind-ing surfaces on the proteins due probably to changes in their conformation. The molecular basis for this unique hydrophilic-amphiphilic transition has not yet been elucidated for any single channel-former. However, structural studies at a molecular genetic level are now underway and considerable progress in this field should be made in the near future.

Although the monomeric native proteins are sensitive to proteolytic degradation, all of the oligomerized protein com-plexes studied to date have, fortunately, been found to be re-markably stable. They withstand not only the action of very high concentrations of non-ionic detergent and deoxycholate, but also resist destruction by proteases at neutral pH (Tranum-Jensen et al, 1978, Bhakdi and Tranum-Jensen, 1978, Füssle et al, 1981). Their isolation from target membranes is therefore usually quite simple – much more so than the isolation of native proteins from serum or from bacterial culture supernatants. All three protein channels to be discussed here were originally isolated from mem-branes after lysis of target erythrocytes with unpurified toxin

or complement components. The general approach has been to treat
cells with crude or partially purified toxin preparations or with
whole serum, and to subsequently isolate the channels from washed
and detergent-solubilized membranes. High concentrations of deoxycholate (250 mM) effects quantitative solubilization of erythrocyte membranes (Biesecker et al., 1979), and a single centrifugation
of membrane solubilisates through linear sucrose density gradients
in a low detergent concentration (e.g. 6-10 mM) can then already
lead to satisfactory purification of many protein channels (Bhakdi
and Tranum-Jensen, 1982, Bhakdi et al., 1983b, Bhakdi et al, 1984).
During this procedure, the large channel structures will be separated from other membrane and membrane-bound proteins. Moreover,
membrane lipids remain floating in the detergent micelles at the
top of the gradients (Helenius and Simons, 1975), so that the
channels are recovered in extensively delipidated form. The isolated channels have regularly been found to be very immunogenic,
and antisera raised against these proteins can subsequently be
used in immunological studies of the oligomerized as well as the
native proteins (e.g. Bhakdi et al, 1978).

Protein oligomerisation can often be induced simply by con-
centrating purified protein preparations and incubation at 37° C
or at higher temperatures. Spontaneous formation of the protein
channels in solution has been observed to occur in this fashion
with S. aureus α-toxin (Arbuthnott et al., 1967), Tetanolysin
(Rottem et al., 1982) and with complement component C9 (Podack
and Tschopp, 1982, Tschopp et al., 1982). On a membrane target,
and at lower, physiological concentrations, membrane "receptors"
or specific binding sites probably serve the important function
of creating the required local protein concentration. In the case
of -SH activated bacterial toxins such as Streptolysin-O, this
function is served by membrane cholesterol (Alouf, 1981). In the
case of C9, which the major channel-subunit of the complement
system, the function is served by membrane-bound C5b-8 (Kolb et al,
1972, Kolb and Müller-Eberhard, 1984, Podack et al., 1982). Such
specific binding sites may not be a general requirement for binding of other channel formers, however. Analogous "receptors" have
for instance not been identified for S. aureus α-toxin, or for
the "pre-terminal" C5b-7 complement complex.

Protein channels have been characterized on a functional basis
by determining the appearance of functional pores in the membrane.
Many experimental systems have been utilized for this purpose, including measurements of release of intracellularly trapped markers
(Giavedoni et al., 1979, Füssle et al., 1981), and conductance
measurements across planar lipid bilayers (Michaels et al., 1976).
Generally, the different experimental approaches have all yielded
data compatible with the concept of true transmembrane pore
formation (see Mayer, 1978, Bhakdi and Tranum-Jensen, 1983c).
Minor discrepancies arising with regard to the true dimensions

of the lesions have probably originated from the specific experimental conditions selected by the different groups of investigators, and from the interpretational difficulties inherent in many such systems (Bhakdi and Tranum-Jensen, 1983c).

STAPHYLOCOCCAL α-TOXIN AND STREPTOLYSIN-O: TWO PROTOTYPES OF CHANNEL-FORMING BACTERIAL TOXINS

Staphylococcal α-toxin

Staphylococcal α-toxin is produced by most pathogenic strains of staphylococci and is considered one of the major factors of staphylococcal pathogenicity (McCartney and Arbuthnott, 1978). The toxin is secreted as a hydrophilic, 3.3S monomer of M_r 34 000 (Bhakdi et al., 1981) with an isoelectric point of approximately 8.5. Upon contact with an appropriate target membrane, the monomers self-associate to form small channels that appear to represent a homogeneous population of 11-12 S hexamers (M_r 200 000; Bhakdi et al., 1981). The latter bind lipid and detergent. They generate circumscribed functional "holes" in the membrane of resealed erythrocyte ghosts whose effective diameter appears to be ∿ 2 nm (Füssle et al, 1981). In the electron microscope, the channels indeed display a central pore of these dimensions (Fig.1). The external diameter of the hexamers measures 8.5-10 nm as determined on the extramembranous portion of the cylinder. The hexamer extends approximately 4 nm into the extramembranous phase, so that the volume of the extramembranously oriented portion of the complex can be estimated to be approximately 200-250 nm^3, which already corresponds to a mass of 160-200 000 daltons. These calculations indirectly indicate that the intramembranous domain of the α-toxin rings may comprise only a small part of the total mass; the walls of the pore within the membrane have not been directly seen by electron microscopy and may in fact be much thinner than those forming the walls of the externally oriented cylinder.

Triggering of the hexamerisation process is not recognizably dependent on the presence of a biochemically defined membrane binding site (Freer et al. 1968, Füssle et al, 1981). Spontaneous hexamer formation occurs in the absence of a lipid bilayer when purified toxin is exposed to specific heating conditions (Arbuthnott et al, 1967) or to deoxycholate detergent (Bhakdi et al, 1981). Hexamers also form when toxin molecules come into contact with human plasma low density lipoprotein (LDL), probably through unspecific triggering of the oligomerisation process by lipid contained in the LDL particle (Bhakdi et al, 1983a). As with all other channel formers, toxin oligomers are hemolytically inactive, probably due to their low solubility in water. Binding and hexamer formation of α-toxin on LDL thus causes toxin inactivation and may represent a significant non-immune defence mechanism of the host towards this toxin.

The efficacy of toxin-binding to cell membrane is low: at toxin concentrations of $3 \times 10^{-8} - 10^{-6}$ M (1-30 µg/ml), less than 5 % of toxin offered to a surplus of cells becomes membrane-bound. We believe that this is due to the absence of specific membrane binders for the toxin. As toxin levels are raised, overall binding will increase to quite abruptly reach levels of 50-70 % of total toxin offered to the cells. Thus, binding of the toxin to cells in this concentration range does not exhibit characteristics of a simple ligand-receptor interaction.

Since specific binders are probably absent, the initial diffusion and attachment of the toxin to the cell surface can probably be influenced by a number of quite unspecific factors including surface charge. It is probably for this reason that different cell species display a very wide variation in overall sensitivity towards cytolytic toxin action. For example, it has long been known that human erythrocytes are lysed at toxin concentrations that are approximately 100 fold higher than those required to lyse rabbit erythrocytes (McCartney and Arbuthnott, 1978). However, we have noted a marked pH-dependence in sensitivity of human red cells towards lytic toxin action. At pH 5-5.5, these cells are lysed by toxin levels approximately five-fold lower than those required at neutral pH. We have suggested that this phenomenon derives from neutralisation of negative charges on the membrane surface which otherwise restrict diffusion of the toxin molecules to the lipidic surface through binding of the positively charged toxin (pI 8.5).

Streptolysin-O

This toxin is a secreted product of group A ß-hemolytic streptococci and represents the prototype of -SH activated bacterial cytolysins (Alouf, 1980). At least 14 other bacterial exotoxins belong to this group and share the following properties. All are reversibly inactivated by atmospheric oxygen. The initial binding of toxin is to membrane cholesterol, and membrane damage can thus be produced in a very wide variety of mammalian cells. In contrast, bacterial membranes which lack cholesterol are not attacked by the toxins. After binding to cholesterol, streptolysin-O (SLO) molecules self-associate in an apparently temperature-dependent process to form very large, curved rod structures (Duncan and Schlegel, 1975) that lie embedded within the bilayer and generate channels.

We have recently isolated SLO from bacterial culture supernatants and identified two hemolytically active forms (unpublished). Native toxin has a M_r of approx. 69 000 and an isoelectric point of approx. 6.1. During purification procedures, it can be proteolytically cleaved to yield a hemolytic 57 000 dalton polypeptide with an isoelectric point of approximately 7.4. Both

toxin forms bind to erythrocyte membranes yielding the characteristic channel structures. SLO-oligomers exhibit marked heterogeneity, and a broad array of structures ranging from C-shaped
curved rods to fully closed rings is observed (Fig. 1). These
complexes insert into the membrane to generate very large, 30-35 nm
defects in the bilayer. Functional studies also reveal the existence
of large hydrophilic pores across such membranes (Buckingham and
Duncan, 1983). The channels can be particularly well visualized
following their re-incorporation into bilayers of pure egg lecithin
(Fig. 1). When C-shaped oligomers become membrane-incorporated in
such a system, the ensuing channels appear lined only in part by
protein (Fig. 1 and Bhakdi et al., 1984). Facing the concave
sides of the protein channel, a sharp edge of lipid appears to
line the residual part of the channel. Insertion of frankly
"incomplete" channels consisting of C-shaped toxin oligomers thus
already appears to create transmembrane pores, probably because of
repellment of lipid by the hydrophilic concave sides of the mem-
brane-inserted complexes. It will be of great interest to eventually determine the state of molecular packing and orientation of
lipids in such membrane regions.

The fact that isolated and extensively delipidated toxin
oligomers can re-associate with pure lecithin serves to underline
the fact that cholesterol, although important in triggering the
oligomerisation process, does not itself significantly contribute
to the structure of the channel. Once exposed, the apolar regions
of the protein complex also exhibit no recognizable specificity
with regard to the type of lipid that can be bound (Bhakdi et al.,
1984).

Initial estimates yield volumes of SLO-oligomers ranging from
approximately 2000-6000 nm^3, corresponding to a range in mass of
1.5 - 5.0 x 10^6 daltons. This corresponds to a heterogeneous population of complexes containing a range of 25-80 molecules of
native toxin. Hemolytic titrations indeed indicate that the presence of 70-125 toxin monomers/cell suffice to generate one functional lesion per cell (unpublished results). It is clear that
such titrations can only give an indication of the true number of
lesions required to lyse a cell. They clearly suggest, however,
that very few (perhaps a single) toxin oligomers formed on a membrane will induce hemolysis.

THE CYTOLYTIC C5b-9(m) COMPLEMENT COMPLEX

The C5b-9(m) complex (the suffix "m" is used to denote the
membrane location of the molecule) forms on and in a membrane
after initiation of both classical and alternative complement
pathways, and is able to damage a wide range of biological membranes, spanning the scale from prokaryotes to mammals. Although
C5b-9(m) is the most complex protein channel recognized at pres-

ent, it was the first to be isolated and characterized at a bio-chemical, immunological and ultrastructural level. Very simple methods were first used to demonstrate its existence on target erythrocyte membranes, and to reveal its similarity to integral membrane proteins (Bhakdi et al, 1975). The complex can easily be isolated in quantity from target erythrocytes without the use of purified components, special reagents or techniques (Bhakdi et al, 1983b). Rabbit antisera raised against the purified complex react with native C5-C9 and with the C5b-9 complex (Bhakdi et al, 1978). Moreover, the complex carries characteristic neoantigenic determinants that permit its immunological differentiation from native C5-C9 components (Kolb and Müller-Eberhard, 1975; Bhakdi et al, 1978; Bhakdi et al, 1983b). Isolated C5b-9(m) recovered from sucrose density gradients can be directly utilized in membrane reconstitution studies and studied in the electron microscope.

Since complement components circulate freely in plasma, it is essential that regulatory mechanisms exist to prevent destruction of innocent cells. Major regulatory mechanisms operate at the level of C3/C3b, and the complement cascade may be arrested if C3b-inactivating mechanisms prevail to save the cell from assault by C5b-9(m) (Fearon, 1980; Kazatchkine and Nydegger, 1982). If inactivation of cell or particle-bound C3b does not occur to the necessary extent, C5 will be cleaved to its active derivative C5b. No further proteolytic cleavage of terminal C6-C9 components has been identified after this stage of the terminal reaction. C6 and C7 spontaneously associate with C5b to form a trimolecular C5b-7 complex (Kolb and Müller-Eberhard, 1972). If this complex forms in a hydrophilic phase, e.g. through complement activation in whole serum by immune complexes or alternative pathway activators, the nascent complex will be inactivated through binding of the serum "S"-protein (Podack and Müller-Eberhard, 1978); this may represent the last regulatory mechanism in the entire complement sequence. SC5b-7 will subsequently bind C8 and C9 so that a cytolytically inactive, water-soluble SC5b-9 complex forms whose biological functions, if any, remain unknown at present (Kolb and Müller-Eberhard, 1975b; Bhakdi and Tranum-Jensen, 1983c; Bhakdi and Roth, 1981).

C5b-7 forming on a target lipid bilayer will, in contrast, insert into the membrane and escape inactivation by the S-protein. It is thus at this stage that hydrophobic regions first appear on a terminal complex (Hammer et al, 1975; Hu et al, 1981). C5b-7 insertion does not, however, create membrane instability or leakiness (Michaels et al, 1976). The complex possesses one binding site (Kolb and Müller-Eberhard, 1972) for the ß-chain of C8 (Monahan and Sodetz, 1981). Binding of C8 appears to create small channels in the bilayer (Michaels et al, 1976), and erythrocytes carrying C5b-8 complexes have been reported to lyse slowly

(Stolfi, 1968). The functional dimensions of C5b-8 channels in erythrocyte membranes have been estimated to be in the order of 0.9 nm (Ramm et al, 1982b). The ultrastructure of neither C5b-7 nor C5b-8 has been established.

The C5b-8 complex serves as the binding substrate for C9 (Kolb and Müller-Eberhard, 1974; Podack et al, 1982). Initial binding of one C9 molecule to C5b-8 probably triggers an auto-catalytic reaction leading to further attachment and self-asso-ciation of C9 molecules within the complex. This causes "widening" of the pore to a maximum of 5-7 nm (Michaels et al, 1976; Giavedoni et al, 1979; Ramm and Mayer, 1980). At a certain, as yet undefined ratio of C9:C5b-8 molecules, defined channel structures are seen in the electron microscope. Analogies may here be drawn to the event of channel formation by -SH activated toxins: C5b-8 serves as the initial receptor triggering the C9-oligomerisation reaction much as cholesterol serves to initially bind SLO. Formation of ul-trastructurally visible channels per se is then the consequence of C9-oligomerisation in the former, and of toxin molecules in the latter case. In analogy to spontaneous oligomerisation occurring with -SH activated toxins (as reported for Tetanolysin, Rottem et al, 1982) and S. aureus α-toxin under specific conditions (Arbuthnott et al, 1967), isolated C9 will also spontaneously oligomerize to form the channel structures characteristic of C5b-9(m) complexes carrying high numbers of C9 (Podack and Tschopp, 1982; Tschopp et al, 1982). These channel structures have been described as hollow protein cylinders rimmed by an annulus at one terminus harbouring an internal pore of 10 nm. The cylinders are vertically oriented to the membrane plane and, when viewed en face on the membrane surface, are seen as the typical ring structures that were originally described by Humphrey and Dourmashkin (1969) as the classical complement "lesions". Membrane reconstitution studies reveal that 4-5 nm of the thin-walled portion of the cylinder distal to the annulus carry the lipid-binding sites which insert into the membrane. Frank interruptions in the continuity of the bilayer are observed at the sites of insertion of the complex, and stain deposits are seen traversing the internal diameter of the channel to enter liposomes (Fig. 2; Bhakdi and Tranum-Jensen, 1978). The micromorphology of such protein cylinders embedded within the bilayer of target erythrocytes has recently been studied by freeze-fracture electron microscopy (Tranum-Jensen and Bhakdi, 1983). The originally proposed model for fully formed C5b-9(m) complexes (Tranum-Jensen et al, 1978; Bhakdi and Tranum-Jensen, 1978) was fully corroborated using this technique. In particular, complementary replicas showed that each EF-face ring corresponded to a hole in the lipid plateau of the PF-face, and etched fractures confirmed the existence of a central, water-filled pore in the mo-lecule (Fig. 2; Tranum-Jenson and Bhakdi, 1983).

It is now recognized that the bulk of the described cylindri-

Fig. 1. A : Fragment of rabbit erythrocyte lysed with S. aureus α-toxin. 10 nm ring-shaped structures are seen over the membrane (arrows). B : Isolated α-toxin hexamers in detergent solution. C : Lecithin liposomes carrying re-incorporated α-toxin hexamers, seen as stubs along the edge of the liposomal membrane and as rings over the membrane (arrows). D : Erythrocyte membrane lysed by strep-tolysin-O showing numerous 25-100 nm long and approximately 7.5 nm broad, curved rods. Most rods are approximately semicicular, often joined in pairs at their ends. Dense accumulations of stain are seen at the concave side of the rods. When these do not form closed pro-files, the stain deposit is partly bordered by a "free" edge of the erythrocyte membrane (arrows). E : Isolated streptolysin-O olig-omers. F : Purified streptolysin-O complexes re-incorporated into cholesterol-free lecithin liposomes. The toxin oligomers form holes in the liposomes. Part of the circumference of such holes appear bordered by a "free" edge of liposomal membrane (unlabelled arrows). P : Lesion seen in profile. Scale bars indicate 100 nm in all frames. Sodium silicotungstate was used as negative stain in frames B-F and uranylacetate in A.

Fig. 2. A : Complement-lysed erythrocytes: C5b-9(m) complexes are seen as numerous circular lesions over the membrane together with some "twinned" forms (bold arrows), and as 10 nm high cylindrical projections along the bent edge of the ghost membrane (arrows). B : Isolated C5b-9(m) complexes in detergent solution. The complex has the basic structure of a 15 nm high, thin-walled cylinder, rimmed by an annulus at one end. The cylinder is seen in various levels of tilt between side views (s) and axial projection (e). C : Selection of C5b-9(m) complexes exhibiting a small appendage (arrows), often seen on the annulus. D : "Poly-C9" formed by pro-longed incubation of purified human C9 in detergent-free buffer so-lution at 37° C as described by Tschopp et al, (1982a). Occasional-ly, small ordered arrays of cylinders are seen (arrows), associated at the putative apolar terminus opposite the annulus. E and F : C5b-9(m) complexes (arrows) re-incorporated into phosphatidylcholine liposomes. Vesicles that escaped incorporation of a complex (aster-isks) are characteristically impermeable to the stain. G : Comple-mentary freeze-etch replicas of complement-lysed sheep erythrocyte. Fracture E-faces (left frame) exhibit numerous ring-shaped struc-tures, representing the intramembranous portion of C5b-9(m) cylin-drical complexes. The rings are complementary to circular defects in the lipid plateau of the inner membrane leaflet (PF-face). A number of complementary lesions are labelled by arrowheads. Inset at upper right shows C5b-9(m) annuli (arrows) on the etched true outer surface (ES) of a proteolytically stripped ghost membrane. 25° rotary shadowing with Pt. Scale bars indicate 100 nm in frames A to G. Sodium silicotungstate was used for negative staining in frames A to F. Figs. 1 and 2 reproduced with permission of The Royal Society, London.

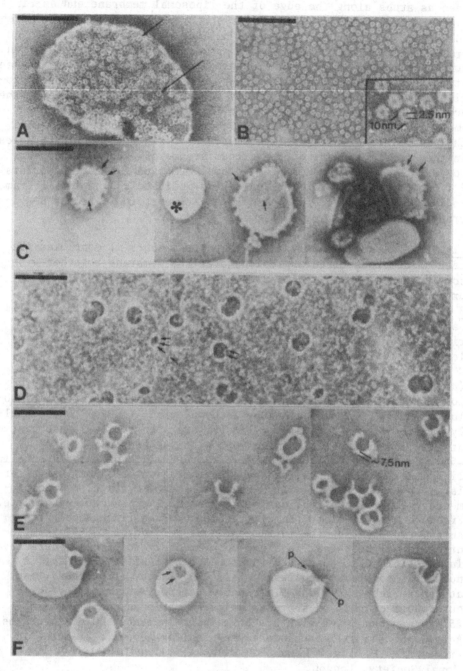

Fig. 1

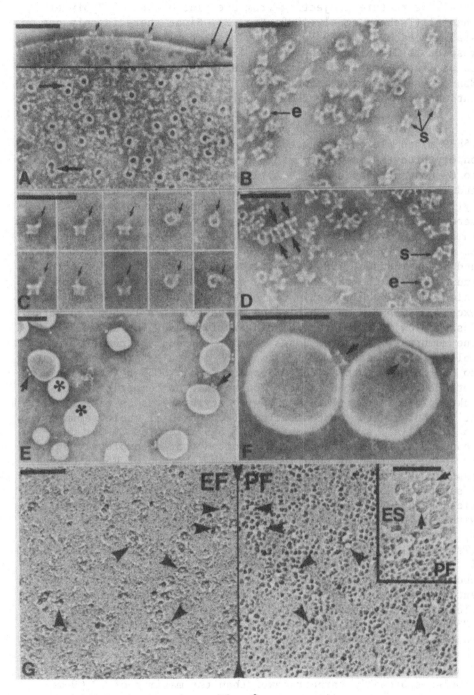

Fig. 2

cal structure is composed of C9 oligomers (Tschopp et al, 1982).
The structure and exact orientation of C5b-8 within such C5b-9(m)
remains unclear. Determinants of C5 and C6 are present on a
"stalk" structure projecting from one side of the C9 "polymer"
channel (Tschopp et al, 1982; Fig. 2). Since there is only one
stalk on each "poly-C9" cylinder, each complex is a monomer with
respect to C5b-8 (Tschopp et al, 1982; Tschopp, 1983). It seems
to us likely that the stalk structure represents but a part of
C5b-8, the other participating in formation of the channel walls,
but obscured as such by the predominating C9 structure.

Recent functional and biochemical studies have shown that
C5b-9(m) complexes generated by the action of whole human serum
on erythrocytes comprise heterogeneous populations with respect
to C9 content (Boyle et al, 1979; Ramm et al, 1982; Bhakdi
and Tranum-Jensen, 1984; Tschopp, 1983), and the typical
cylindrical structure of C5b-9(m) discussed above is characteristic only of those complexes carrying relatively high
numbers of C9 molecules. A major cause of C5b-9(m) heterogeneity
is a naturally occurring, relative shortage of C9 in serum (Bhakdi
and Tranum-Jensen, 1984). Thus, serum concentrations of both C8
and C9 are in the range of 70-80 µg/ml, equivalent to two molecules C9 for each molecule C8. At high cell concentrations and
excess of C5b-8 membrane binding sites relative to applied serum
dosage, low C9-C8 average binding ratios ensue (C9:C8 = 2-3:1 on
the membrane). As serum doses given to a constant number of target
cells are increased, more and more C9 molecules are free to bind
to C5b-8 and higher C9:C8 ratios are found. SC5b-9 formation does
not occur as a bystander reaction so that no competition for C9
takes place in the fluid-phase with erythrocytes as target cells.
At very high serum concentrations (e.g. 5-10 ml whole serum given
to 10^9 cells), a maximal average of 6-9 molecules C9 per cell-
bound C8 is found. It has been reported that a completely built
C9 channel formed by purified C9 in the absence of C5b-8 has a
mass of approximately 10^6 and is composed of 12(16) molecules C9
(Tschopp, 1983). One such channel bound to a C5b-8 monomer would
yield a C5b-9(m) complex with the subunit composition $(C5b-8)_1 C9_{12}$
with a M_r of 1.5-1.6 x 10^6. This probably represents the maximal
M_r of a completely formed, unit lesion of normal dimensions
(Tschopp, 1983). Since a maximal average C9:C8 ratio of only 6-8:1
is found in C5b-9(m) preparations, however, it is apparent that
such "complete" complexes can only represent a minority of the
entire population. On the target membrane, an array of other complexes exist with compositions probably covering the range
$(C5b-8)_{1-2}$ - $(C5b-8)_1 C9_{12}$. Close scrutiny of individual ring-
shaped lesions on the surface of target erythrocytes indeed reveals that most complexes exhibit defects of closure (Fig. 2;
Tranum-Jensen and Bhakdi, 1983; Tschopp, 1983). Although such
complexes probably harbour fewer than the maximum of 12 C9 molecules, they would still exhibit the typical cylindrical structure

when viewed in profile. Furthermore, many complexes exhibit aberrant forms, rings of smaller diameter (probably also containing fewer C9 molecules) abound within any random population of C5b-9(m) complexes, and even under conditions of C9 excess a large number of terminal complexes of ill-defined morphology exist on an erythrocyte membrane. It is not known which number of C9 bound to C5b-8 is critical for the appearance of the ultrastructurally defined cylinder forms, nor is it clear at which C9:C8 ratio the largest (maximal) functional pore (5-7 nm) appears. At present, the collective data suggest that the majority of channel-like structures has the composition $(C5b-8)_1 C9_{6-9}$ corresponding to a M_r range of $1-1.3 \times 10^6$. A dimer nature with respect to C5b-8 has been claimed in the past (Biesecker et al., 1979; Podack et al., 1980; Podack et al, 1982), but since our initial criticism of these data was voiced (Bhakdi and Tranum-Jensen, 1981), other functional (Ramm et al, 1982a) and structural studies have appeared (Tschopp et al, 1982; Tschopp, 1983) that clearly speak against the dimer model. We adhere to our original proposal that the unit lesion is a monomer with respect to C5b-8, and believe that the earlier structural data taken to support the dimer model (Podack et al, 1980) require re-investigation. The concept of lesion heterogeneity deriving from differing numbers of C9 molecules attached to C5b-8 monomers also is in contrast to the model of heterogeneity due to the parallel existence of monomer and dimer complexes as proposed by Podack et al (1982). However, our data and model are in complete accordance with those of Tschopp (1983).

CONCLUDING REMARKS

A relatively simple chain of events can be envisaged to underlie the process of membrane penetration by channel-forming proteins. The initial reaction leading to formation of the first oligomers (dimers?) is a process obviously exhibiting very slow kinetics in a hydrophilic environment. Once formed, however, these oligomers trigger a second, autocatalytic reaction that is fast, leading to generation of the channels. The oligomerisation process may be initiated through protein-binding to specific substrates. The mechanisms responsible for protein-binding in the absence of such identifiable membrane receptors are not understood.

Membrane insertion per se may be a spontaneous process driven simply by the energetically favoured hydrophobic-hydrophobic interactions. With regard to the mode of pore formation, two basic mechanisms may be envisaged. Firstly, lipid (and membrane proteins) may be expelled at the channel sites. Alternatively, a "force-aside" mechanism could cause lateral displacement of membrane constituents. In the latter case, there would be no necessity for expulsion and release of integral membrane proteins and lipids into the environment. Although the former model for channel formation has been favoured in the past (for discussion, see Bhakdi and Tranum-Jensen,

1983c), recent data from our laboratory tend to support the latter (unpublished data). Repellment of lipid (and membrane protein) may be initiated by the insertion of "incomplete", non-circularized oligomeric structures with exposure of hydrophilic surfaces within the membrane plane, such as appears to occur with the majority of streptolysin-O complexes. Complete circularization of the complexes is thus probably not even necessary for generation of functional transmembrane pores. These arguments probably also hold for C5b-9(m) complexes, where generation of lesion heterogeneity through differential binding of C9 shows obvious analogies to heterogeneity of the streptolysin-O channels.

The concept of membrane damage by channel-formers is thus now well documented and many other protein systems will probably eventually be found to operate in a similar fashion. The subject is becoming of increasing interest to immunologists since channel-formation also seems to represent an important mechanism of cellular cytotoxicity (e.g. Simone and Henkart, 1980; Dourmashkin et al., 1980; Dennert and Podack, 1983; Henkart et al, 1984). It is easy to anticipate that cell biological and pathophysiological aspects will now become most fruitful fields to explore. Obvious questions relate to the fate of membrane-bound channels, and to secondary effects possibly mediated by the proteins.

ACKNOWLEDGEMENTS

We thank Margit Pohl and Marion Muhly for outstanding technical assistance. Our studies were supported by the Deutsche Forschungsgemeinschaft (Bh 2/1-3,4,5 and SFB 47).

REFERENCES

Alouf, J.E., 1980, Streptococcal toxins. Pharmac. Ther. 11: 661

Arbuthnott, J.P., Freer, J.H. and Bernheimer, A.W., 1967, Physical states of staphylococcal α-toxin. J. Bacteriol. 94: 1170

Bhakdi, S., Bjerrum, O.J., Rother, U., Knüfermann, H. and Wallach, D.F.H., 1975, Detection of the terminal complement complex and its similarity to "intrinsic" erythrocyte membrane proteins. Biochim. Biophys. Acta 406: 21

Bhakdi, S., Bjerrum, O.J., Bhakdi-Lehnen, B. and Tranum-Jensen, J., 1978, Complement lysis: evidence for an amphiphilic nature of the terminal membrane C5b-9 complex of human complement. J. Immunol.121: 2526

Bhakdi, S. and Tranum-Jensen, J., 1978, Molecular nature of the complement lesion. Proc. Natl. Acad. Sci. US 75: 5655

Bhakdi, S., Füssle, R. and Tranum-Jensen, J., 1981, Staphylococcal α-toxin: oligomerisation of hydrophilic monomers to form amphiphilic hexamers through contact with deoxycholate. Proc. Natl. Acad. Sci. US, 78: 5475

Bhakdi, S. and Roth, M., 1981, Fluid-phase SC5b-8 complex of human complement: generation and isolation from serum. J. Immunol. 127: 576

Bhakdi, S. and Tranum-Jensen, J., 1981, Molecular weight of the membrane C5b-9 complex of human complement: characterization of the terminal complex as a C5b-9 monomer. Proc. Natl. Acad. Sci. U.S. 78: 1818

Bhakdi, S. and Tranum-Jensen, J., 1984, On the cause and nature of C9- related heterogeneity of C5b-9 complexes generated on erythrocyte membranes through the action of whole human serum. J. Immunol., in press

Bhakdi, S., Füssle, R., Utermann, G. and Tranum-Jensen, J., 1983 a, Binding and partial inactivation of S. aureus α-toxin by human plasma low density lipoprotein. J. Biol. Chem. 258: 5899

Bhakdi, S., Muhly, M. and Roth, M., 1983 b, Isolation of specific antibodies to complement components. Methods in Enzymology, 93: 409

Bhakdi, S. and Tranum-Jensen, J., 1983 c, Membrane damage by complement. Biochim. Biophys. Acta 737: 343

Bhakdi, S., Tranum-Jensen, J. and Sziegoleit, A., 1984, Structure of streptolysin-O in target membranes. In: Bacterial Protein Toxins, (Alouf, J. and Jeljaszewicz, J., eds.) pp. 173-180, Academic Press London

Biesecker, G., Podack, E.R., Halverson, C.A. and Müller-Eberhard, H.J., 1979, C5b-9 dimer: isolation from complement-lysed cells and ultrastructural identification with complement-dependent membrane lesions. J. Exp. Med. 149: 448

Boyle, M.D.P., Gee, A.P. and Borsos, T., 1979, Studies on the terminal stages of immune hemolysis. VI. Osmotic blockers of differing Stokes' radii detect complement-induced transmembrane channels of differing size. J. Immunol. 123: 77

Buckingham, L. and Duncan, J.L., 1983, Approximate dimensions of membrane lesions produced by Streptolysin S and Streptolysin-O. Biochim. Biophys. Acta 729: 115

Dennert, G. and Podack, E.R., 1983, Cytolysis by H-2 specific T killer cells. J. Exp. Med. 157: 1483

Dourmashkin, R.R., Deteix, P., Simone, C.B. and Henkart, P., 1980, Electron microscopic demonstration of lesions on target cell membranes associated with antibody-dependent cellular cytotoxicity. Clin. Exp. Immunol. 43: 554

Duncan, J.L. and Schlegel, R., 1975, Effect of Streptolysin-O on erythrocyte membranes, liposomes and lipid dispersions - a protein-cholesterol interaction. J. Cell Biol. 67: 160

Fearon, D.T., 1980, Identification of the membrane glycoprotein that is the C3b receptor of the human erythrocyte, polymorphonuclear leukocyte, B-lymphocyte and monocyte. J. Exp. Med. 152: 20

Freer, J.H., Arbuthnott, J.P. and Bernheimer, A.W., 1968, Interaction of staphylococcal α-toxin with artificial and natural membranes. J. Bacteriol. 95: 1153

Füssle, R., Bhakdi, S., Sziegoleit, A., Tranum-Jensen, J., Kranz,

T. and Wellensiek, H.J., 1981, On the mechanism of membrane damage by S. aureus α-toxin. J. Cell Biol. 91:83

Giavedoni, E.B., Chow, Y.M. and Dalmasso, A.P., 1979, The functional size of the primary complement lesion in resealed erythrocyte membrane ghosts. J. Immunol. 122: 240

Hammer, C.H., Nicholson, A. and Mayer, M.M., 1975, On the mechanism of cytolysis by complement: evidence on insertion of C5b and C7 subunits of the C5b, 6, 7 complex into the phospholipid bilayer of erythrocyte membranes. Proc. Natl. Acad. Acad. Sci. U.S. 72: 5076

Helenius, A. and Simons, K., 1975, Membrane solubilization by detergents. Biochim. Biophys. Acta 415: 29

Henkart, P., Millard, P.J., Reynolds, C.W. and Henkart, M.P., 1984, Cytolytic activity of purified cytoplasmic granules from cytotoxic rat. LGL tumors. J. Exp. Med., in press

Hu, V., Esser, A.F., Podack, E.R. and Wisnieski, B.J., 1981, The membrane attack mechanism of complement: photolabeling reveals insertion of terminal proteins into target membrane. J. Immunol. 127: 380

Humphrey, J.H. and Dourmashkin, R.R., 1969, The lesions in cell membranes caused by complement. Adv. Immunol. 11: 75

Kazatchkine, J. and Nydegger, U.E., 1982, The human alternative complement pathway. Prog. Allergy 30: 193

Kolb, W.P., Haxby, J.A., Arroyave, C.M. and Müller-Eberhard, H.J., 1972, Molecular analysis of the membrane attack mechanism of complement. J. Exp. Med. 135: 549

Kolb, W.P. and Müller-Eberhard, H.J., 1974, Mode of action of C9: adsorption of multiple C9 molecules to cell-bound C8. J. Immunol. 113: 479

Kolb, W.P. and Müller-Eberhard, H.J., 1975 a, Neoantigens of the membrane attack complex of human complement. Proc. Natl. Acad. Sci. US 72: 1687

Kolb, W.P. and Müller-Eberhard, H.J., 1975 b, The membrane attack mechanism of complement. Isolation and subunit composition of the C5b-9 complex. J. Exp. Med. 141: 724

Mayer, M.M., 1978, Complement, past and present. Harvey Lect. 72: 139

McCartney, C. and Arbuthnott, J.P., 1978, Mode of action of membrane-damaging toxins produced by staphylococci. In: Bacterial toxins and cell membranes. (Jeljaszewicz, J. and Wadström, T., eds) Academic Press, Inc. New York p. 89

Michaels, D.W., Abramovitz, A.S., Hammer, C.H. and Mayer, M.M., 1976, Increased ion permeability of planar lipid bilayer membranes after treatment with the C5b-9-cytolytic attack mechanism of complement. Proc. Natl. Acad. Acad. Sci. US 73: 2852

Monahan, J.B. and Sodetz, J.M., 1981, Role of the ß-subunit in interaction of the eighth component of human complement with the membrane-bound cytolytic complex. J. Biol. Chem. 256: 3258

Podack, E.R. and Müller-Eberhard, H.J., 1978, Binding of desoxycholate, phosphatidylcholine vesicles, lipoprotein and of the

S-protein to complexes of terminal complement components. J. Immunol. 121: 1025

Podack, E.R., Esser, A.F., Biesecker, G. and Müller-Eberhard, H.J., 1980, Membrane attack complex of complement: a structural analysis of its assembly. J. Exp. Med. 151: 301

Podack, E.R. and Tschopp, J., 1982, Polymerization of the ninth component of complement. Proc. Natl. Acad. Sci. US 79: 574

Ramm, L.E., Whitlow, M.B. and Mayer, M.M., 1982 a, Transmembrane channel formation by complement: functional analysis of the number of C5b6, C7, C8 and C9 molecules required for a single channel. Proc. Natl. Acad. Sci. US 79: 4751

Ramm, J.E., Whitlow, M.B. and Mayer, M.M., 1982 b, Size of the transmembrane channels produced by complement proteins C5b-8. J. Immunol. 129: 1143

Rottem, S., Cole, R.M., Habig, W.H., Barile, M.F. and Hardegree, M.C., 1982, Structural characteristics of tetanolysin and its binding to lipid vesicles. J. Bacteriol. 152: 888

Simone, C.B. and Henkart, P., 1980, Permeability changes induced in erythrocyte ghost targets by antibody-dependent cytotoxic effector cells: evidence for membrane pores. J. Immunol. 124: 952

Stolfi, R.L., 1968, Immune lytic transformation: a state of irreversible damage generated as a result of the reaction of the eighth component in the guinea-pig complement system. J. Immunol. 100: 46

Tranum-Jensen, J., Bhakdi, S., Bhakdi-Lehnen, B., Bjerrum, O.J. and Speth, V., 1978, Complement lysis: ultrastructure and orientation of the C5b-9 complex on target sheep erythrocyte membranes. Scand. J. Immunol. 7: 45

Tranum-Jensen, J. and Bhakdi, S., 1983, Freeze-fracture analysis of the membrane lesion of human complement. J. Cell Biol. 97: 618

Tschopp, J., Müller-Eberhard, H.J. and Podack, E.R., 1982, Formation of transmembrane tubules by spontaneous polymerization of the hydrophilic complement protein C9. Nature 298: 534

Tschopp, J., Podack, E.R. and Müller-Eberhard, H.J., 1982, Ultrastructure of the membrane attack complex of complement. Detection of the tetramolecular C9-polymerizing complex C5b-8. Proc. Natl. Acad. Sci. US 79: 7474

Tschopp, J., 1983, Ultrastructural analysis of the assembly of the membrane attack complex. Immunobiology 164: 307

DISCUSSION

Martz: Are nucleated cells generally less susceptible to these toxins than are red cells, perhaps because of repair mechanisms?

Bhakdi: Yes, nucleated cells can repair such damage, as shown by Ramm et al (J. Immunol. 131:1411), and also by Schlager and colleagues (Crit Rev Immunol. 3:165). We have always thought that endocytosis would be the most natural means for such repair, and alpha toxin lesions can be repaired quite efficiently by nucleated cells. That it not true, however, for streptolysin O, which forms such huge lesions that the cell probably does not have time for repair, and the cellular contents egress directly through the lesion.

Young: Have you tried freeze-fracture studies on C5b-8 lesions?

Bhakdi: Many times, but these structures are terribly difficult to analyze and we haven't found them yet.

Young: Is the spontaneous oligomerization of alpha toxin calcium dependent?

Bhakdi: Not at all.

Berke: Why was it necessary to have the cells lysed beforethe freeze-etching studies, since if the hole created by the C5b-9 is sufficient for lysis it should be posible to detect them prior to the lysis.

Bhakdi: It is not necessary to lyse the cells. The lysis is secondary to swelling caused by water influx, and hemoglobin is probably released in cracks in the membrane.

Weiss: In a target like gram-negative bacteria, where lipid bilayers seem accessible, do complexes like C5b-7 and C5b-8 play a double role: not only promoting oligomerization of the membrane attack complexe, but also creating membrane perturbing effects which might promote insertion?

Bhakdi: This would be a question of belief, because you can't prove it by experiment. I don't think the C5b-7 alters the structure of bacterial outer membranes to make such insertions more likely.

Podack: I would like to comment on that. I think this suggestion is correct in that you can show that C9, on red cells as well as bacteria, requires C5b-8 in order to polymerize. C9 alone, under conditions where it does polymerize, will not insert into the membrane.

Bhakdi: There are many possibilities to explain why poly-C9 won't bind that wouldn't involve a change in the membrane structure. For example, simple charge effects--C9 is a very acid molecule, with a pI of 4.6, and the bacterial surface will not let it get near.

Herberman: Could you comment on diptheria toxin, in which it has been claimed that in addition to the channel the actual toxicity is due to the A chain?

Bhakdi: In the case of such toxins, which require endocytosis to reach the lysosome, it apears that the B chain is forming some sort of channel, although the structure of the channel is not known. They may not be related to the type of channels I have discussed. They may be transient and very specific, just allowing the A chain to be released from the lysosome and get into the cytoplasm. I have always speculated that maybe the B chain is inserted into the membrane and repelling the lipids, such as seems to happen in the partial Streptolysin O lesions and probably also incomplete C9 complexes.

Herberman: So there isn't a well-defined channel?

Bhakdi: There is a well defined functional channel that can be observed in black lipid membranes.

IgE-DEPENDENT PLATELET CYTOTOXICITY AGAINST HELMINTHS

Michel Joseph, Claude Auriault, Monique Capron,
Jean-Claude Ameisen, Véronique Pancré, Gérard Torpier,
Jean-Pierre Kusnierz, Gérard Ovlaque and André Capron

Centre d'Immunologie et de Biologie Parasitaire
(Unité mixte INSERM U167-CNRS 624), Institut Pasteur
P.O. Box 245, 59019 Lille, France

INTRODUCTION

During the last decade, a growing interest has been devoted to parasite immunology, and, more precisely, to the analysis of effector mechanisms against helminths. These works have led to entirely new concepts in cellular immunology, among which the promotion of the eosinophils to the full status of cytotoxic effectors toward several species of trematodes and nematodes, or the description of receptors for IgE on cells other than mast cells and basophils, such as lymphocytes, eosinophils, macrophages and monocytes, the interaction of IgE with its specific receptor on the cell membrane being associated, in most cases, with highly efficient activation processes.

In fact, in humans and animals, the killing mechanisms, described in vitro, generally involve cellular and humoral factors, in which neutrophils, eosinophils - with an accessory role for mast cells -, monocytes and macrophages have all been shown to exhibit cytotoxic properties against schistosome larvae, in association with antibody of various isotypes or with the complement. These observations make antibody-dependent cellular cytotoxicity (ADCC) to appear as a major function in the killing of one or another stage of the parasite cycle (1).

The experiments reported here show that blood platelets, also, express cytotoxic properties against metazoan parasites, and more particularly against schistosomes, in an IgE-dependent process, and that these blood elements specifically bind the IgE isotype (2).

CYTOTOXICITY OF PLATELETS AGAINST SCHISTOSOMES

In the course of the rat infection with <u>Schistosoma mansoni</u> , a physiological concentration of platelets showed increasing killing capabilities, in the presence of either immune rat serum (Figure 1, doted bars), or normal serum (open bars), or even heat-inactivated foetal calf serum (hatched bars), with a maximum when rats expressed a high level of immunity to reinfection. The very low number, if not the absence, of contaminating leukocytes in our preparations was unable to induce, by itself, such a lethal effect. Human platelets from patients with schistosomiasis also gave high percentages of larval death in the presence of serum from either infected patients or healthy donors (Figure 1, "Infected donors").

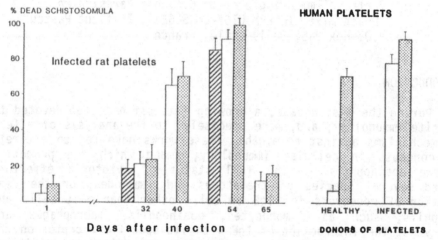

Fig. 1. Anti-schistosome cytotoxicity of platelets from infected rats or human patients (Legend in the text above).

Platelets isolated from normal individuals (humans or rats) could be induced into cytotoxic effectors by incubation with the serum of infected subjects (Figure 1, "Healthy donors"), in very narrow correlation, in the rat, with the anti-schistosome immune status of the donors (Figure 2). In the same time, the number of platelets in the blood of infected rats also increased, up to three times the normal level at the 6th week post-infection. Both parameters, cytotoxicity and thrombocytosis, then rapidly decreased after reaching the maximum value (Figure 3).

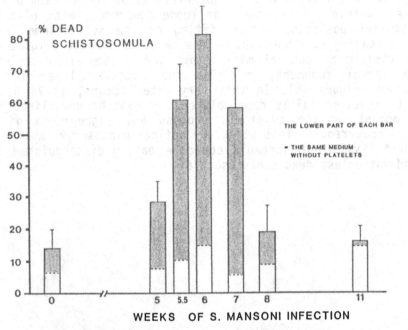

Fig. 2. Anti-schistosome cytotoxicity of platelets from normal rats
incubated in the serum of normal or infected animals.

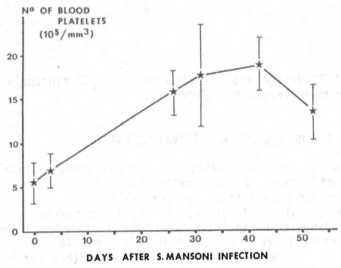

Fig. 3. Thrombocytosis in Fischer rats during experimental infection
by Schistosoma mansoni.

Optical and ultrastructural observations of the killing process presented, within 2 h, pictures of loose adherence, with platelets in equatorial position, and a lifting of the schistosome double membrane, leading to a bubbling of the parasite surface (Figure 4a), clearly visible by optical microscopy, and a complete dissolution of the larval tegument, reaching the muscular layer of the schistosome (Figure 4b). In this very late picture, at 24 h, the platelets appeared mainly degranulated. It must be underlined that at no moment of the cytotoxic process any aggregation of the platelets occurred. At this stage, by optical microscopy, mobile and refringent living schistosomula could be easily distinguished from dark and motionless dead schistosomula.

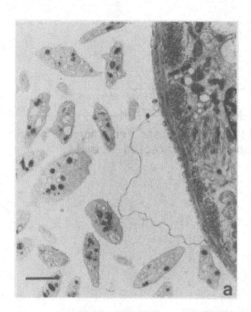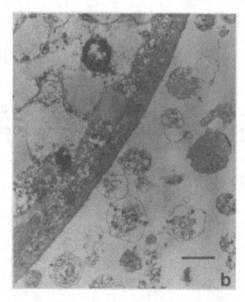

Fig. 4   a) 2h-damage and b) 24h-damage of schistosomula by immune serum-activated rat platelets.

IDENTIFICATION OF IgE AS THE ACTIVATING FACTOR

Regarding the possibility to induce normal platelets into cytotoxic effectors, an activating factor, in the serum, was investigated and proved to be IgE (Figure 5) :
- it was heat-labile and not restored by fresh serum;
- it was adsorbed on anti-IgE but not on anti-IgG immunosorbent;
- it was competitively hindered to bind to platelets by a ten-fold excess of aggregated IgE, up to a thousand-fold excess aggregated IgG being inefficient in this respect.
- the use of a polyclonal antibody directed against the receptor for

IgE on human lymphocytes, an immune serum prepared and kindly donated by Dr H.L. Spiegelberg in La Jolla (3), inhibited the cytotoxicity induced into normal platelets by the serum of infected individuals (Figure 5).

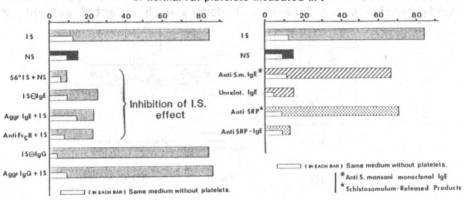

Anti-schistosome activity
of normal rat platelets incubated in :

Fig. 5.   Fig. 6.

The involvement of IgE in the activating process was confirmed by the use of a monoclonal anti-schistosome IgE, produced in our laboratory by Claudie Verwaerde, which induced high levels of cytotoxicity (Figure 6). Similarly, the serum of rats immunized with schistosome-released products, containing the major allergens of this parasite, also induced the platelet killing activity which was abrogated by IgE immune adsorption (4).

These in vitro observations have been interestingly corroborated by in vivo experiments, based on the intravenous passive transfer of immune platelets to naive animals, conferring a high degree of protection toward a challenge infection, when the same number of normal platelets was inefficient.

Taken together, the findings reported here implied the existence of a receptor specific for the Fc fragment of IgE on the surface of platelets. Preliminary results by flow cytofluorometry indicated that between 10 and 20 % of the platelets showed a positive labelling in normal individuals. This percentage was increased up to 50 % in schistosome-infected rats and in patients with schistosomiasis or with IgE-dependent allergic pathologies (5).

27

SUPEROXIDE ANION AND HYDROGEN PEROXIDE GENERATION

Regarding the cytocidal mediators of the killing mechanism described here, we investigated whether a close contact was needed or not. For this purpose, we used Boyden chambers and 0.2 μm polycarbonate filters (Nuclepore, Pleasanton, CA) to ensure the separation between the platelets and the target larvae. In these conditions, the cytotoxic process could be achieved with only a difference in the speed of action according to the distance between both partners. Such an effect was observed either by immune rat platelets (Figure 7), or by normal rat platelets with the serum of infected rats, or by human platelets from patients with schistosomiasis, or from normal donors with infected patient sera.

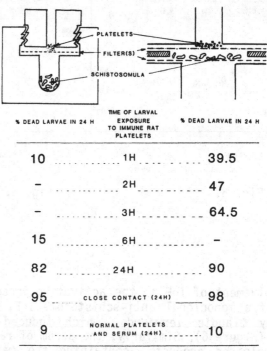

% DEAD LARVAE IN 24 H	TIME OF LARVAL EXPOSURE TO IMMUNE RAT PLATELETS	% DEAD LARVAE IN 24 H
10	1H	39.5
–	2H	47
–	3H	64.5
15	6H	–
82	24H	90
95	CLOSE CONTACT (24H)	98
9	NORMAL PLATELETS AND SERUM (24H)	10

Fig. 7. Anti-schistosome cytotoxicity of platelets through 0.2 μm nuclepore filters

Among the soluble mediators of this cytotoxicity, cationic proteins could be excluded, at least as the main agent, since platelets from patients with Gray platelet syndrome (obtained through Prof Jacques Caen, Hôpital Lariboisière, Paris), which specifically lack alpha-granules containing these proteins, killed schistosomula as efficiently as normal platelets. Thus, we investigated oxygen metabolites by chemiluminescence, using the amplifying technic described by Whitehead and coworkers (6), who observed that a mixture of luminol and luciferin is much more light-emitting than each of the reagents alone. The authors used this method to measure peroxidase in immunoenzymatic assays, by adding hydrogen peroxide to the reaction. We inverted the constituents by introducing horseradish peroxidase into the platelet suspensions, hydrogen peroxide being provided by the platelets themselves. Such a procedure allowed the detection of oxygen metabolites produced at higher rates by platelets from rats immune to schistosomes when triggered by schistosome antigens or by anti-IgE, than when incubated with anti-IgG or unrelated antigens (Figure 8).

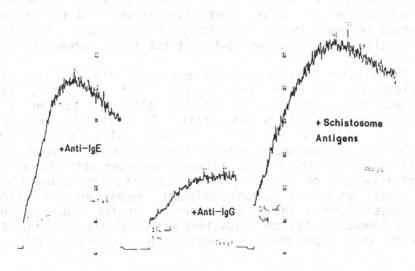

Fig. 8. Chemiluminescence of platelets from a rat infected with S. Mansoni for 50 days

Similar observations were made with human platelets from asthmatic patients : chemiluminescence was significantly higher with anti-IgE or the allergens specific of the patient sensitivity, than with anti-IgG or unrelated allergens. Platelets from healthy donors were totally insensitive to all these reagents. Furthermore, in the situation of platelets from asthmatic patients, or with platelets from normal donors passively sensitized with the serum of asthmatics, an anti-schistosome cytotoxicity was also obtained by addition of anti-IgE or specific allergens, i.e. in the very conditions of triggering which produced chemiluminescence.

These results provide good evidence that the killing mediators - this is the key of the cytotoxic process - were generated by the interaction of surface-bound IgE antibodies with their specific ligands (specific of the parasite target with platelets bearing anti-schistosome IgE, specific of the allergens with platelets bearing allergic IgE)(5).

29

CONCLUSION

All together, and considered in the general concept of IgE-dependent ADCC, mediated by various phagocytes, these observations demonstrate that the anti-schistosome cytotoxicity can be induced in vitro by specific cytophilic antibody of the IgE isotype into normal macrophages (7), eosinophils (8), and now platelets. In the three populations, the cytotoxic process can be inhibited by IgE immune adsorption but not by IgG adsorption, by competition with non specific aggregated IgE but not IgG, by preincubation with antibody directed toward the Fc epsilon specific receptor of these cells, but not by anti C3b receptor, and finally the cytotoxicity is induced in all three populations by monoclonal anti-schistosome IgE. Some recent observations by Azizul Haque and Jean-Yves Cesbron, in our laboratory, indicate that this platelet cytotoxicity is also active against first stage larvae of filarial worms.

The precise physico-chemical nature of the IgE receptor on platelets is now under investigation. But preliminary results associate this structure to the low affinity receptor already identified and analysed on other cells. It is clearly distinct from the high affinity receptor on mast cells and basophils.

The direct interaction between IgE and platelets reported here, the striking activation which follows, together with the existence of IgE receptors on several cell populations, open a new field to the investigation of immune effector mechanisms in different infectious diseases and a new approach to the understanding of various immunopathological situations where IgE are involved (9). It is with that hope that we entered in this fascinating area.

ACKNOWLEDGMENTS

The authors are greatly endebted to Prof J. Caen for supplying platelets from patients with Gray platelet syndrome, to Dr H.L. Spiegelberg for providing Fc epsilon receptor poly-clonal antibody, to Mrs C. Verwaerde and M. Damonneville for the gift of rat anti-schistosome monoclonal IgE and rat anti-schistosome-released product antiserum, respectively. They are particularly grateful to Mr H. Vorng for his expert tech-nical assistance and to Mrs A.M. Schacht for her skilful preparation of mouse monoclonal IgG anti-human IgE. They thank Prof J.P. Dessaint for his help in the word processing of this text.

REFERENCES

1. A. Capron, J.P. Dessaint, A. Haque and M. Capron, Antibody-dependent cell-mediated cytotoxicity against parasites. Progr. Allergy, 31:234 (1982).
2. M. Joseph, C. Auriault, A. Capron, H. Vorng and P. Viens, A new function for platelets : IgE-dependent killing of schistosomes. Nature, 303:810 (1983).
3. H.L. Spiegelberg, Structure and function of Fc receptors for IgE on lymphocytes, monocytes and macrophages. Adv. Immunol. 35:61 (1984).
4. C. Auriault, M. Damonneville, C. Verwaerde, R. Pierce, M. Joseph, M. Capron and A. Capron, Rat IgE directed against schistosomula-released products is cytotoxic for Schistosoma mansoni schistosomula in vitro. Eur. J. Immunol., 14:132 (1984).
5. M. Joseph, J.C. Ameisen, J.P. Kusnierz, V. Pancré, M. Capron and A. Capron, Participation du récepteur pour l'IgE à la toxicité des plaquettes sanguines contre les schistosomes. C.R. Acad. Sci. Paris, 298:55 (1984).
6. T. Whitehead, G. Thorpe, T. Carter, C. Groucutt and L. Kricka, Enhanced luminescence procedure for sensitive determination of peroxidase-labelled conjugates in immunoassay. Nature, 305:158 (1983).
7. J.P. Dessaint, A. Capron, M. Joseph, C. Auriault and J. Pestel, Macrophage-mediated IgE ADCC to helminth parasites and IgE-dependent macrophage activation, in: "Macrophage-mediated antibody-dependent cellular cytotoxicity," H.S. Koren, ed., Marcel Dekker Inc., New York (1983).
8. M. Capron, H.L. Spiegelberg, L. Prin, H. Bennich, A.E. Butterworth, R.J. Pierce, M.A. Ouaissi and A. Capron, Role of IgE receptors in effector function of human eosinophils, J. Immunol. 132:462 (1984).
9. A. Capron, J.P. Dessaint, M. Capron and M. Joseph, IgE receptors on different cell lines and their role in triggering different immunological mechanisms, in: "Proc. XII Congr. Eur. Acad. Allergol. Cin. Immunol.," U. Serafini and E. Errigo, eds. O.I.C. Medical Press, Firenze, Italy (1983).

DISCUSSION

Dennert: I have a problem understanding the IgE dependent platelet system you described with respect to the in vivo differences in shistosomiasis immunity between man, mouse and rat. In humans and mice there seems to be little or no immunity to chronic shistosomiasis infection. In rats there is an excellent immunity to such shistomosomiasis, even when the rats are thymectomized so that their antibody systhesis is largely suppressed. What then, is the physiologicalrelevance of the platelet ADCC you described in relation to these three species.?

Joseph: The in vivo relevance is certainly a crucial but unresolved question. The problem is that these in vitro mechanisms are balanced in vivo by escape mechanisms which I have not described here. Even in humans and mice there is demonstrable immunity against infection, although it is weak.

Nathan: It seems to me that we have to think about different anatomic compartments for different stages of the disease. Clearly in vivo the platelet mechanism would operate only when the parasites reside in the vascular compartment, not during skin penetration or the centers of cell-rich granulomata.

Dennert: I agree, it is a question of whether there is immunity to reinfection.

Bhakdi: What is the molar concentration of IgE in serum?

Joseph: Due to the polyclonal IgE stimulation produced by these parasites, the total IgE concentration is about 1 ug/ml, but the specific anti-parasite IgE is 10-20% of this amount. This would correspond to well under 1 nM.

Bhakdi: If the binding affinity of the receptor is $10^{-7}M$, the extent of saturation of the receptor is very small.

Joseph: We would say that this is compatible with the physiological role of IgE. It is only in special situations such as parasitic infections or allergy that the IgE levels are regulated, and the low receptor affinity would then allow the cells to acquire the IgE most physiologically relevant to the host response.

Bonavida: Could you tell us more about the nature of the cytotoxic mediators produced by platelets, especially in terms of target cell specificity.

Joseph: In addition to helminths and schistosomes, we now have evidence that other parasites are also killed, for example, microfilaria. Prof. Viance, in Montreal, has shown that trypanosomes are killed by platelets, but there is no evidence on the factors involved. We really know little about the nature of the mediators of these cytotoxic effects on parasites. We do know that oxygen metabolites are produced, but that is all we can presently say.

Bonavida: Can any IgE trigger the response?

Joseph: Yes, the specific ligand binding to any IgE bound to the surface can trigger the platelet. In the lab this can be done with anti-IgE.

Springer: Is the $10^{-7}M$ affinity constant of the receptor for monomeric or divalent IgE?

Joseph: The affinity for monomers is very much lower, the value of $10^{-7}M$ is for dimers and small polymers.

Springer: It would seem that if the purpose of the IgE receptors on these platelets is to destroy microorganisms, it would be an advantage not to be saturated by circulating monomeric IgE, but still allow binding by particles with multiple ligands giving high-afinity interactions.

Joseph: We have shown with macrophages that activation occurs with aggregated IgE or IgE immune complexes, but not by monomeric IgE. This is the work of Dessin and Metzger.

Granger: Under the conditions where you observed chemiluminescence, can you detect superoxide or H_2O_2 production?

Joseph: It is known that platelets do produce low levels of these mediators, but we found the chemiluminescence assay much more convenient. Herberman: Do you have any evidence that the oxidative burst is in fact responsible for the ADCC that you are seeing?

Joseph: We did see inhibition of the cytotoxicity with catalase and with cytochrome c, so we feel that the oxidative burst is involved, although it may not be the only source of damage. Cationic proteins do not seem to be involved, as I mentioned.

KILLING OF GRAM-NEGATIVE BACTERIA BY NEUTROPHILS: ROLE OF O$_2$-INDEPENDENT SYSTEM IN INTRACELLULAR KILLING AND EVIDENCE OF O$_2$-DEPENDENT EXTRACELLULAR KILLING

Jerrold Weiss, Michael Victor, Linda Kao, and
Peter Elsbach

Departments of Medicine and Microbiology
New York University School of Medicine
New York, New York, 10016

INTRODUCTION

The cytotoxic capabilities of the neutrophil have long been recognized, particularly in relation to this cell's function against invading microorganisms (1). Two events central to the mobilization of the cytotoxic function of the neutrophil are: 1) the respiratory burst, a prompt and marked rise in O$_2$ consumption generating, de novo, several toxic metabolites of reduced O$_2$ (2); and 2) degranulation, the fusion of cytoplasmic granules with plasma membrane sites proximate to the target delivering pre-existing cytotoxic proteins into the space surrounding the microbe (3). Both granule proteins and O$_2$ metabolites can be released outside the neutrophil and damage extracellular tissues and large non-ingested cells and parasites (4). However, substantial extracellular killing of bacteria has not been found under normal circumstances. Hence, it is generally believed that intracellular sequestration of the bacterium is required for effective killing by neutrophils (5).

Work in our laboratory has focussed on the mechanism(s) of killing of certain species of gram-negative bacteria (e.g., Escherichia coli, Salmonella typhimurium) by neutrophils. An important feature of this process revealed in earlier studies is the limited structural and functional disorganization that accompanies bacterial killing (6). This suggested that, despite the vast cytotoxic arsenal of neutrophil, only a few (or perhaps even a single agent(s) initially participate in inflicting a discrete, yet lethal lesion. The fact that disrupted neutrophils, incapable of forming toxic O$_2$ metabolites, are as actively bactericidal as intact neutrophils prompted a search for preformed substances that could conceivably account for the bactericidal activity of the intact cell toward these gram-negative bacteria (7). This led to the isolation of a single protein that not only accounts for the bactericidal activity of crude cell-free fractions but also, as will be described below, may play a principal role in the killing of ingested E.coli and S.typhimurium by intact neutrophils (8). In addition, we will show that, at least for one strain of E.coli, extracellular (non-ingested) bacteria can also be killed but apparently in an O_2-dependent fashion.

PROPERTIES OF BACTERICIDAL/PERMEABILITY-INCREASING PROTEINS

The bactericidal protein we isolated is referred to as the bactericidal/permeability-increasing protein (BPI), so named for the effects it imparts on susceptible bacteria. BPI has been purified from both rabbit and human polymorphonuclear leukocytes (PMN)(8). The two species of BPI are closely similar in all properties examined, including (sub)cellular localization, molecular structure, and biological action (8). Both proteins are present only in neutrophilic (heterophilic in rabbit) PMN and are localized in cytoplasmic granules. The two proteins are similar in molecular size (50-60 Kd), both are highly cationic (pI $\geq$ 9.6) and each protein exhibits hydrophobic properties. Foremost in their similarity is their specific and potent (LD$_{50}$:$\sim$10^{-8}M vs. 10^7 bacteria/ml) action toward several species of gram-negative bacteria.

The specificity of BPI action is determined mainly at the bacterial surface by the selective and avid interaction of BPI with the gram-negative bacterial outer membrane, the unique outer envelope layer of these microorganisms (9). Major determinants of the surface properties of these bacteria are the lipopolysaccharides (LPS), which are localized almost exclusively in the outer leaflet of the outer membrane (Fig1;9). LPS contains a cluster of negatively charged groups at the base of the polysaccharide chain adjacent to the hydrophobic lipid A moiety (Fig.1). These sites contain tightly bound divalent cations (Mg^{2+},Ca^{2+})(9,10) which are needed to maintain the structural stability of the outer membrane (11). The cationic BPI competes with Mg^{2+} and Ca^{2+} for the surface anionic sites, competing most effectively when the polysaccharide chain of LPS is short (8,12). When these charge-charge interactions are followed by hydrophobic interactions between BPI and, probably, lipid A (8,13), the LPS layer is disrupted (14) and several alterations, principally affecting the outer membrane, are almost immediately ($\leq$15s) apparent (8,13). These changes include: 1) an increase in outer membrane permeability to small, normally impermeant, hydrophobic substances such as actinomycin D; 2) degradation of outer membrane phospholipids (15) and peptidoglycan; and 3) cessation of biosynthesis of a major outer membrane protein, omp F, that forms pores needed for uptake of small hydrophilic molecules (e.g. nutrients) (Fig. 1; 9). By contrast, normal biosynthesis of virtually all other proteins and other macromolecules

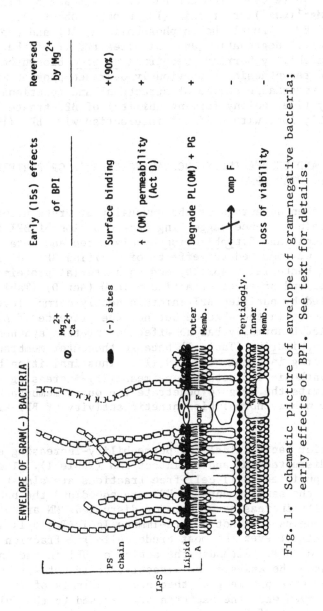

Fig. 1. Schematic picture of envelope of gram-negative bacteria;
early effects of BPI. See text for details.

continues for at least 30 min, as does K^+ transport, indicating that the biochemical machinery and energy-producing apparatus associated with the inner membrane remain intact. This localization of BPI's effects to the outer envelope layers reflects the superficial location of most of the bound BPI (8,12,13). Approximately 90% of the bound BPI can be removed from the bacterial surface by high concentrations of $Mg^{2+}(Ca^{2+})$ or trypsin (13, unpubl. observ.). Removal of surface-bound BPI abruptly halts phospholipid (16) and peptidoglycan (unpubl. observ.) degradation and initiates repair of the outer membrane permeability barrier (requiring de novo biosynthesis of LPS (14)) and resynthesis of previously degraded phospholipids (16). Despite this remarkable degree of structural and functional integrity, the viability (i.e. colony-forming ability) of BPI-treated bacteria is irreversibly lost within 15s of interaction with BPI (13).

BACTERICIDAL AND PERMEABILITY-INCREASING EFFECTS OF PURIFIED BPI, DISRUPTED AND INTACT PMN

We have taken advantage of the unusually discrete nature of BPI's action to obtain evidence suggesting participation of BPI in the killing of E.coli and S.typhimurium by disrupted and intact PMN. For this purpose, we compared the effects of purified BPI, disrupted and intact PMN on bacterial viability and on bacterial protein synthesis in the absence and presence of actinomycin D (Act D) (Table I). Bacteria killed by purified BPI maintain nearly normal levels of protein synthesis in the absence but not the presence of Act D (Table I). Act D normally has no effect on protein synthesis by E.coli or S.typhimurium (Table I) because the outer membrane blocks entry of the drug into the cell (9,11). Thus inhibition by Act D of protein synthesis reflects the permeability-increasing effect of BPI which permits the drug to penetrate the outer membrane and inhibit the otherwise nearly normal biosynthetic activity of BPI-killed bacteria.

Very similar bactericidal and permeability-increasing effects are produced by disrupted PMN and by intact PMN (Table I). The activities of crude and purified (BPI) cell-free fractions are almost exactly the same when the same amounts of BPI are added and the bactericidal and permeability-increasing effects of disrupted PMN are blocked by anti-BPI antibodies (but not by pre-immune IgG) (Table I) indicating that the effects of even the most crude cell-free fraction is due to the action of BPI. Although the action of BPI in the intact neutrophil cannot be assessed as directly, it is noteworthy that the discrete outer envelope lesions that are a hallmark of BPI action are also manifest even when the bacteria are exposed to the full antibacterial equipment of the intact PMN.

Table I. Bactericidal and permeability-increasing activities of purified BPI, disrupted and intact PMN. The values shown represent the mean of data compiled from previously published and unpublished experiments with several strains of E.coli and S.typhimurium. See references 12 and 17 for further details of experimental procedures.

Addition to Bacteria:	Bacterial Viability	^{14}C-amino acids → TCA ppt	
		-ActD	+ActD
	(% of bact. incub. alone)		
None	100	100	105
Purified BPI	< 1	90	10
Disrupted PMN	< 1	70	5
" + anti-BPI IgG	106	90	100
Intact PMN	5	80	8

39

Based on these and related findings, we have concluded that BPI is the principal pre-existing bactericidal agent in PMN toward E.coli, S.typhimurium, and certain other species of gram-negative bacteria (8,17). To indirectly assess its effectiveness in the intact neutrophil, we have measured bacterial killing under conditions in which the formation of the other major group of cytotoxic substances elaborated by intact PMN, those derived from the respiratory burst, is blocked. This is accomplished either by depleting O$_2$ from suspensions of normal PMN or by use of abnormal PMN (e.g. from patients with chronic granulomatous disease (CDG) that inherently are unable to mount a respiratory burst (2).

Table II shows that prior flushing of cell suspensions with N$_2$ almost completely eliminates the respiratory burst normally provoked when bacteria are added to PMN indicating the effectiveness of O$_2$ depletion. N$_2$ flushing does not reduce PMN killing of BPI-sensitive S.typhimurium MR10 (Table II). After 30 min incubation of 20 Salmonellae/PMN, only 5% of the added Salmonella remain viable outside the PMN either under room air or N$_2$. Brief sonication to lyse PMN and release intracellular bacteria does not increase the number of viable bacteria measured indicating no intracellular survival of Salmonella either in the presence or absence of O$_2$. By contrast, the ability of PMN to kill BPI-resistant Staphylococcus epidermidis is greatly diminished under N$_2$ (Table II). Increased bacterial survival under N$_2$ is apparent only after sonication indicating that ingestion is normal but intracellular killing of Staphylococci is impaired. The same results are obtained when the Salmonellae and Staphylococci are together added to the PMN: killing of the Salmonellae is equally effective under room air or N$_2$ but killing of Staphylococci is nearly abolished under N$_2$.

The effectiveness of O$_2$-independent killing of Salmonella by PMN is equally apparent under conditions of maximum bacterial challenge and also when a more virulent strain of S. typhimurium is tested. Testing from 5 bacteria/PMN to 160 bacteria/PMN, no difference in killing of either the rough(MR10) or the more virulent smooth (MS395) strain is detected under room air or N$_2$ (17). In both the presence and absence of O$_2$, roughly 70-80 MR10 or 30-40 MS395 are killed/PMN (17). Under no conditions are viable bacteria detected inside the PMN (17).

These findings indicate that O$_2$-independent bactericidal system(s) alone are sufficient to kill all ingested Salmonella, whether an avirulent or virulent (mouse-model) strain is tested. Okamura and Spitznagel have reported very similar findings using six different strains of S. typhimurium and aerobic or anaerobic human PMN (18). The possibility that traces of residual respiratory burst activity after N$_2$ flushing are actually responsible for the efficient killing of ingested Salmonella is unlikely for several reasons: 1) intracellular killing of S. epidermidis is greatly

Table II. Effect of N_2 flushing on bactericidal and respiratory burst activities of rabbit PMN. See reference 17 for further experimental details.

Incubation conditions		Bacterial survival (%)		Resp. Burst*
Bacteria	N_2	-sonic.	+sonic.	(fold stimul.)
S.typhimurium MR10	-	5	3	14
(20/1)	+	6	6	0.5
Staph.epidermidis	-	18	24	5
(10/1)	+	19	71	0.1
S.typhimurium MR10	-	4	4	
(20/1)	+	1	1	
+				
Staph.epidermidis	-	13	29	
(10/1)	+	19	86	

*Hexose monophosphate shunt ($[1-^{14}C]$glucose $\rightarrow$ $^{14}CO_2$).

impaired by N_2 flushing; 2) the _Salmonella_ strains used produce both superoxide dismutase and catalase (17) which should protect against the small increments of O_2 metabolism; and 3) leukocytes from a patient with CGD killed the smooth strain of _S. typhimurium_ nearly as effectively as did normal leukocytes.

The effectiveness of O_2-independent killing of _S. typhimurium_ MS395 is particularly striking in view of the greater resistance of that bacterium to killing by isolated (cell-free) BPI (12). However, this and other smooth strains of _S. typhimurium_ and _E. coli_ are effectively killed when higher (3-10-fold) concentrations of BPI are provided. BPI content in PMN is approx. 0.1 mg/10^8 cells (determined by radioimmunoassay) suggesting that concentrations of BPI within the phagocytic vacuole may approach 5 mg/ml. This concentrated setting may render differences in affinity of BPI for rough and smooth strains unimportant and provide such favorable conditions for the action of BPI that its activity can match any rate of ingestion, even of relatively resistant smooth strains (17).

BINDING OF BPI TO INGESTED E. COLI: EVIDENCE FOR O_2-INDEPENDENT
INTRACELLULAR KILLING AND O_2-DEPENDENT EXTRACELLULAR KILLING

If BPI acts within the intact neutrophil, it must attach to
ingested susceptible bacteria. To determine whether binding of BPI
to intracellular bacteria indeed takes place, we employed immunofluorescence to visualize surface-bound BPI. For these studies, we used
E. coli S15 which form somewhat longer rods than other strains of
E. coli and S. typhimurium we had available making visualization
of the bacteria easier. E. coli killed by either crude or purified
(BPI) cell-free fractions are brightly fluorescent when treated with
rabbit anti-BPI serum and, after washing, rhodamine-labeled swine
(anti-rabbit Ig) antibodies. This staining is specifically due to
the reaction of anti-BPI antibodies with BPI bound to E. coli because
no staining is seen when BPI-killed E. coli are treated with pre-
immune serum nor when either serum is used to treat E. coli not exposed to BPI.

To examine E. coli incubated with intact PMN by immunofluorescence, the same procedure was carried out except that the cell
suspensions were first sonicated to disperse the bacteria. Heparin
was added to prevent binding of BPI to E. coli during the disruption
of the PMN (19).

These experiments yielded two surprising results: first,
following 60 min incubation of 10 E. coli/PMN in room air, nearly
all bacteria are killed but only about half show fluorescent staining;
second, following similar incubations under N_2, again only half of
the bacteria are stained and also only 50% are killed. In contrast
to the increased survival under N_2 of S. epidermidis (Table II),
the viable E. coli form colonies both before and after sonication
suggesting that increased survival of E. coli under N_2 is extracellular.

This suspicion was confirmed by separation of PMN-associated
and extracellular E. coli by low-speed sedimentation of PMN. Nearly
all viable E. coli recovered from O_2-depleted cell suspensions are
extracellular. Uptake of E. coli by PMN is very similar under room
air and N_2 but, at maximum, only about 50% of the added E. coli are
PMN-associated. These PMN-associated E. coli are efficiently killed
under both room air and N_2; most are killed within 5 min and nearly
all are dead after 30 min. The other 50% of E. coli that remain
extracellular are also nearly completely killed under room air
(after an initial delay of 15 min) but not when O_2 is replaced by N_2.

Thus, in room air, nearly equal numbers of E. coli S15 are killed
inside and outside the PMN. O_2-depletion does not appreciably
reduce killing of PMN-associated E. coli but nearly abolishes killing
of extracellular bacteria. We conclude, therefore, that PMN can

kill E. coli S15 by O_2-independent intracellular mechanisms and by O_2-dependent extracellular means.

Examination of PMN-associated and extracellular E. coli by immunofluorescence with anti-BPI serum reveals bright fluorescent staining of E. coli recovered in the PMN pellet after as little as 5 min incubation (Fig.2B) but no staining of extracellular E.coli at any time (up to 60 min) (Fig.2C). This staining is specifically due to reaction of anti-BPI antibodies with bound BPI since no staining is seen following pre-immune serum treatment. BPI binds to E. coli within the intact neutrophil and not during the disruption of the PMN by sonication that is carried out to disperse the bacteria; whole suspensions of E. coli and PMN sonicated without prior incubation show little or no bacterial fluorescence (Fig.2A).

Thus BPI binds rapidly to ingested E. coli. The absence of BPI on extracellular bacteria confirms that these bacteria were not ingested and, therefore, in room air were killed by extracellular mechanisms.

SUMMARY

To summarize, our studies have revealed two mechanisms of killing of E. coli and S. typhimurium by neutrophils(Fig.3).

For many strains of these two bacterial species, ingested bacteria are efficiently killed by O_2-independent mechanisms. Intracellular killing depends not on de novo generation of toxic products of the respiratory burst but rather on intracellular delivery to pre-existing cytotoxic proteins. The principal O_2-independent bactericidal system toward these bacteria appears to be BPI which rapidly binds to ingested bacteria and whose discrete action closely resembles the initial lesions produced by the intact neutrophil. In addition, at least for one strain of E. coli (S15), extracellular bacteria can be killed in an O_2-dependent fashion.

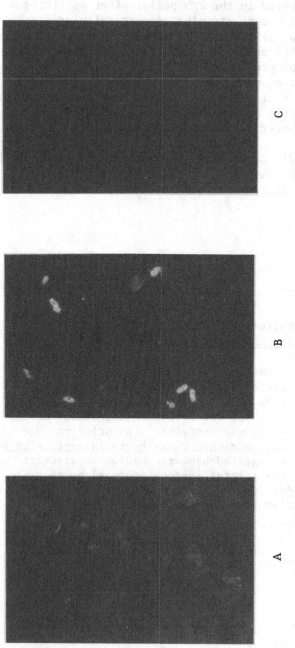

A   B   C

Fig.2. Immunofluorescent staining of E.coli S15 incubated with intact PMN. A) Whole cell suspensions (0 min); B) PMN pellet (5 min); C) extracellular supernatant (30 min). PMN pellet and extracellular supernatant were separated by centrifugation (100xg;10 min). All samples were sonicated to lyse PMN and disperse bacteria, dried and fixed on a microscope slide, treated with rabbit anti-BPI serum and, after washing, treated with rhodamine-labeled swine (anti-rabbit Ig) IgG. Sodium heparin (50 units/ml) was added before sonication to prevent attachment of BPI to E.coli during disruption of PMN. E.coli S15 are 1-2 microns in length.

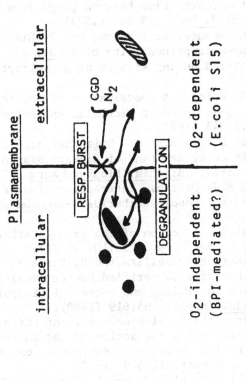

Fig.3. Schematic summary of findings on killing of E. coli and S. typhimurium by neutrophils. Shaded intracellular bacterium represents BPI-coating.

REFERENCES

1) Metchnikoff, E. "Lectures on the Comparable Pathology of Inflammation" (translated by F.A. Starling and E.H. Starling) Kegan, Paul, Trench, Truber, London (1893).

2) Babior, B.M. O2-independent microbial killing by phagocytes. New Eng. J. Med. 298:659 (1978).

3) Hirsch, J.G. and Z.A. Cohn. Degranulation of polymorphonuclear leukocytes following phagocytosis of microorganisms. J. Exp. Med 112:1005 (1960).

4) Clark, R.A. Extracellular effects of the myeloperoxidase-hydrogen peroxide-halide system. Adv. Inflamm. Res. 5:107 (1983)

5) Densen, P. and G.L. Mandell. Gonococcal interactions with polymorphonuclear neutrophils: Importance of the phagosome for bactericidal activity. J. Clin. Invest. 62:1161 (1978).

6) Elsbach, P. On the interaction between phagocytes and micro-organisms. N. Engl.J. Med. 289:846 (1973).

7) Beckerdite, S., C. mooney, R. Franson, and P. Elsbach. Early and discrete changes in permeability of E.coli and certain other gram-negative bacteria during killing by granulocytes. J. Exp. Med. 140:396 (1974).

8) Elsbach, P. and J. Weiss. A reevaluation of the roles of the O2-dependent and O2-independent microbial systems of phagocytes. Rev. Infect. Dis.5:843 (1983).

9) Lugtenberg, B. and L. van Alphen. Molecular architecture and functioning of the outer membrane of Escherichia coli and other gram-negative bacteria. Biochim. Biophys. Acta 737:51 (1983).

10) Schindler, M. and M.J. Osborn. Interaction of divalent cations and polymixin B with lipopolysaccharide. Biochemistry 18:4425 (1979).

11) Leive, L. The barrier function of the gram-negative bacterial envelope. Ann. N.Y. Acad. Sci. 235:109 (1974).

12) Weiss, J., S. Beckerdite-Quagliata,and P. Elsbach. Resistance of gram-negative bacteria to purified bactericidal leukocyte proteins. Relation to binding and bacterial lipopolysaccharide structure. J. Clin. Invest. 65:619 (1980).

13) Weiss, J., M. Victor,and P. Elsbach. Role of charge and hydrophobic interactions in the action of the bactericidal/permeability0increasing protein of neutrophils on gram-negative bacteria. J. Clin. Invest. 71:540 (1983).

14) Weissl J., K. Muello, M. Victor, and P. Elsbach. The role of lipopolysaccharides in the action of the neutrophil bactericidal/permeability-increaing protein on the bacterial envelope. J. Immunol. 132:3109 (1984.

15) Weiss, J., S. Beckerdite-Quagliata, and P. Elsbach. Determinants of the action of phospholipases A on the envelope phospholipids of Escherichia coli. J. Biol. Chem. 254:10010 (1979).

16) Weiss, J., K. Schmeidler, R.C. Franson, S. Beckerdite-Quagliata, and P. Elsbach. Reversible envelope effects during and after killing of Escherichia coli by a highly purified rabbit poly-morphonuclearleukocyte fraction. Biochim. Biophys. Acta 436: 154 (1976).

17) Weiss, J., M. Victor, D. Stendahl, and P. Elsbach. Killing of
     gram-negative bacteria by polymorphonuclear leukocytes. Role
     of an O_2-independent bactericidal system. J. Clin. Invest.
     69:959 (1982).

18) Okamura, N. and J.K. Spitznagel. Outer membrane mutants of
     Salmonella typhimurium LT-2 have lipopolysaccharide-dependent
     resistance to bactericidal activity of anaerobic human neutro-
     phils. Infect. Immun. 36:1086 (1982).

DISCUSSION

Podack: Is there any evidence for polymerization of the BPI, and do you find it any other cells?

Weiss: Regarding the first question, largely no, although there is some evidence from early studies with rabbit BPI that the 50kd molecule might be composed of subunits. Regarding the second question, we have looked particularly at other blood cells and find BPI only in PMN.

Young: Is BPI hemolytic to red blood cells?

Weiss: No.

Adams: On the independence of BPI and oxygen, we have found in our macrophage system that oxygen can be active at very low levels, e.g., 10^{-6} to 10^{-7}M, particularly in cooperation with a lytic cofactor. So can you take the two bacterial strains and determine if there is a requirement for trace of reactive oxygen species by doing a dose-response titration of ROI in the presence and absence of BPI.

Weiss: That's a fair question. The removal of the last traces of oxygen so that the respiratory burst becomes supressed is difficult. We have not done the experiment you suggested. We have measured BPI activity under the same kind of anaerobic conditions that we generate the cells, and we see no difference, even though the oxidative burst is reduced to less than 5%. This level of oxygen depletion is very effective in abolishing the killing of Staphococcus epidermitus and also the extracellular killing of E. coli. The strains that we use, particularly Salmonella, but E. coli as well, have significant amounts of superoxide dismutase and catalase which should be effective in scavenging small amounts of oxidatgive metabolites. Finally, we have been able to reproduce the results I discussed with the cells of patients with CGD.

Nathan: Have you found any disease or difficiency state of BPI?

Weiss: No.

Nathan: How specifically does BPI inflict its irreversible injury to viability?

Weiss: We're not sure. We have been intrigued with the recent observation that it blocks formation of the outer membrane porin, which is clearly required for viability. But there are problems with taking that too seriously. For example, there is a

reservior of the presynthesized porin. One can also obtain
mutants of ombeth which have only 1% of normal levels and still
have nearly normal growth capabilities. But ombeth is subject to
regulation by various environmental stimuli, e.g. osmotic
conditions, and the mechanisms of this regulation have been
worked out in great detail and appear to involve regulatory
proteins located in the zones of adhesion between inner and outer
membranes. The first step in BPI induced irreversible loss in
viability could occur here.

Nathan: Have you identified any resistant strains where
the resistanace is not due to the failure of BPI to bind?

Weiss: No.

Nathan: Does BPI have any effects on non bacterial cells?

Weiss: We are impressed by its specificity. It really
only works on Gram-negative bacteria, which probably reflects the
unique character of their envelope.

Seaman: If the CGD cells will kill Salmonella typhurium,
will the monocytes from those patients do it?

Weiss: Good question, but I don't know specifically.
There is an intriguing analogy, starting 10-15 years ago in
studies on mechanisms of virulence and intraphagocytic survival
of Salmonella typhum. About 1970 Miller and coworkers showed
that virulent strains of S. typhi were ingensted in equal amounts
as wereavirulent strains, but unlike the latter, the virulent
strains muted the normal oxidative burst triggered by ingestion
of the bacteria. Based on that it was proposed that the
oxidative burst was an important factaor in the virulence of
those organisms. However, about a decade later, Mandel and
coworkers repeated these experiments in neutrophils and measured
additional parameters such as bacterial killing. They reproduced
the results on the oxidative burst, but found that the two
strains were equally effectively killed. We would say this is no
surprise, but in a mononuclear cell with no BPI those cells may
be at risk.

Young: The PMN granules also contain other protein
species, isolated under similar conditions to BPI, on of which is
a 28kd protein called by some workers chymotrypsin-like protein.
Johnsson and Venge have shown that this is very hemolytic. Have
you looked at this protein for bacterial killing?

Weiss: Those laboratories studied a group of 4-5 cationic
proteins with chymotruptic activity many years ago. They kill a
wide range of cells, including E. coli and Staph aureus. They

differ from BPI in several important respects. For one, they require as much as 50-fold more protein to kill E. coli. Secondly, killing is accompanied by much more diffuse target cell damage.

Young: Could you give us the relative quantities of those two proteins in the granules?

Weiss: There are 3-5-fold more of the chymotryptic proteins.

Bhakdi: Could you explain how you distinguish between extracellular and intracellular killing?

Weiss: Our primary means of differentiating these is by viability before and after sonication. If the viability is the same before and after sonication, we conclude that viable bacteria were extracellular. Subsequently we have used other means to verify this.

Granger: Could BPI be an enzyme, for example a lipase?

Weiss: Lipases were in fact dear to our hearts before we discovered BPI. BPI and phospholipase A2 copurify through many steps, and the permeability effects we observed were mirrored by phospholipid degradation. We therefore thought that BPI was itself a lipase or that the two worked in close collaboration. However we have now completely separated the two proteins by further purification, and BPI maintains its activity without the phospholipase A2. Furthermore one can produce a strain of bacteria which lacks its own phospholipid degrading activities (which are important contributors to the phospholipid degradation we normally measure), and under those conditions there is no measureable phospholipid degradation but BPI remains bacteriocidal.

ABERRANT OXYGEN METABOLISM IN NEOPLASTIC CELLS

INJURED BY CYTOTOXIC MACROPHAGES

Donald L. Granger[1], Albert L. Lehninger[2],
and John B. Hibbs, Jr.[3]

[1] Department of Medicine, Duke University
School of Medicine, Durham, NC 27710
[2] Department of Physiological Chemistry,
Johns Hopkins University School of Medicine,
Baltimore, MD 21205
[3] Veterans Administration Medical Center and
Department of Medicine, University of Utah
College of Medicine, Salt Lake City, UT 84148

INTRODUCTION

The focus of this workshop is to explore the mechanisms by which leukocytes injure other cells. Macrophages are particularly unique cells to study for two reason. First, cytotoxicity may not always be manifested as a lytic event. The early work of Evans and Alexander clearly demonstrated the profound and long-term antimitotic effect macrophages exert on neoplastic targets (1). When death does occur it may be many hours following the arrest of cell division. In no other effector-target cell interaction is the complete cessation of reproduction so dissociable from cell death and such a paramount feature of cell injury. Secondly, the efficiency and spectrum of macrophage-mediated cytostasis is remarkable. Under appropriate in vitro conditions virtually all added cells of a given target cell line are prevented from dividing. Furthermore, of the numerous neoplastic cell types which have been studied, none are capable of dividing in the presence of macrophages which have differentiated to the cytotoxic state (2). Our contribution to this conference deals with macrophage cytostasis. We have studied metabolic changes which occur in neoplastic cells upon contact with mouse peritoneal cytotoxic macrophages (CM) in vitro. These studies followed an observation that macrophage-injured neoplastic cells developed an unusual carbohydrate dependence. It is possible that understanding changes which occur in target cells upon CM-induced injury may provide insight into defining the biochemical mechanism(s) by which CM exert their universal antimitotic action.

INJURY OF L1210 LEUKEMIA CELLS BY CYTOTOXIC MACROPHAGES: CYTOSTASIS WITHOUT LYSIS

In general, studies on macrophages cytotoxicity have focused on death of neoplastic cells as a measure of cell injury. The transformed cell lines used as targets for macrophage killing have been selected on the basis of susceptibility to lysis rather than propensity to cause malignant disease. We set out in search of highly malignant cell types which might be resistant to macrophage-induced cytolysis. It was observed that lymphoblastic leukemia line 1210 (L1210) cells were not killed by CM under culture conditions where other transformed cell types were readily lysed (3). However, L1210 cells were clearly injured by CM since target cell division was totally arrested. This result of CM-induced injury (i.e., cytostasis not progressing to cytolysis) had been observed by Krahenbuhl et al. for a murine breast carcinoma cell line, EMT-6 (4). The phenomenon has subsequently been substantiated by Cook et al. who surveyed a variety of cell lines transformed by different oncogenic viruses (5).

L1210 cells continue to divide for about 4-6 hours following initial exposure to CM, then target cell division stops (Figure 1). During the ensuing 70-90 hours these cells fail to divide but remain viable. This result cannot be due to the combined effects of division of a portion of target cells and death of another portion because the total number of L1210 cells remains constant while measurement of cell death by isotope release reveals that very few CM-injured L1210 cells die (6). After 20 hours coculture, L1210 cells were separated from CM, washed, and recultured in fresh medium. Despite removal from CM, injured L1210 cells failed to divide during a subsequent 50-hour culture period (Figure 2). Once CM-induced cytostasis is established, the effect is independent of macrophages and persists long beyond the initial coculture period. Macrophage-induced cytostasis is not the result of depletion of a nutrient such as arginine (7) since L1210 cell division remains inhibited upon resupplying with fresh nutrients (Figure 2). Additionally, it was found that the medium from CM-L1210 cell cocultures supported exponential growth of uninjured L1210 cells (Figure 3). These same arguments apply in ruling out the possibility that CM-induced cytostasis in this system results from the elaboration of a macrophage product into the culture medium which inhibits L1210 cell division (e.g., thymidine [8]).

The ultimate fate of CM-injured cells was studied. L1210 cells were cocultured with CM for 20 hours, then separated from macrophages, and recultured for prolonged periods with daily nutrient replenishment. At 60-80 hours following removal of CM, L1210 cell

division recommenced with the usual 12-13 hour generation time (9).
Experiments using CM-injured L1210 cells cultured individually
revealed that at least 50% of these cells recover the capacity for
cell division. Macrophage-induced injury in this experimental
system is a reversible process (9). This same phenomenon had been
noted by Krahenbuhl et al. in earlier studies (4).

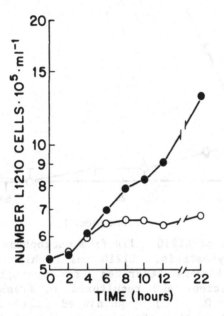

Figure 1: Induction of L1210 cell division arrest by CM. L1210
cells were culture alone (o) and with CM (o). At the
times shown cell counts were made. Viability remained
greater than 95% in both types of cultures.

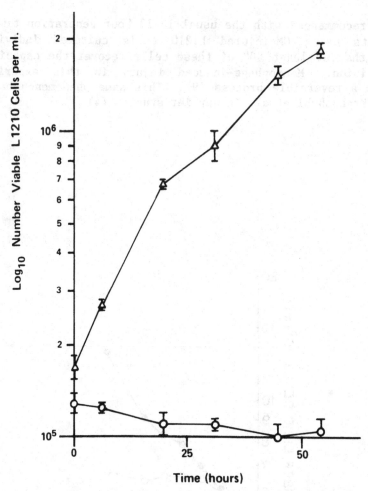

Figure 2: Separation of L1210 cells from macrophages does not reverse cytostasis. L1210 cells which had been exposed to CM (o) were separated from macrophages, washed by centrifugation, and recultured in fresh medium at Time (hours) = 0. ( ) = uninjured L1210 cells which were handled in exactly the same way, except that they had not been exposed to CM.

OXIDATIVE PHOSPHORYLATION IS INHIBITED IN NEOPLASTIC CELLS INJURED BY CYTOTOXIC MACROPHAGES

It was found that once L1210 cells had been injured by CM (i.e., by exposure to CM for 15-20 hours), they developed an absolute requirement for a hexose. If CM-injured L1210 cells separated from macrophages were cultured in glucose-free medium, nearly all

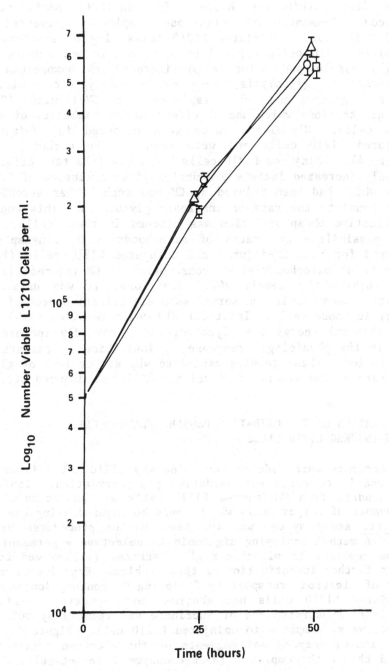

Figure 3: Medium from CM–L1210 cell cocultures supports multiplication of uninjured L1210 cells. Mediums from 20 hour
cultures of CM alone (o) or CM+L1210 cells ( ) were
centrifuged to remove cells and then used to resuspend
fresh L1210 cells for the growth curve measurements shown.
( ) = fresh culture medium.

cells died within 2-4 hours. In contrast, media containing
D-glucose, D-mannose or D-fructose completely prevented injured
L1210 cell death. Uninjured L1210 cells (log or stationary phase
cells) or L1210 cells exposed to noncytotoxic macrophages remained
totally viable and actually proliferated in hexoseless medium.
Inhibitors of glycolysis, such as 2-D-deoxyglucose blocked the
effect of glucose and led to rapid death of CM-injured L1210 cells
at concentrations which had no effect on the viability of uninjured
L1210 cells. Glycolysis rates were measured in CM-injured and
uninjured L1210 cells and were found to be markedly different
(Figure 4). Uninjured L1210 cells had a clear Pasteur effect, i.e.,
markedly increased lactate production after exclusion of O_2. L1210
cells which had been injured by CM had much higher aerobic glycolysis equal to the rate of anaerobic glycolysis. This would occur
if oxidative phosphorylation was blocked in these cells. To test
this possibility the rates of mitochondrial O_2 consumption were
measured for both CM-injured and uninjured L1210 cells (Table 1).
The rate of mitochondrial O_2 consumption in CM-injured L1210 cells
was inhibited by nearly 90%. Therefore, it was unlikely that
oxidative phosphorylation served as a significant source of chemical
energy in these cells. Injured L1210 cells remained viable, producing chemical energy via glycolysis at a markedly increased rate.
This is the physiologic response to inhibition of oxidative phosphorylation. These results explained why either lack of glycolytic
substrate or inhibitors of glycolysis killed CM-injured L1210 cells.

LOCALIZATION OF THE OXIDATIVE PHOSPHORYLATION DEFECT
IN CM-INJURED L1210 CELLS

Attempts were made to determine why L1210 cells injured by CM
were unable to carry out oxidative phosphorylation. Isolation of
mitochondria from CM-injured L1210 cells was unsuccessful because
the number of target cells which could be injured using the standard
in vitro assay system was too few for the procedures ordinarily
used. A method employing digitonin to selectively permeabilize the
plasma membrane to mitochondrial substrates (11) proved to be the
key to further investigation of this problem. Experiments measuring
rates of electron transport by following O_2 consumption showed that
CM-injured L1210 cells had abnormal mitochondria. Oxidation of
NAD-linked substrates and of succinate was reduced by 90% and 80%,
respectively, compared to uninjured L1210 cells (Figure 5). Assays
for selected enzymes and segments of the electron transport chain
showed that both complex I (NADH-coenzyme Q reductase) and complex
II (succinate-coenzyme Q reductase) had markedly reduced activities.
Yet electron transport from cytochrome c to O_2 occurred at a high
rate, only slightly below the rate for uninjured L1210 cells (Figure
5). Moreover, CM-injured L1210 cells permeabilized to glycerophosphate oxidized this substrate at a rate indistinguishable from
that of uninjured L1210 cells under state 3 conditions (Figure 6).

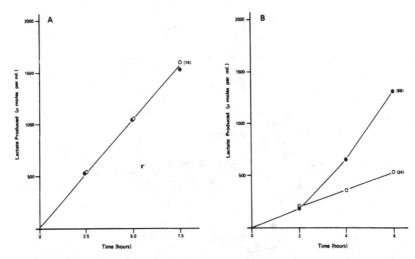

Figure 4: Glycolysis rates for CM-injured and uninjured L1210 cells. Aerobic (o) and anaerobic (o) glycolysis for L1210 cells which had been exposed to CM for 20 hours (Panel A) or uninjured L1210 cells (Panel B). Numbers in parentheses are maximal rates of lactate produced (nanomoles per hour per 10^5 L1210 cells).

Table I: Endogenous Respiration of CM-injured L1210 Cells

No. of experiments	L1210 cells cultured with:[*]	O_2 consumption[+]
		$\mu l/hr \cdot 10^6$ cells
6	Alone	7.4±0.3
4	Alone + ET (200 ng/ml)	7.2±0.4
2	Alone + MAF (10% vol/vol)	7.2±0.9
4	SM	6.9±0.7
6	CM	1.1±0.1
2	CM (MAF)	1.7±0.4
3	Alone (oligomycin inhibited)[§]	0.9±0.1
3	Alone (antimycin A inhibited)[§]	0.3±0.1

[*] For these experiments, L1210 cells were cultured alone or with macrophages for 24-40 h before respiration measurements.

[+] Values are the mean±SEM for the number of experiments shown.

[§] The effects of oligomycin and antimycin A were determined by injection into the respiration vessel to a final concentration of 0.1 and 0.01 μM, respectively. Previous experiments showed that these concentrations produced maximal inhibition of uninjured L1210 cell respiration at 2 x 10^6 cells/ml.

ET	= endotoxin
MAF	= macrophage activating factor from sodium periodate stimulated lymphocytes
SM	= stimulated macrophages (peritoneal macrophages from mice given sterile proteose peptone ip 3 days before harvest)
CM (MAF)	= macrophages activated by to the cytotoxic state by addition to MAF to the culture medium

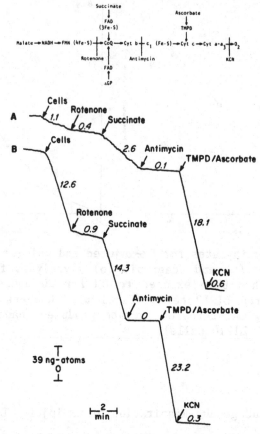

Figure 5: Addition of mitochondrial substrates to CM-injured L1210 cells permeabilized with digitonin. Polarographic traces of CM-injured cells (A) and uninjured cells (B) permeabilized with 0.005% digitonin in 0.25 M sucrose solution containing 5 mM K-malate, 2 mM KP_i, 10 mM $MgCl_2$, 2 mM ADP and 10 mM K-HEPES, pH 7.1. Numbers are rates of O_2 consumption in nanogram atoms per minute per million cells. A scheme of the mitochondrial electron transport chain is given above for reference.

Injured L1210 cells oxidizing glycerophosphate exhibited acceptor control, demonstrating indirectly that this oxidation was coupled to phosphorylation of ADP (Figure 5). While oxidative phosphorylation, fueled by glycerophosphate, occurred under conditions where CM-injured L1210 cells were made permeable to this substrate present in the incubation medium, experiments with intact L1210 cells under in vitro culture conditions revealed no evidence of either endogenous

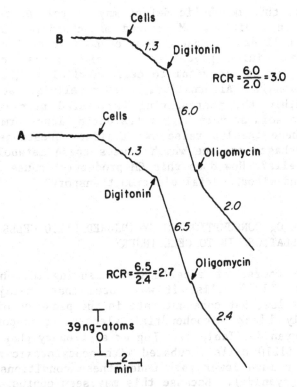

Figure 6: Oxidation of glycerophosphate by CM-injured L1210 cells permeabilized with digitonin. Polarographic traces of CM-injured L1210 cells (A) and uninjured L1210 cells (B) oxidizing -glycerophosphate, 10 mM, in the medium described in Figure 5, but with 100 nanomolar rotenone present. Oligomycin added (final concentration = 100 nanomolar) to inhibit the mitochondrial ATPase.

$$\text{Acceptor control ratio (ACR)} = \frac{\text{State 3 rate (no oligomycin)}}{\text{State 4 rate (with oligomycin)}}$$

production or mitochondrial oxidation of glycerophosphate. This agreed with the previous finding that intact CM-injured L1210 cells were incapable of carrying out oxidative phosphorylation and hence relied totally on glycolysis for ATP production (6).

From these studies it was clear that CM-induced injury led to selective defects in the respiratory chain of target L1210 cells, namely high level inhibition of complexes I and II. Since nearly all mitochondrial electron flow funnels through these enzyme complexes, CM-induced inhibition paralyzes oxidative phosphorylation. Time course experiments revealed that inhibition of complex I began shortly before the arrest of target cell division, leaving open the possibility that this metabolic defect may be related to the cyto-static event. In addition, CM-induced mitochondrial injury could lead to target cell death because some neoplastic cell types may be incapable of sustaining glycolysis at high rates required for energy-consuming processes vital to cell survival (e.g., ATP-driven ion translocations). Alternatively, intracellular acidification could occur within the nonrespiring CM-injured neoplastic cells, producing lactic acid at very high rates during long-term incubation (1-3 days). These results raise two critical questions: What do cytotoxic macrophages produce which causes these metabolic defects in neoplastic cells? How does this CM product(s) cause shutdown of ,cell division and mitochondrial electron transport?

NONMITOCHONDRIAL O_2 CONSUMPTION IN CM-INJURED L1210 CELLS AND ITS POTENTIAL RELATIONSHIP TO CELL INJURY

During the course of experiments measuring mitochondrial O_2 uptake in intact L1210 cells, it was noted that CM-injured cells consumed O_2 at a low, but constant rate in the presence of inhibitors which completely block mitochondrial electron transport, namely antimycin A or cyanide (Table 2). Log or stationary phase uninjured L1210 cells or L1210 cells incubated with noncytotoxic macrophages consumed O_2 at a much lower rate under these conditions (i.e., in the presence of cyanide). Because this may seem confusing, a short clarification may be useful. For intact L1210 cells growing under in vitro culture conditions mitochondrial O_2 uptake accounts for 96% of all oxygen consumed (6). The residual non-mitochondrial O_2 uptake (measured with cyanide or antimycin A present) is very low, being about 0.2-0.3 nanogram atoms per minute per million cells (Table 2). Macrophage injury reduced L1210 cell mitochondrial respiration by about 90% (6). Therefore, whole cell O_2 uptake is low since the great majority of the oxygen consumed is mitochondrial. However, non-mitochondrial O_2 uptake (cyanide or antimycin A present) is increased 3-5 fold in L1210 cells injured by CM, compared to uninjured L1210 cells (Table 2). Thus, CM-induced injury results in inhibition of mitochondrial and induction of non-mitochondrial respiration in L1210 target cells. It is important to point out that inhibition of mitochondrial respiration in and of itself is not sufficient to produce the cyanide-insensitive O_2 uptake observed for CM-injured L1210 cells. For example, inhibition of both complexes I and II in uninjured L1210 cell mitochondria with rotenone and theonyltrifluoroacetone, respectively, did not lead to increased cyanide-insensitive O_2 consumption above the rate obtained in the presence of cyanide alone.

When injured L1210 cells are removed from CM following the coculture incubation, some macrophages invariably dislodge from the culture vessel surface and contaminate the injured L1210 cell suspensions. However, the cyanide-insensitive O_2 uptake was not due to these contaminating macrophages because after they were removed

Table II: Cyanide Insensitive O_2 Uptake in L1210 Leukemia Cells Injured by Cytotoxic Macrophages

Incubation conditions prior to O_2 uptake measurements[a]	O_2 consumption rate[b] (nanogram atoms $O \cdot min^{-1} \cdot 10^{-6}$ cells)
1. L1210 cells cocultured with CM for:	
4 hours	0.30
12 hours	1.46
20 hours	1.10 ± 0.09[c]
2. L1210 cells cocultured with CM for 20 hours; then separated from CM and contaminating CM removed by successive steps of adherence to plastic dishes[d]	1.02
3. CM cultured with L1210 for 20 hours; L1210 cells removed, disgarded and then CM detached with rubber policeman and CM O_2 consumption was measured[e]	0.22
4. L1210 cells cocultured with noncytotoxic macrophages for 20 hours[f]	0.31
5. L1210 cells cultured alone:	
log phase cells	0.24 ± 0.02[c]
stationary phase cells	0.21

a. L1210 cells were cultured together with macrophages or alone and then at the times given they were separated from macrophages by rinsing, washed by centrifugation, and resuspended in fresh culture medium for O_2 uptake measurements.
b. Cells were suspended at approximately 5×10^6 per ml in culture medium (pH 7.4) containing 2.5 mM NaCN. Total volume was 1.3 ml in a continuously stirred chamber equipped with a Clark-type oxygen electrode. T = 37°C.
c. Mean ± standard error of mean for 8 separate experiments.
d. L1210 cells removed from CM by rinsing were re-incubated in culture medium without serum in plastic dishes for 30 minutes. This was repeated twice. The final L1210 cell suspension contained less than 1% contaminating cells from the CM monolayers.
e. This shows the rate of cyanide insensitive O_2 uptake of approximately 10 times the number of CM ordinarily present in the L1210 cell suspensions harvested by rinsing from CM monolayers.
f. Peritoneal macrophages from mice injected 3 days previously with 1.0 ml sterile 10% proteose peptone.

by successive stepwise adherence to plastic, there was no diminution of the rate of cyanide-insensitive respiration for the purified injured L1210 cells (Table 2). Furthermore, CM, detached with a rubber policeman, showed very little cyanide-insensitive respiration under these conditions (Table 2). The appearance of injured L1210 cell cyanide-insensitive O_2 uptake correlated with the development of CM-induced cytostasis and inhibition of oxidative phosphorylation. The onset is between 4 and 12 hours after exposure to CM [Table 2, Figure 1 and (10)]. Using a method of continuous recording, the O_2 consumption with cyanide present continues at a constant rate for at least 3 hours in stirred CM-injured L1210 cell suspensions. The reaction requires that injured L1210 cells be intact because disruption with detergent or by sonication completely stops cyanide-insensitive O_2 uptake. Inhibition also occurs if injured L1210 cells are permeabilized with 0.005% digitonin, suggesting that a cytosolic component required for this reaction may leak into and be diluted by the suspending medium. The oxygenase inhibitors, azide salicylhydroxamate, indomethacin and nordihydroguaiacetate, had no effect.

CONCLUSIONS

As L1210 cells are injured by CM, they acquire an oxygen-consuming reaction which is not due to the activity of mitochondrial cytochrome oxidase, that is, it is not affected by cyanide. Consequently, this reaction becomes extremely interesting because its possible products, O_2^- and H_2O_2, can directly or indirectly cause cell injury (12). These reduction intermediates may themselves damage cell components or O_2^- and H_2O_2 may react to produce the hydroxyl radical. The latter specie is highly reactive and can damage membranes, proteins and nucleic acids (12). Generation of oxygen intermediates by CM-injured L1210 cells could relate to the inhibition of mitochondrial electron transport. It has been shown that O_2-dependent lipid peroxidation causes inhibition of the electron transport complexes, most notably complexes I and II, in liver mitochondria (13). While it is well-known that leukocytes, including CM, produce superoxide upon appropriate stimulation (14), it may also be that macrophages in some way cause target cells to generate O_2 intermediates endogenously.

ACKNOWLEDGEMENTS

We thank Olive Sherman and David Claris for preparing the manuscript. This work was funded in part through a grant from the NIH (CA35893).

REFERENCES

1. Evans, R., and P. Alexander. 1976. Mechanisms of extracellular killing of nucleated mammalian cells by macrophages. In D. S. Nelson (ed.), Immunology of the Macrophage. New York: Academic Press, 535-76.
2. Hart, I. R., and I. J. Fidler. 1981. The implications of tumor heterogeneity for studies on the biology and therapy of cancer metastasis. Biochem. Biophys. Acta. 651:37-50.
3. Hibbs, J. B., Jr., and Granger, D. L. 1982. Activated macrophage-induced respiratory inhibition in neoplastic cells: Identification of lytic and nonlytic neoplastic cell phenotypes. In O. Forster (ed.), Heterogeneity of Macrophages. New York: Academic Press.
4. Krahenbuhl, J. L., L. H. Lambert, and J. S. Remington. 1976. The effects of activated macrophages on tumor target cells: Escape from cytostasis. Cell. Immunol. 25:279-93.
5. Cook, J. L., J. B. Hibbs, Jr., and A. M. Lewis, Jr. 1980. Resistance of simian virus 40-transformed hamster cells to the cytolytic effect of activated macrophages: A possible factor in species-specific viral oncogenicity. Proc. Natl. Acad. Sci. (U.S.A.) 77:2886-9.

6. Granger, D. L., R. R. Taintor, J. L. Cook, and J. B. Hibbs, Jr. 1980. Injury of neoplastic cells by murine macrophages leads to inhibition of mitochondrial respiration. J. Clin. Invest. 65:357-70.

7. Currie, G. A. 1978. Activated macrophages kill tumor cells by releasing arginase. Nature (London) 273:758-9.

8. Stadecker, M. J., J. Calderon, M. J. Karnovsky, and E. R. Unanue. 1977. Synthesis and release of thymidine by macrophages. J. Immunol. 119:1738-43.

9. Granger, D. L., and J. B. Hibbs, Jr. 1981. Recovery from injury incurred by leukemia cells in contact with activated macrophages. Federation Proc. 40:761 (abstract).

10. Granger, D. L., and A. L. Lehninger. 1982. Sites of inhibition of mitochondrial electron transport in macrophage-injured neoplastic cells. J. Cell Biol. 95:527-35.

11. Fiskum, G., S. W. Craig, G. L. Decker, and A. L. Lehninger. 1980. The cytoskeleton of digitonin-treated rat hepatocytes. Proc. Natl. Acad. Sci. (U.S.A.) 77:3430-4.

12. McCord, J. M., and I. Fridovich. 1978. The biology and pathology of oxygen radicals. Ann. Int. Med. 89:122-7.

13. Narabayashi, H., K. Takeshige, and S. Minakami. 1982. Alteration of inner-membrane components and damage to electron transfer activities of bovine submitochondrial particles induced by NADPH-dependent lipid peroxidation. Biochem. J. 202:97-105.

14. Badwey, J. A., and M. L. Karnovsky. 1980. Active oxygen species and the functions of phagocytic leukocytes. Ann. Rev. Biochem. 49:695-726.

THE CELL BIOLOGY OF TUMOR CELL CAPTURE BY ACTIVATED MACROPHAGES

D.O. Adams and S.D. Somers

Departments of Pathology and Microbiology-Immunology
Duke University Medical Center
Durham, North Carolina 27710

INTRODUCTION

Mononuclear phagocytes represent an important cellular element in the destruction of emerging and established neoplasms in vivo (1). Over the past several years, several distinct types of tumor cell kill by macrophages have been identified and examined in detail (2). This multiplicity of destructive modes is not surprising, since mononuclear phagocytes possess over 30 defined receptors on their surface and secrete over 75 distinct molecules (3). At least 10 of these receptors and over 20 of these molecules are potential candidates for recognizing and destroying tumor cells respectively (2,3). Thus, a general paradigm for cellular kill by macrophages has emerged: recognition of a tumor cell by one or more receptors, transduction of a signal from these receptors, and secretion of one or more injurious molecules to effect target injury and destruction (2,3). This paradigm is consistent with data available in the three systems of macrophage-mediated destruction of tumor cells now studied in some detail. In all three, kill may be divided into two stages: a) recognition and b) lysis (TABLE 1).

One of the most interesting forms of destruction is macrophage-mediated tumor cytotoxicity (MTC), which does not require antibodies for target recognition (2). This form of lysis, first described over a decade ago by Evans and Alexander (4) and by John Hibbs and colleagues (5), involves the selective lysis of neoplastic but not non-neoplastic cells by activated but not types of other macrophages. Over the past several years, we have analyzed this form of lysis in some detail (3,6,7). MTC, like other forms of kill, is completed in two stages: a) recognition and b) lysis. The lytic step is effected by secretion of lytic substances, including a novel cytolytic protease (for review, see 8). In this chapter, we shall focus on recent studies analyzing the recognition step.

Recognition in MTC, as detailed below, is manifested by a vigorous cell-cell interaction between activated macrophages and neoplastic target cells. This encounter results in the formation of strong and selective adhesion between the two cell types, which has been termed binding. The characteristics of selective binding, the development of competence for binding during macrophage activation, the multiple stages in establishment of binding, and the consequences of such binding will be described in this chapter.

TWO TYPES OF TARGET BINDING BY MACROPHAGES

We have observed two general types of binding interactions between macrophages and target cells (2,9). First, a low-level binding (i.e., 4-15% of added targets bound overall or 2-8 x 10^4 targets bound/10^6 macrophages) is observed between inflammatory macrophages and either neoplastic cells, lymphocytes or lymphoblasts. However many targets are added to such monolayers, the binding cannot be saturated. Second, a high-level and selective binding (i.e., 35 to 60% of added targets or 18-30 x 10^4 targets/10^6 macrophages) is observed between activated macrophages and a wide range of nonadherent, neoplastic targets. To date, over 20 neoplastic cell lines of disparate origins have been found to bind significantly to macrophages activated in vivo or in vitro (2). These two types of binding differ significantly from one another in many regards (Table II).

BINDING AS A RECEPTOR-MEDIATED EVENT

The selective macrophage-tumor cell binding resembles the binding between ligands and cellular receptors in several regards (see Table II). Of these, three bear further comment. The usual method for quantifying specific binding between ligand and receptor is to determine binding of the radiolabelled ligand in the presence of a large excess of unlabelled ligand. When we used similar methods, we found the binding of tumor targets to inflammatory macrophages to be entirely non-specific, while the binding to activated macrophages to be mostly specific (9). The binding of lymphocytes to both types of macrophages is almost entirely non-specific (9). Second, binding of tumor cells by activated macrophages initiates execution of two functions by the macrophages - initiation of cytolysis and secretion of CP (10). When BCG-activated macrophages are pulsed with tumor cells or with plasma membranes from such cells, the macrophages secrete an augmented amount of CP and do so much more rapidly than unpulsed macrophages. Induction of augmented secretion is selective, in that only tumor targets augment secretion (10). Lastly, such binding is quite selective (see above).

INDUCTION OF CAPACITY FOR SELECTIVE BINDING

The ability to complete selective binding of tumor cells is an acquired property of macrophages. Specifically, only macrophages in the last two stages of activation (i.e., primed macrophages and activated macrophages) can complete selective binding; resident peritoneal macrophages and inflammatory macrophages cannot (11).

The capacity for augmented binding is induced principally, if not entirely, by lymphokines (12). Exposure of young mononuclear phagocytes from sites of inflammation (i.e., responsive macrophages), though not of resident peritoneal macrophages, to lymphokine(s) induces, competence for selective binding. This effect is dose-dependent and optimal induction of binding requires 8-12 hours of interaction between macrophages and lymphokines. Only lymphokine(s) appear to be required and a requirement for any additional signal, including endotoxin, has not been established. Of interest, the requirements and kinetics of induction closely resemble those for induction of priming for cytolysis.

Recent evidence from numerous laboratories indicates that γ-interferon is an extremely potent macrophage activating factor (for review, see 13). We too have found this to be the case (11,14). Specifically, we have found that interaction of responsive (i.e., inflammatory) macrophages with γ-interferon induces two changes: a) competence for selective binding and b) preparation or priming for release of CP upon addition of a second signal such as endotoxin (11). The dose and cellular requirements for this induction, as well as the kinetics and sensitivity of inbred strains of mice, mimic precisely those with crude lymphokine preparations containing MAF (11,14). Thus, competence for selective binding of tumor cells can be readily induced in vitro over 6-8 hours by exposure of appropriate macrophages to crude MAF or to γ-interferon (11,14). Over this period of time, numerous biochemical changes, which include an extensive remodeling of surface membrane proteins, are also induced (for review, see 3).

It has recently been established that macrophages, like other cells, have a specific receptor for γ-interferon on their surface (15). The intracellular events, which transpire at a biochemical level, between engagement of this receptor and the functional alterations and membrane changes described above, however, remain obscure. We have recently found that these changes can be pharmacologically mimicked (14). In addition to the well known cyclic AMP pathway of signal transduction, a pathway involving phosphoinositol metabolism has recently received considerable interest (16). In this mechanism of signal transduction, metabolism of phosphoinositol is initiated by engagement of a surface receptor, which leads to formation of inositol triphosphates and diacylglycerol. The former of these two compounds is now thought to initiate intracellular calcium fluxes, probably from the endoplasmic reticulum, while the latter is a direct stimulant of protein kinase C (PKc) (16). Together the stimulation of protein kinase C and initiation of intracellular calcium fluxes can initiate a wide variety of cellular functions (16). These effects can be pharmacologically mimicked by addition of the calcium ionophore A23187 plus PMA (a potent stimulant of PKc) to cells (16).

We have recently discovered that macrophages can be fully primed for cytolysis in vitro by addition of these two pharmacologic agents, while capacity for selective binding is fully induced by PMA alone (14). These changes require 6-8 hours and thus mimic exactly the time course of macrophage priming induced by pure γ-interferon. The data therefore suggest that γ-interferon acts to prepare macrophages for tumor cell binding, in part, by initiation of intracellular calcium fluxes and stimulation of protein kinase C.

CELL BIOLOGY OF BINDING

The cell biology of selective binding is illuminated by comparing the binding of tumor cells by activated macrophages with that by inflammatory macrophages (9,17). The binding of targets to BCG-activated macrophages is time-dependent, and maximum binding occurs only after 2-3 hours of interaction. The binding of targets to inflammatory macrophages, however, reaches its maximum rapidly within 15 minutes. Treatment of BCG-macrophages with 2-deoxyglucose, iodoacetic acid, sodium azide, cochicine or cytochalasin B, at concentrations sufficient to reduce phagocytosis of IgG-coated sheep red blood cells significantly, abrogates selective tumor cell binding (9,17). By contrast, these inhibitors do not reduce the low-level binding of target cells to inflammatory macrophages.

We have recently studied the forces required to dislodge targets bound to macrophages (17). The complete interaction of neoplastic targets with activated macrophages occurs in at least two steps. First, a weak interaction (i.e., one disrupted by application of 100 g or $< 10^{-5}$ dyn per target cell) occurs very rapidly (i.e., in ~ 10 min.) after probe cells are brought into contact with any type of macrophage; the probe cells can be either tumor cells or lymphocytes. If the macrophages are activated and the probe cells are neoplastic, the weak interactions are converted with time (i.e., over 60-120 min.) to a much stronger bonding$_4$ (i.e., one stable by applications of up to 1800 g or $> 10^{-4}$ dyn per cell) It is interesting to note that the metabolic requirements for developing strong binding are exactly those for developing selective binding as described above (17). By contrast, the development of weak binding has essentially no metabolic requirements and proceeds at 4°C.

These data consistent with the following model. Weak cell-cell interactions, presumably due to weak bonds such as van der Wahl's forces or electrostatic charges, are formed between most cells in culture (18). These weak bonds are easily disrupted by low g forces. In the case of activated macrophages and neoplastic cells, a selective, receptor-mediated, recognition system comes into play. This receptor-mediated system initiates a series of events, which culminate over 60 to 120 minutes in formation of stable bonds and hence strong binding between the two cell types. It should be noted that the metabolic requirements of this system depend on the recognition system involved rather than the macrophage-target pair. Evidence for this contention comes from the observation that the same tumor cells, when coated with antibody and added to activated macrophages, are strongly bound at 4°C within 15 minutes (17).

PMA has proven a useful probe to unravel the complex sequence of events that convert weak to strong binding. PMA at extremely small doses (i.e. 1 ng/ml) augments selective binding (19). This augmentation, which occurs in less than 10 minutes, is effective only if the macrophages have an already established capacity for selective binding (i.e., if the macrophages are primed or activated). In this circumstance, the total capacity for trypsin-sensitive and hence selective binding is increased by ∼ two-fold. The effect is due to changes in the macrophages; and no alterations is seen in capture of lymphocytes by activated macrophages or of any cell type by inflammatory macrophages. Treatment of macrophages with PMA bypasses most of the metabolic requirements described above. That is to say, binding develops very rapidly and is not blocked by inhibitors of microtubules, microfilaments, or methylation reactions; the requirement for metabolic activity as manifested by need for incubation 37°C is, however, maintained. Studies with trypsinization of the macrophages before and after addition of PMA indicate that the increased binding results from a PMA-induced eversion of cryptic, trypsin-sensitive binding sites to the surface of the macrophages. These data thus suggest that this reorganization normally occurs during selective binding and that PMA bypasses the need for this eversion by inducing it before the actual capture begins (19).

These initial studes on the cell biology of binding do not yet permit formation, in precise detail, of how stable attachment between tumor cells and activated macrophages is achieved. Our current working _hypothesis_ is that the contact between many diverse cell pairs leads to rapid but weak attachment between the two cell types. Activated macrophages possess trypsin-sensitive receptors in the plasma membrane that recognize surface components contained within the plasma membrane of tumor cells. The interaction between these structures and the putative receptor on macrophages, in cooperation with microtubules and microfilaments in the macrophages, leads to the gradual development of stable attachments of the tumor cells to the activated macrophages. We are criticaly examining this hypothesis at present and are attempting to define those capacities possessed by activated macrophages which permit the development of such binding.

RELATIONSHIP OF TARGET BINDING TO CYTOLYSIS

All evidence currently available indicates that selective binding of neoplastic cells is an essential part of macrophage-mediated cytolysis (for review in detail, see 2,10). To review these studies briefly, the selectivity of such binding mimics that of cytolysis (i.e , only neoplastically transformed cells are bound by and susceptible to destruction by activated macrophages). The addition of unlabelled tumor cells or of tumor cell membranes inhibits selective binding and cytolysis proportionately. BCG-elicited macrophages from A/J mice are genetically deficient in their capacity to bind neoplastic cells and are incapable of effecting macrophage-mediated cytolysis (22). Abrogation of binding abrogates cytolysis. Binding of targets to macrophages, howeer, does not necessarily lead to target destruction. In sum, the selective binding of targets to activated macrophages is necessary, but not sufficient for completion of macrophage-mediated cytolysis.

Binding appears to serve at least three major functions in macrophage-mediated cytolysis (reviewed in 2,10). First, selective binding appears to be the recognition mechanism by which activated macrophages discriminate between neoplastic cells and their non-transformed counterparts. Second, such binding triggers the release of lytic substances from the macrophages. Third, the strength and duration of such binding and the extremely close physical apposition between macrophages and bound targets may well serve to protect and concentrate the secreted lytic mediators in the space between macrophages and targets.

70

DISCUSSION

One of the more intriguing problems in immunology is analysing the biological basis of cell-cell interactions. The selective binding between activated macrophages and neoplastic cells has proven to be an excellent model for addressing some of the critical questions in this rapidly emerging field. Already, one model (i.e., the binding interaction), like the overall cytolytic reaction, can be divided into multiple substeps. As we learn more of these steps, how they are effected in molecular terms and how macrophages gain competence for completing them, we should begin to gain insight into the fascinating language of cell-cell communication.

REFERENCES

1. D. O. Adams and R. Snyderman., A possible modification of the immune surveillance hypothesis: Do macrophages destroy nascent tumors?, J. Nat'l. Cancer Inst., 62:1341 (1979).

2. D. O. Adams and P. Marino, Activation of Mononuclear Phagocytes for Destruction of Tumor Cells As A Model For Study of Macrophage Development, in: "Contemporary Hematology-Oncology", A. S. Gordon, R. Silber and LoBue, J., eds., Plenum Publishing Corp., New York (1984).

3. D. O. Adams and T. A. Hamilton, The Cell Biology of Macrophage Activation, Ann. Review of Immunol. 2:283 (1984).

4. P. Alexander and R. Evans, Endotoxin and Double-Stranded RNA Render Macrophages Cytotoxic, Nature New Biol. (London), 232:76 (1971).

5. J. B. Hibbs, L. H. Lambert and J. S. Remington, In Vitro nonimmunologic destruction of cells with abnormal characteristics by adjunant activated macrophages, Proc. Soc. Exp. Biol. Med., 139:1049 (1972).

6. D. O. Adams, W. Johnson and P. A. Marino, Mechanisms of target recognition and destruction in macrophage-mediated tumor cytotoxicity, Fed. Proc., 41:2212 (1982).

7. W. J. Johnson, S. D. Somers and D. O. Adams, Activation of Macrophages for Tumor Cytotoxicity, in: "Contemporary Topics in Immunobiology", Vol. 14, pp. 127-146, D. O. Adams and M. G. Hanna, eds., Plenum Press, New York (1984).

8. W. J. Johnson, R. H. Goldfarb and D. O. Adams, Secretion of a Novel Cytolytic Protease by Activated Murine Macrophages: Its Properties and Role in Tumor Cytolysis, in: "Lymphokines", S. Mizell and E. Pick, eds., Academic Press, New York (1984) (In press).

9.   S. D. Somers, P. A. Mastin and D. O. Adams, The binding of tumor cells by murine mononuclear phagocytes can be divided into two, qualitatively distinct types, J. Immunol., 141:2086 (1983).

10. W. Johnson, C. Whisnant and D. O. Adams, The binding of BCG-activated macrophages to tumor-targets stimulates secretion of cytolytic factor, J. Immunol., 127:1787 (1981).

11. W. J. Johnson, P. A. Marino, R. D. Schreiber and D. O. Adams, Sequential activation of murine mononuclear phagocytes for tumor cytolysis: Differential expression of markers by macrophages in the several stages of development, J. Immunol., 131:1038 (1983).

12. P. A. Marino and D. O. Adams, The capacity of activated murine macrophages for augmented binding of neoplastic cells: Analysis of induction by lymphokine containing MAF and kinetics of the reaction, J. Immunol., 128:2816 (1982).

13. R. Schreiber, Identification of γ-Interferon as Murine Macrophage Activating Factor for Tumor Cytotoxicity, Cont. Topics Immunobiol., 13:174 (1984).

14. S. D. Somers, J. Weiel, T. Hamilton and D. O. Adams, Activation of murine mononuclear phagocytes for tumor cell destruction by phorbol myristate acetate and calcium ionophore, manuscript submitted (1984).

15. A. Celada, P.W. Gray, E. Rinderknecht and R.D. Schreiber, Evidence for a γ-Interferon Receptor That Regulates Macrophage Tumoricidal Activity, J. Exp. Med., 160:55 (1984).

16. Y. Nishizuka, The Role of Protein Kinase C in Cell Surface Signal Transduction and Tumor Promotion, Nature, 308:693 (1984).

17. S. D. Somers, C. C. Whisnant and D. O. Adams, Binding of tumor cells by activated macrophages: Formation of firm cell-cell attachment develops in two stages, manuscript in preparation (1984).

18. R. Bongrand, C Capo, and R. Depieds, Physics of Cells Adhesion, Prog. Surface Science, 12:217 (1982).

19. S. Somers and D. O. Adams, Enhancement of selective tumor cell binding by activated murine macrophages in response to phorbol myristate acetate, manuscript submitted (1984).

20. D. O. Adams, J. G. Lewis and W. J. Johnson, Multiple Modes of Cellular Injury by Macrophages: Requirement for Different Forms of Effector Activation, in: "Progress in Immunology V", Academic Press Japan, Inc. (1984).

DISCUSSION

Henney: Do you need some LPS present in order for macrophages to kill targets?

Adams: In the mouse system, you do. That does not act at
the binding level at all. The data is published and is clear
that LPS is one trigger for the release of cytolytic proteases.
It is also a powerful stimulator of phosphorylation in these
cells. We would make the argument that this kind of binding occurs and that after that two signals are delivered to the
macrophage, the binding signal and LPS, and that these together
cause release of the lytic molecules which lead to target damage.

Henney: What is the role of gamma interferon in the
selective binding and lysis?

Adams: There is a large body of evidence that gamma
interferon is a potent activating agent. Joe Oppenheim has found
that one of the interleukins can have the same effect, Monty
Meltzer has found a 22kd factor from a continuous T cell line
that has that effect, and Josh Fidler has similar data in human
systems. Therefore gamma interferon is a very potent MAF.

Ortaldo: Do you have any data to show that your strong and
weak receptors are simliar?

Adams: I doubt that weak binding is due to a receptor at
all.

Ortaldo: Have you been able to inhibit the strong binding
with any subcellular target structures?

Adams: In the last six months we have found a useful assay
which would allow us to test that, but at this time we do not
have any soluble preparations from tumor cells which will block
the binding. So I have no molecular information.

Sitkovsky: Can you generate macrophage resistant tumor
cell lines, which would be expected if a specific binding event
is required?

Adams: Hans Schreiber and Jim Urban have produced very
nice lines of that character. But our current assay is limited
to testing non-adherent cells, and we would like to test to see
if we can identify target structures such as I was referring to
on adherent tumor cells.

Hiserodt: Is there any evidence for a role for the Fc
receptor or Mac-1 in the strong binding?

Adams: No. A variety of evidence would suggest that neither the Fc not C3 receptors are involved in this recognition.

Herberman: On the question of an LPS requirement, there is evidence that LPS may not be absolutely required. Luigi Varesio from our group had evidence that gamma interferon alone would activate, while Steve Russell had maintained that LPS was absolutely required. They have just done some comparative experiments which have revealed that their differences may largely attributable to the mouse strains involved. C57Bl/6, which Varesio had worked with, could be activated by gamma interferon alone in both labs, while the C3H, which Russell had used previously used, tends to require much more LPS as a second signal.

Adams: One gets to a problem of LPS detection. I can only say that in our hands, those batches of gamma interferon which could activate turned out to contain LPS.

Nathan: There are now available monoclonal antibodies against the macrophage fibronectin receptor, and also fibronectin peptides which inhibit this binding. Have you had an opportunity to test these reagents in your system?

Adams: No, not yet.

DESTRUCTIVE INTERACTIONS BETWEEN MURINE MACROPHAGES, TUMOR CELLS, AND ANTIBODIES OF THE IgG$_{2a}$ ISOTYPE

William J. Johnson, Zenon Steplewski, Hilary Koprowski and Dolph O. Adams

Depts. of Pathology, and Microbiology-Immunology
Duke Univ. Medical Center, Durham, N.C
Wistar Institute
Philadelphia, PA

INTRODUCTION

Accumulated evidence from several laboratories indicates that murine antibodies of the IgG$_{2a}$ isotype are particularly potent in producing inhibition and destruction of murine tumors growing in situ (1-3) and of human tmors implanted in nude mice (4). Such antibodies can interact with macrophages to kill tumor cells in vitro (4,5), and macrophages have been implicated in the tumor destruction induced by IgG$_{2a}$ antibodies in vivo (3,4,5,6). Given this evidence, we examined the lytic interrelationships between macrophages, tumor cells, and anti-tumor antibodies of the IgG$_{2a}$ isotype in some detail. We here summarize the evidence that this interaction results in a potent antibody-dependent cell-mediated cytotoxicity (ADCC) reaction, distinct in several regards from that usually effected by macrophages and pertinent to the destruction of growing neoplasms in vivo.

BASIC CHARACTERISTICS OF IgG$_{2a}$-MEDIATED ADCC BY MACROPHAGES

To initiate these studies, we examined the interaction between human colorectal carcinoma cells, monoclonal antibodies (MAb) directed against the tumor cells, and murine peritoneal macrophages in a combination previously reported to result in tumor cell injury in vitro (4). Specifically, murine peritoneal macrophages elicited by thioglycollate broth were co-cultured with the SW-1116 colorectal tumor cells and examined by phase microscopy (7,8). In the presence of antitumor antibodies of either the IgG$_{2a}$ (i.e., the 17-1-A MAb) or IgG$_{2b}$ (i.e., the 480-1-4 MAb) isotype, the tumor cells

75

rapidly clustered about the macrophages and became bound to them. No destruction of the tumor cells was seen after six hours. After 24 to 48 hours, the tumor cells cultured with macrophages alone, with the IgG_{2b} MAb plus macrophages, or either MAb alone had grown extensively throughout the culture dishes. In the presence of macrophages plus MAb of the IgG_{2a} isotype, however, the tumor cells had virtually disappeared.

These observations were confirmed and extended upon subsequent analysis of this interaction using $[^3H]$-TdR labeled tumor cells (7,8). Destruction of tumor cells was again found to be a relatively slow process, resulting from lysis and requiring 24-48 hours for maximum release of lable. Again, only antibodies of the IgG_{2a} isotype were effective. Of particular interest, TG-elicited macrophages were much more efficacious than BCG-activated macrophages in mediating this form of lysis (i.e., lysis of 60 to 80% over 48 hrs versus lysis of 10 to 20% over the same period).

We wondered if this marked difference could be related specifically to the stage of activaton of the macrophages (7,8). As macrophages progress through different stages of activation (i.e., resident, responsive, primed and activated) to complete direct lysis of tumor cells, they acquire objective markers which distinguish populations of macrophages in the various stages (9). When macrophages in all of the stages of activation were tested, only certain populations of macrophages in the responsive or primed stages (i.e., only primed or responsive macrophages elicited by certain stimuli) were capable of mediating IgG_{2a}-dependent ADCC. To test this conclusion critically, we took populations of responsive or primed macrophages and added the signal or signals appropriate to activate them fully. Concomitant with acquisition of direct tumoricidal activity was loss of the ability to mediate IgG_{2a}-dependent ADCC. This loss was not due to a down-regulation of Fc receptor number or affinity (10).

These basic conclusions have now been confirmed and extended with multiple other combinations of targets and antibodies (10). In each, the TG-elicited inflammatory macrophages were more efficient in lysing the tumor cells than the BCG activated macrophages. The requirement for antibodies of the IgG_{2a} isotype, however, has not been maintained absolutely; antibodies of the IgG_{2b}, IgG_1, and IgG_3 isotypes and are also efficacious, though often to a lesser degree (10).

CELL BIOLOGY OF CYTOLYSIS

The binding and lysis of tumor cells in the presence of antibodies of the IgG_{2a} isotype is mediated by FcRI on the macrophages (8). This is evidenced by inhibition with prior

76

trypsinization of the macrophages and by failure to inhibit with a MAb directed against FcRII. Populations of macrophages which effect the slow lysis bind IgG_{2a}-coated tumor cells comparably to macrophages which cannot. Indeed, IgG_{2b} coated tumor cells are also bound well by lytic or non-lytic macrophages. By use of various temperatures for example, the overall lytic reaction could be divided into two steps: a) target binding and b) target lysis. These and other lines of evidence thus indicate that binding of antibody-coated tumor cells to macrophages, though essential for lysis, is not sufficient and that activation is expressed at the lytic rather than the binding step.

Since reactive oxygen intermediates have been demonstrated to be involved in the rapid lysis of antibody-coated tumor cells by murine macrophages (11), we investigated the role of these substances in IgG_{2a}-dependent ADCC. Macrophages cultured in an anaerobic environment or in glucose-free medium for 48 hrs maintained their viability and phagocytic capacity but showed a 60% decrease in their ability to mediate IgG_{2a}-dependent lysis. Furthermore, TG broth itself, which is a potent scavenger of H_2O_2, effectively inhibited lysis by ~ 60-70%. Released ROI from the macrophages thus appear to be a major mediator of IgG_{2a}-dependent ADCC.

RELEVANCE OF IgG_{2a}-MEDIATED ADCC IN VIVO

Growth of the SW-1116 colorectal carcinoma in nude mice is suppressed by systemic administration of an antitumor Mab's of the IgG_{2a} isotype but not by those of other isotypes (4). In order to examine the role of macrophages in this regression, the tumors were disaggregated and the intratumoral macrophages analyzed (12). Tumors were taken from young nude mice injected seven days earlier with 1×10^7 SW-1116 cells subcutaneously and either the 17-1-A Mab of the IgG_{2a} isotype or the 480-1-4 Mab of the IgG_{2b} isotype intraperitoneally; additional control tumors were taken from mice given no antibody. All tumors grew progressively save those from mice given the 17-1-A MAb, which were rejected. When the resulting macrophage populations from the tumors were compared, the overall number of cells in control tumors was greater than in rejecting tumors, but the number of macrophages was greater and the number of tumor cells less in the latter tumors. The ratio of macrophages to tumor cells was 1.6 to 1.0 in rejecting tumors, while in control tumors the ratio was 0.26 to 1.0 (12). Macrophages from the progressing tumors were not cytolytic in the presence of IgG_{2a} Mab, but macrophages from regressing tumors were. Furthermore, by use of objective markers (12), the latter macrophages were found to be in the responsive stage.

CONCLUSIONS

The lysis of tumor cells by macrophages in the presence of antibodies has heretofore been observed to be a rapid process, which is mediated by macrophages activated for direct lysis of tumor cells (13-15). We have now observed that macrophages in the presence of certain antibodies, polyclonal or monoclonal antibodies of the IgG_{2a} isotype predominantly, produce a distinct form of destruction. The overall reaction is generally slow and is distinguished by the fact that the macrophages must be of specific phenotypes which are not competent for direct lysis. The requirement for such macrophages has been extensively and critically tested and is thus the hallmark of this distinct form of macrophage-mediated form of ADCC.

Further evidence suggests that at least two alterations in intratumoral macrophages are necessary to result in the regression of a tumor after systemic treatment with antibodies of the IgG_{2a} isotype. First, the number of macrophages relative to the number of tumor cells must increase significantly. Second, the macrophages must be activated to mediate the slow or IgG_{2a}-dependent form of ADCC. Taken with data from other studies of this form of immunotherapy, the data further imply that immunotherapy utilizing monoclonal antibodies may be limited by the number of available macrophages and by the activation state of such macrophages. It is now important to define how the presence of IgG_{2a} antibodies at a tumor site produce an influx of macrophages and their activation for IgG_{2a}-mediated ADCC.

REFERENCES

1. T. J. Matthews., J. J. Collins, G. J. Roloson, Thiel, H-J., and D. P. Bolognesi, Immunologic control of the ascites form of murine adenocarcinoma 755. IV. Characterization of the protective antibody in hyperimmune serum, J. Immunol. 126:2332 (1981).

2. C. C. Badger and I. D. Bernstein, Therapy of murine leukemia with monoclonal antibody against a normal differentiation antigen, J. Exp. Med. 157:828 (1983).

3. M. E. Key and J. S. Haskill, Antibody-dependent cellular cytotoxicity (ADCC): A potential anti-tumor defense mechanism in situ in a murine mammary adenocarcinoma, in: "Macrophage-mediated Antibody Dependent Cytotoxicity," H. S. Koren, ed., Marcel Dekker and Co., New York (1984).

4. D. Herlyn and H. Koprowski, IgG2a monoclonal antibodies inhibit human tumor growth through interaction with

effector cells, <u>Proc. Natl. Acad. Sci. USA</u> 79:4761 (1982).

5. A. J. Langlois, T. J. Matthews, G. J. Roloson, H.-J. Thiel, J. J. Collins and D. P. Bolognesi, Immunologic control of the ascites form of murine adenocaricnoma 755. V. Antibody-directed macrophages mediate tumor cell destruction, <u>J. Immunol.</u> 126:2337 (1981).

6. R. J. Johnson, R. F. Siliciano and H. S. Shin, Suppression of antibody-sensitized tumor cells by macrophages: insufficient supply or activation of macrophages within large tumors, <u>J. Immunol.</u> 122:379 (1979).

7. D. O. Adams, J. G. Lewis and W. J. Johnson, Multiple Modes of Cellular Injury by Macrophages: Requirement for Different Forms of Effector Activation, <u>in</u> "Progress in Immunology V," Academic Press Japan, Inc., pp. 1009-1118 (1984).

8. W. J. Johnson, Z. Steplewski, T. J. Matthews, H. Koprowski and D. O. Adams, A Distinct Cytolytic Interaction Between Murine Macrophages, Tumor Cells, and Antibodies of the IgG_{2a} Isotype. Manuscript submitted (1984).

9. W. J. Johnson, P. A. Marino, R. D. Schreiber and D. O. Adams, Sequential activation of murine mononuclear phagocytes for tumor cytolysis: differential expression of markers by macrophages in the several stages of development, <u>J. Immunol.</u> 131:1038 (1983).

10. W. Johnson and D. O. Adams. Unpublished (1984).

11. C. Nathan and Z. A. Cohn, Role of oxygen-dependent mechanisms in antibody-induced lysis of tumor cells by activated macrophages, <u>J. Exp. Med.</u> 152:198 (1980).

12. D. O. Adams, T. Hall, Z. Steplewski and H. Koprowski, Tumors undergoing rejection induced by monoclonal antibodies of the IgG_{2a} isotype contain increased numbers of macrophages activated for a distinctive form of antibody-dependent cytolysis <u>Proc. Natl. Acad. Sci., USA</u> 81:3506 (1984)

13. C.F. Nathan, L. H. Brukner, G. Kaplan, J. Unkeless and Z. A. Cohn, Role of activated macrophages in antibody-dependent lysis of tumor cells, <u>J. Exp. Med.</u> 152:183 (1980).

14. H. S. Koren, S. J. Anderson, and D. O. Adams, Studies on the antibody-dependent cell-mediated cytotoxicity (ADCC) of thioglycollate-stimulated and BCG-activated peritoneal macrophages, <u>Cell. Immunol.</u> 57:51 (1981).

15. W. J. Johnson, D. Bolognesi, and D. O. Adams, Antibody dependent cytolysis (ADCC) of tumor cells by activated murine macrophages is a two step process:

quantification of target binding and subsequent target lysis, <u>Cell. Immunol</u>. 83:170 (1984).

SECTION 2. MECHANISTIC FEATURES SHARED BY CTL AND NK CELLS

INTRODUCTION

In the past few years, most studies aimed at characterizing NK cells have agreed that these cells fall into a morphologically distinct class of lymphocyte, the large granular lymphocyte (LGL). It is also clear that these cells also mediate most of the lymphocyte antibody-dependent cytotoxic (ADCC) activity. The LGL thus account for the cytotoxic activity of lymphocytes in unimmunized animals, and are clearly distinct from the cytotoxic T lymphocytes (CTL) which arise after immunization with foreign tissue or viruses. Several early studies of the NK cytotoxic mechanism were interpreted to suggest basic differences in the lytic mechanism between these two classes of lymphocoytes in addition to the clear differences in their recognition systems. Recently, however, a number of lines of evidence suggest that the post target binding events may be similar in both the LGL-mediated and CTL-mediated mechanisms. First, detailed mechanistic studies such as those previously presented by Targan (Mechanisms of Cell-Mediated Cytotoxicity, p. 389) show close parallels in the two cases. Secondly, cytoplasmic granules have been implicated in both types of lymphocyte cytotoxicity by morphological studies as reviewed by Zagury, et al. and Henkart and Henkart (Mechanisms of Cell-Mediated Cytotoxicity, p. 149 and p. 227), and by the contribution of Dennert, et al in this section. Further evidence for a role for such granules in both CTL and LGL cytotoxicity comes from the demonstration of their cytolytic properties as shown by the contributions of Podack, et al. and Henkart, et al. in this section.

Studies of the inhibition of CTL and NK cytotoxicity by antibodies prepared against killer cell cytoplasmic extracts have led Hiserodt to suggest that a common cytotoxic pathway operates in these two cell types, as described in the fourth chapter of this section. The relationship of these cytoplasmic components to granules is not presently known.

A final line of research which has suggests a close relationship between these two cell types has been the study of cytotoxic cells cultured in IL-2. Several laboratories have reported that the characteristic MHC restricted target cell recognition pattern of CTL undergoes a spontaneous shift to an

NK-like pattern with time in culture. It could be argued that
these developmental relationships suggest a common basic mechanism for the NK cell and the CTL. Other studies such as that
presented in this section by Grimm, et al. indicated that T cells
grown in IL-2 acquire a cytotoxicity which is unique, i.e, neither CTL nor LGL but sharing some properties with each.

REORIENTATION OF THE GOLGI APPARATUS AND THE
MICROTUBULE ORGANIZING CENTER: IS IT A MEANS
TO POLARIZE CELL-MEDIATED CYTOTOXICITY?[1]

Gunther Dennert[+], Abraham Kupfer[*],
Carol Gay Anderson[+] and S. J. Singer[*]

[+]University of Southern California
School of Medicine
Los Angeles, CA 90033

[*]Department of Biology
University of California
San Diego, CA 92037

INTRODUCTION

Cell-mediated cytolysis is one of the central mechanisms of immune defense and has therefore attracted much attention. The recent availability of cloned cell lines with cytolytic activity[1,2] had been instrumental in understanding some of the events that lead to target cell lysis. Using negative staining and thin sectioning electronmicroscopy with clones of natural killer cells (NK) and specific H-2 restricted cytotoxic T cells (TK), we have shown that the effector cells secrete tubular structures that are inserted into target cell membranes, presumably leading to target cell destruction[3,4]. Previous studies by others pointed to the importance of an intact secretory system in the killer cell and the potential participation of granules in the cytolytic reaction. It was therefore hypothesized that target cell binding triggers the onset of secretion of cytolytic components from the killer cell[5,6]. An interesting observation in this respect was that target cell lysis by specific TK cells appears to be a highly polarized reaction. For instance, TK cells with anti-H-2^b specificity will lyse TK cells of H-2^b haplotype that express anti-H-2^d

[1]This work was supported by USPHS grants CA 15581, CA 19334, and CA 37706 and the American Cancer Society Grant IM-284 to G.D. and USPHS grant AI-06659 to S.J.S.

specificity but not vice versa[7]. The action of cytolytic components therefore seems to be polarized towards the bound target. Among the organelles that may play a role in a directed secretion of cytolytic components is the Golgi apparatus (GA), presumably the packaging plant for the dense granules[8]. Another organelle which may play a role is the microtubule organizing center (MTOC) which is the region of the interphase cell from which the intracellular microtubules emanate[9]. We were prompted to study the localization of these two important organelles in effector cell-target couples by the results of previous studies that had been carried out with cells undergoing directed migration[10,11]. By double "immunofluorescent labeling" of the GA[12] and MTOC, it was first shown that the GA and MTOC were always co-localized near the nucleus of a cell, and furthermore that upon stimulating a cell to move, the GA and MTOC were rapidly and coordinately repositioned to face the leading edge of the cell[10]. The function served by this reorientation is apparently to direct the insertion of new membrane mass derived from the GA into the leading edge[11], as part of the overall mechanism of cell propulsion. We reasoned that such a GA/MTOC reorientation might also occur inside cytotoxic effector cells as part of the killing mechanism. Accordingly, we carried out immunofluorescence experiments to determine the localization of the GA[12] and MTOC within pairs of cloned effector cells and their targets. The results indicated[13,14] that the binding of susceptible target cells to killer cells induces a rapid GA/MTOC reorientation inside the killer cell towards the target binding site, which very likely serves to direct the secretion of cytolytic components towards the target cell.

MTOC and GA are Localized Close to Each Other in Cytolytic Effector Cells

In several experiments with cloned NK[13] and TK cells[14] conjugated to their respective targets, it was observed, using antibodies specific for either tubulin or for the membranes of the GA[12], that at the resolution of the light microscope both organelles are localized close together near the cell nucleus. An analogous co-distribution has been observed in every cell type so far examined[10,15]; it is, in fact, a very old observation that the pair of centrioles in an interphase cell (which forms part of the MTOC) is located proximal to the GA[16], although the significance of this observation has not been appreciated heretofore[15]. The association of the GA and MTOC in killer cells allowed us to stain either one or the other organelle under the assumption that the two organelles reposition coordinately in the effector cell. In the following experiments, either the MTOC or the GA were stained with a fluorescein-conjugated probe so that the effector cells could be distinguished by rhodamine-labeling with anti Thy-1 antibody.

Are MTOC and GA Repositioned in Effector-Target Cell Conjugates?

We conjugated a number of different NK clones, previously described and characterized[17], with S194 (H-2^d) targets and observed that at an early time after conjugation (20 minutes) about 70% of the effector cells have their MTOC oriented toward the target cell, while at 30 minutes essentially all the NK cells have the MTOC oriented toward the target contact area. These results suggested that the GA/MTOC orientation in the NK-target conjugate is initially random and that a time-dependent reorientation occurs after NK-target binding[13]. The GA/MTOC were randomly distributed in the target cell independent of the length of incubation. Using H-2^b anti H-2^d clones as effectors and H-2^d (S194) tumor cells as targets[14], we found that in almost all killer-target conjugates the GA/MTOC were oriented toward the target cell at the earliest times examined. These results are related to those previously obtained with heterogeneous cell populations containing cytotoxic effector cells. Bykovskaja et al.[18] had shown by thin section electron microscopy of T killer-target pairs that shortly after conjugation the GA in the killer cell was randomly positioned with respect to the target binding site, while at later times the GA was oriented towards the binding site. Geiger et al.[19], using immunofluorescence observations to localize the MTOC in similar T killer-target pairs, observed at early times after cell mixing that the MTOC was always oriented towards the bound target.

All of these results are consistent with the conclusion that the GA/MTOC inside the effector cell is oriented towards the bound target, but two quite different mechanisms for this orientation are conceivable. In one, the target becomes bound at a random site on the surface of the effector cell, and this results in a signal that induces the rapid reorientation of the GA/MTOC inside the effector cell to face the target. In the other[19], a specialized domain pre-exists on the surface of the effector cell, which is opposed to its GA/MTOC, and the target binds to this specialized domain.

The Effect of Altered Microtubule Assembly Status on the GA and on Target Cytolysis

In order to help discriminate between these two possibilities, effector cells were treated in one of two ways to alter the assembly status of their microtubules. One way involved the complete disassembly of the microtubules by treatment with nocodazole. This results in the elimination of an MTOC structure dectectable by immunofluorescent labeling for tubulin, and also results in the complete dispersion of elements of the GA from their normal compact perinuclear organization into the cell periphery[15,16]. The second way involved following the treatment with nocodazole with a mixture of nocodazole and taxol. Under these circumstances[20], an "abortive" MTOC forms; i.e., a structure is observed by immunofluorescent labeling for tubulin which is perinuclear and from which short strands of microtubules emanate. The bulk of the tubules, however, remain disassembled and, most significant for our purposes, the elements of the GA that were dispersed into the cell periphery by the initial nocodazole treatment, remain dispersed upon replacement with nocodazole/ taxol[15]. The dispersion of GA elements by nocodazole, with or without subsequent nocodazole/taxol treatment, appears remarkably enough to have little if any effect on GA functions[21].

In NK and TK cells that were treated with nocodzaole, followed by nocodazole/taxol, and then conjugated with target cells, the binding of the two cells appeared normal, but the "abortive" MTOC was randomly oriented with respect to the target binding site even after prolonged incubation. Assay of cytolytic activity of such conjugates revealed that cytotoxicity was either completely or severely inhibited (Table 1). These results showed

Table 1. Effect of Nocodazole on NK and TK Mediated Cytolysis and its Reversibility by Con A

Effector Cells	Targets	Treatment of Effectors	% Cytolysis at 4 h 10:1	3:1	1:1
NK B61B10	YAC-1	-	30	2	7
NK B61B10	YAC-1	Noc → Noc	7	2	2
NK B61B10	YAC-1	Noc → Medium	23	11	3
TK B61B10	S194	-	161	49	28
TK B61B10	S194	Noc → Noc	53	35	14
TK B61B10	S194	Noc → Medium	51	43	26
NK B61B10	YAC-1	-	15	7	3
NK B61B10	YAC-1	Con A	26	13	5
NK B61B10	YAC-1	Noc → Noc	<1	<1	<1
NK B61B10	YAC-1	Noc → Noc + Con A	12	6	3
TK B61E6	S194	-	81	72	49
TK B61E6	S194	Con A	83	68	45
TK B61E6	S194	Noc → Noc	17	4	<1
TK B61E6	S194	Noc → Noc + Con A	43	19	12

several important points: i) NK and TK cells are able to bind to their targets even when the microtubules are completely disassembled by nocodazole; ii) binding of NK and TK to their targets occurs at sites on the effector cells that are randomly positioned with respect to the abortive MTOC formed in nocodazole/taxol; and iii) no reorientation of the abortive MTOC occurs in the effector cells after target binding.

Reassembly of Microtubules from the MTOC Results in the Recompaction of the GA, GA/MTOC Reorientation in the Effector Cell, and Subsequent Target Cell Lysis

Removal of nocodazole or nocodazole/taxol from the effector cells bound to their targets resulted in the rapid reappearance of microtubules emanating from the MTOC, and was followed invariably by the orientation of the MTOC towards the target binding site[13,14]. In other studies[15], it has been shown that the normal reassembly of microtubules that occurs after removal of these drugs results in the recompaction of the previously dispersed elements of the GA into a compact perinuclear configuration that is again co-localized with the MTOC. Assay of the cytolytic activity of both NK and TK cells that were first treated with nocodazole and subsequently returned to normal medium showed that the activity was either substantially or completely recovered (Table 1). These results show that: i) an intact and normal microtubule-MTOC system is required to induce the MTOC reorientation towards the bound target; and ii) the signal from the bound target cell that induces the reorientation of the MTOC in the effector cell persists for long periods of time and despite microtubule disassembly or reorganization in the effector cell.

Does GA/MTOC Reorientation in the Effector Cell Serve as a Focusing Mechanism?

In normal cells, as discussed above, the MTOC and GA are compact organelles that are co-localized. Thus, they become reoriented together upon suitable signalling to the effector cell. Disassembly of the microtubules results in a complete dispersion of elements of the GA into the cell periphery, without, however, significant impairment of their secretory or membrane insertion functions[21]. The effect of microtubule disassembly on cytolytic activity[13,14] can therefore be interpreted as being due to a "de-focusing" of GA-derived secretion. In the normal cell, the coordinate reorientation of the compact GA/MTOC towards the target binding site focuses the cytolytic secretory process to that site; dispersion of the GA elements de-focuses it.

These considerations may explain the finding that inhibition of cytolysis by microtubule-depolymerizing drugs is often more pronounced in the NK compared to the TK system (Table 1). In TK-target conjugates, binding usually appears to be more intimate and to involve a larger surface area than in NK-target conjugates. This suggestion is consistent with the fact that cytolysis by TK cells usually cannot be enhanced by the lectin Con A, while NK cytolysis is always dramatically increased (Table 1). Therefore, despite the complete dispersion of GA elements in a nocodazole-treated TK cell, the large surface area of TK-target cell binding may allow sufficient secretion derived from the dispersed GA elements to arrive at the bound target to produce significant lysis, but not in the case of the nocodazole-treated NK cell. If this were correct, then increasing the intimacy and surface area of binding of killer cells to targets by Con A in the presence of nocodazole should partially reverse the inhibition of cytolysis produced by nocodazole alone. Results in Table 1 show that this is indeed the case for both TK and NK.

These results show that neither an intact MTOC, nor a compact perinuclear GA, are absolutely essential to the expression of cytolytic activity by NK or TK cells. Rather they suggest that, in the normal cytolytic interaction, the coordinate reorientation of the co-localized compact GA/MTOC greatly increases the efficiency of cytolysis, presumably by focusing secretory activity derived from the GA to the bound target.

Cell Surface Antigens on the Target Provide the Signals for MTOC-GA Reorientation

Binding of cytolytic effector cells to lysable targets leads to the repositioning of the MTOC and GA towards the target binding site [13,14]. A question then is whether binding of effector cells to any target regardless of its lysability will lead to GA/MTOC reorientation. NK cells were conjugated with two non-lysable target cells, YAC-8, a YAC-1 derivative which binds NK cells, and BCN, a derivative of 10ME which is also a NK binder[22]. In both cases, there was no target cytolysis nor was there MTOC reorientation observed (Table 2). This suggested that nonlysable targets bound to NK cells do not induce MTOC reorientation. In an attempt to reproduce this finding for the TK system, we took advantage of the observation that soybean agglutinin (SBA)-mediated agglutination of TK cells with targets to which they do not bind with their receptors results in cytolysis only if the targets are treated with neuraminidase (NASE)[23]. An H-2[b] anti H-2[d] TK clone was incubated with normal, NASE or SBA-treated H-2[d] (S194), H-2[b] (EL4) or H-2[k] (C1.18.4) targets. Control groups did not receive either NASE or SBA treatments. Results (Table 2) showed that the syngeneic H-2[b] target EL4 was lysed in the presence of SBA, particularly when treated with NASE. In the cases

88

Table 2. Correlation Between Cytolysis and MTOC/GA Repositioning

Effector Cells	Targets	Treatment of Targets	% Cytolysis at 4 h			MTOC/GA Repositioning
			10:1	3:1	1:1	
NK B61B10	YAC-1	-	35	21	15	+
NK B61B10	YAC-8	-	<1	<1	<1	-
NK B61B10	BCN	-	<1	<1	<1	-
TK B6CG11 ($H-2^b$ $\alpha H-2^d$)	S194 ($H-2^d$)	-	63	38	20	+
TK B6CG11 ($H-2^b$ $\alpha H-2^d$)	EL4 ($H-2^b$)	-	6	3	2	-
TK B6CG11 ($H-2^b$ $\alpha H-2^d$)	EL4 ($H-2^b$)	NASE	5	1	1	-
TK B6CG11 ($H-2^b$ $\alpha H-2^d$)	EL4 ($H-2^b$)	SBA	42	31	18	+
TK B6CG11 ($H-2^b$ $\alpha H-2^d$)	EL4 ($H-2^b$)	SBA + NASE	74	61	39	+
TK B6CG11 ($H-2^b$ $\alpha H-2^d$)	C1.18.4 ($H-2^k$)	-	3	<1	<1	-
TK B6CG11 ($H-2^b$ $\alpha H-2^d$)	C1.18.4 ($H-2^k$)	SBA	2	<1	<1	-
TK B6CG11 ($H-2^b$ $\alpha H-2^d$)	C1.18.4 ($H-2^k$)	SBA + NASE	9	3	<1	-
TK B6CG11 ($H-2^b$ $\alpha H-2^d$)	C1.18.4 ($H-2^k$)	Con A	11	7	<1	-

in which cytolysis occured, MTOC reorientation was observed. In contrast, in the Cl.18.4 system none of the conditions induced either cytolysis or MTOC reorientation. Hence in the cases examined, binding of killer cells to targets that are not lysed does not result in MTOC reorientation. This clearly shows that binding of a killer cell to a target is not sufficient to induce reorientation. A specific signal from the target is required to induce reorientation and so far this signal has only been demonstrated on "lysable" targets.

CONCLUSIONS

The events that precede target cytolysis are schematically summarized in Figure 1. Effector and target cells collide, followed by binding of the cells to each other. This first step requires the presence of Mg^{++}. In both NK and TK cells, binding appears to be random with regard to the position of the MTOC and GA. Next, a signal from the target to the killer results in a reorientation of the GA/MTOC complex towards the target binding site. This GA/MTOC reorientation may result in granular traffic towards the cell-cell binding site and may be the mechanism by which a directed secretion of cytotoxic molecules towards the target is accomplished. The apparently random binding of effector cells and targets, supported by the finding that both NK and TK cells are able to bind to several targets simultaneously, strongly argues against the presence of a distinct target receptor region on the effector. But it is of course possible that once this region is involved in the secretion of cytolytic components, it becomes resistant to cytolytic attack.

EVENTS LEADING TO TARGET CELL LYSIS

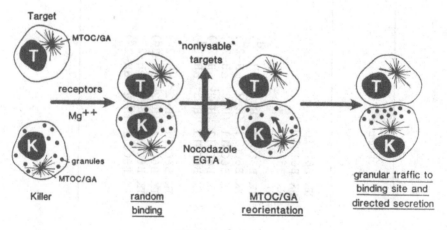

Figure 1

90

GA/MTOC reorientation can be inhibited in several ways. For instance, the absence of Ca^{++} inhibits both reorientation and cytolysis (unpublished results). It therefore appears that Ca^{++} may play a role in at least two stages of the cytolytic process since it is also required for granule-mediated target cell lysis[24]. An interesting speculation would be that a K^+ flux leaving the cell and a Ca^{++} influx into the cell[25] precede reorientation. GA/MTOC reorientation requires a specific signal from the target and at the present time we can only speculate upon which membrane determinants may serve this function. Since the failure to lyse a target also resulted in a failure to signal GA/MTOC reorientation, one could speculate that nonlysable targets are nonlysable because they do not possess the determinants which serve to provide a reorientation signal. On the other hand, it is well known that targets may have largely differing susceptibility to antibody plus complement and cell-mediated cytolysis. It is therefore not excluded that targets do exist that are not lysed yet possess the reorientation signal determinant.

Our finding that GA/MTOC reorientation in both the NK and TK system precedes cytolysis corroborates previous reports suggesting that lysis in the NK and TK systems follow similar mechanisms[5,18]. Moreover, GA/MTOC reorientation may constitute one of the underlying mechanisms that are responsible for the unidirectional cytolytic activity of effector T cells that are conjugated to effector T cells with a third party specificity[7]. Whether other mechanisms such as membrane resistance to the cytolytic attack also play a role in this effect has to be borne out by future experiments.

REFERENCES

1. G. Dennert and M. De Rose, Continuously proliferating T killer cells specific for H-2^b targets: selection and characterization, J. Immunol. 116:1601 (1976).
2. G. Dennert, Cloned lines of natural killer cells, Nature (Lond) 287:47 (1980).
3. E. R. Podack and G. Dennert, Cell-mediated cytolysis: assembly of two types of tubules with putative cytolytic function by cloned natural killer cells, Nature (Lond.) 302:442 (1983).
4. G. Dennert and E. R. Podack, Cytolysis by H-2 specific T killer cells. Assembly of tubular complexes on target membranes, J. Exp. Med., 157:1483 (1983).

5. O. Carpen, I. Virtanen, and E. Saksela, Ultrastructure of human natural killer cells: nature of the cytolytic contacts in relation to cellular secretion, J. Immunol. 128:2691 (1982).

6. O. Carpen, I. Virtanen, and E. Saksela, The cytotoxic activity of human natural killer cells requires the intact secretory apparatus, Cell. Immunol. 58:97 (1981).

7. P. Golstein, Sensitivity of cytotoxic T cells to T cell mediated cytotoxicity, Nature 252:81 (1974).

8. M. G. Farquhar and G. E. Palade, The Golgi apparatus (complex) - (1954-1981) - from artifct to center stage, J. Cell. Biol. 91:77s (1981).

9. J. D. Pickett-Heaps, The evolution of the mitotic apparatus: an attempt at comparative ultrastructural cytology in dividing plant cells, Cytobios. 1:257 (1969).

10. A. Kupfer, D. Louvard, and S. J. Singer, Polarization of the Golgi apparatus and the microtubule-organizing center in cultured fibroblasts at the edge of an experimental wound, Proc. Nat. Acad. Sci. USA 79:2603 (1982).

11. J. E. Bergmann, A. Kupfer, and S. J. Singer, Membrane insertion at the leading edge of motile fibroblasts, Proc. Nat. Acad. Sci. USA 80:1367 (1983).

12. D. Louvard, H. Reggio, and G. Warren, Antibodies to the Golgi complex and the rough endoplasmic reticulum, J. Biol. Chem. 92:92 (1982).

13. A. Kupfer, G. Dennert, and S. J. Singer, Polarization of the Golgi apparatus and the microtubule organizing center within cloned natural killer cells bound to their targets, Proc. Natl. Acad. Sci. USA. 80:7224 (1983).

14. A. Kupfer and G. Dennert, Reorientation of the microtubule organizing center and the Golgi apparatus in cloned cytotoxic lymphocytes triggered by binding to lysable target cells (submitted).

15. A. A. Rogalski and S. J. Singer, Association of elements of the Golgi apparatus with microtubules, J. Cell Biol., in press.

16. E. Robbins and N. K. Gonatas, Histochemical and ultrastructural studies on HeLa cell cultures exposed to spindle inhibitors with special reference to the interphase cell, J. Histochem. Cytochem. 12:704 (1964).

17. J. F. Warner and G. Dennert, Establishment and cloning of cell lines with natural killer activity in lymphokine-containing media. In Lymphokines, S. Mizel, editor, New York, Academic Press, Vol. 6, p. 165 (1982).

18. S. N. Bykovskaja, A. N. Rytenko, M. O. Rauschenbach, and A. F. Bykovsky, Ultrastructural alteration of cytolytic T lymphocytes following their interaction with target cells. I. Hypertrophy and change of orientation of the Golgi apparatus, Cell Immunol., 40:164 (1978).

19. B. Geiger, D. Rajen, and G. Berke, Spatial relationships of microtubule-organizing centers and the contact area of cytotoxic T lymphocytes and target cells, J. Cell Biol., 95:137 (1982).

20. M. De Brabander, G. Geuens, R. Nuydens, R. Willebrords, and J. De Mey, Microtubule stability and assembly in living cells: the influence of metabolic inhibitors, taxol and pH, Cold Spring Harbor Symp. Quant. Biol., 46:227 (1981).

21. A. A. Rogalski, J. E. Bergmann, and S. J. Singer, The effect of microtubule assembly status on the intracellular processing and surface expression of an integral protein of the plasma membrane, J. Cell Biol., in press.

22. G. Dennert, G. Yogeeswaran, and S. Yamagata, Cloned cell lines with natural killer activity. Specificity, function and cell surface markers, J. Exp. Med., 153:545 (1981).

23. T. P. Bradley and B. Bonavida, Mechanism of cell-mediated cytotoxicity at the single cell level. Importance of target cell structures in cytotoxic T lymphocyte-mediated antigen nonspecific lectin-dependent cellular cytotoxicity, J. Immunol., 129:2352 (1982).

24. P. Henkart, P. Millard, M. Henkart, and C. Reynolds, Internat. Symp. on Natural Killer Cells, Kyoto, Japan (Abstract) (1983).

25. J. H. Russel, and C. B. Dobos, Accelerated $^{86}Rb^+(K^+)$ release from the cytotoxic T lymphocyte is a physiologic event associated with delivery of the lethal hit, J. Immunol., 131:1138 (1983).

DISCUSSION

G. Berke: Perhaps let me start by saying that I'd like to congratulate you on this work with natural killers. It confirms our CTL studies published two years ago in the Journal of Cell Biology [Geiger et al., 95:137, 1982] which were done with the idea in mind of finding the mechanism (inaudible) in the Kuppers and Henney experiments.

C. Ware: Correct me if I'm wrong, but in the pictures showing staining with anti-Thy-1, was that more dense in the region of contact?

G. Dennert: Its an interesting question whether you see more Thy-1 or H-2 in these areas. We've done a number of experiments without being able to get any really conclusive results.

J. Hiserodt: I was wondering if you've ever considered an alternative to the actual movement of the MTOC or Golgi -- one could explain it as a simple membrane movement of the effector cell just to the other side of the target, which would switch the orientation without actually moving the cytoplasmic contents of the cell.

G. Dennert: Yes, that's a very important point, which came immediately out. What you see during video focus is that during the contact of NK and target, you see a very rapid movement within the cell of the nucleus. You do not see MTOC or Golgi because we don't have any [vital] stains, but because of this movement of the nucleus within the effector cell, we think that the MTOC and Golgi reorient, rather than this kind of rolling movement of the cells against each other.

E. Podack: I might just call to your attention what I showed this morning, the staining of the granules, and the positioning into the (inaudible) regions. There seems to be a very temporal correlation with what you showed with the MTOC, which would suggest maybe that the real purpose of this reorientation is to bring the granules into the contact zone.

G. Dennert: Yes, that's why we did it.

P. Henkart: I'd like to call attention to the results of Daniel Zagury, who came to the first Workshop, and in fact published two papers in French which unfortunately few of us read. The first was published in 1977, and the second shortly thereafter. He clearly showed by EM sectioning the reorientation phenomenon involving the granules directly. He had statistics which showed this, too. I think that his contribution was one that's sometimes overlooked.

In the experiment that Geiger and Berke did, there was an interpretation of a preorientation already in the binding capacity of the cell. I'd like to ask whether you can agree that this issue is now resolved -- the conditions of your experiment would allow reorientation?

G. Dennert: Yes, and in fact we tried the same experiment that Geiger did. The reorientation was so fast that you can't see it. At the earliest time we looked at these conjugates we see them already reoriented.

G. Berke: I think one experiment is missing in either of our studies. That is to show that when a CTL is attached to two target cells, it will kill the one that is close to the MTOC. I think this could resolve the issue.

G. Dennert: That experiment has been done, in fact, we did it. The problem is that what you really had to do is time lapse photography of a killer which binds to several target cells, and you have to see whether the MTOC goes around and shoots each of them to pieces. What you see is that the MTOC tends to be oriented towards the living cells, and the dead ones have no MTOC (inaudible). Sometimes you see the MTOC oriented towards blebbing cells which are dying. But it is difficult, because you have no staining for the MTOC.

G. Berke: I think Colin had a very good point, whether we are dealing with an orientation because a secretory mechanism is required at the site of interaction, or, is it merely because virtually every organelle of the cell happens to be at that site. The nucleus is usually distal to the contact site. If one is to envisage the contact site as interdigitating fingers, for forming those interdigitating fingers you need a great deal of mechanobiology. That is, activity of the cytoskeletal system. Not only does one see the microtubule organizing center at that region, but as you may recall as Ryser presented at the last meeting, virtually all the actin is located at that site. This is a site where we need a great deal of membrane folding, and this perhaps is the reason why we need the MTOC at that region. I think every other organelle can be located only on this side, because there is no room on the distal side. To me it seems that the MTOC moves back and forth but not really around the cell. So it may have to do with strengthening and building up the ties between the two cells.

G. Dennert: I think its an interesting possibility. The only thing I can say that in situations where we use Con A we do not get reorientation, but we get much stronger binding, although its not the same type of binding.

J. Ding-E Young: Has anyone measured intracellular free calcium of NK cells or lymphocytes during killing or during stimulation.

G. Berke: Reuven Tirosch in our lab has looked using Quin-2 as a calcium probe, and he was able to demonstrate elevation of the cytosolic free calcium, which I'll be presenting later.

J. Ding-E Young: We recently showed with Quin-2 that one can inhibit phagocytosis by macrophages, and I was wondering if one could use Quin-2 not as a measuring probe, but as a buffering probe, instead of EGTA. Would it block reorientation?

G. Dennert: We are presently doing this, but we haven't finished it yet.

G. Berke: Actually, with Quin-2 its tricky because if you put it outside at micromolar concentrations, it will accumulate at millimolar concentrations [inside] because its trapped and hydrolyzed inside. And another point is that the use of EGTA to chelate the calcium is pretty dangerous because it chelates both calcium and magnesium. I think one needs to use magnesium EGTA to leave the magnesium available.

R. Tirosch: It should be noticed that MTOC orientation looks very much like some other cellular phenomena, like motility. You could view in a pair of bound cells that the MTOC is directed towards the growing cone of the cells and this might correlate the motile behaviour of the killer cell, maybe also of the target cell, with respect to the function of the cytolytic mechanism. Indeed I recollect that Ryser and (inaudible) presented this at a previous meeting and showed quite clearly a polarization of the actin-myosin system in the killer cell. I'd like also to mention that if one watches carefully, under the microscope, during the action of the CTL and its target, one can visualize a mobile interaction where you can see the killer coming into the target, and then you can see relaxation. This is best observed when you use lymphoblasts rather than PEL [peritoneal exudate lymphocytes]. I would like to ask you, from this point of view, if you find a difference in the mode of interaction of NK cells with targets with respect to being pressed into the target cell or vice versa. Because I found the description of Zagury quite interesting from the point of view that it appears opposite from what I usually find in CTL-target interaction. Namely, with the NK cells you get the target pressing into the killer, whereas with the CTL it is the opposite. Did you find this?

G. Dennert: I think in the T cell system you have more of this interdigitation, and in the NK you have more envelopment, so I'd say that's correct.

(<u>unidentified</u>): If you see this type of 50-50 effect with the NK cells, what do you get after you activate them. The reason I ask you is because work I'm doing with (inaudible) showed that if you use purified LGL's with Elizabeth Grimm's and Ben Bonavida's single cell assay virtually all the binder cells could go on and kill. So this would speak to Colin's question, because, if you use interferon activated killer cells, and you see the same 50-50 arrangement, and then you can follow those, and they all go on and kill, this would argue against dissociation occurring.

<u>G</u>. <u>Dennert</u>: All these cells are what one would call activated because they produce their own gamma interferon, and there's also gamma interferon in the Con A supernatant in which they're grown.

(<u>unidentified</u>): Do you know what percentage of your initial binders go on and kill?

<u>G</u>. <u>Dennert</u>: Yes, about 70%.

(<u>unidentified</u>): Is there anything that excludes the possibility that the MTOC reorients as a consequence of target cell injury, for example in response to a factor released from the early injured target cell, rather than as a prerequisite for injury?

<u>G</u>. <u>Dennert</u>: Not really, other than that its very fast in the T killer system. That doesn't really exclude it, but it makes it unlikely.

CYTOLYTIC T-CELL GRANULES: BIOCHEMIMCAL

PROPERTIES AND FUNCTIONAL SPECIFICITY

Eckhard R. Podack*, Paula J. Konigsberg*, Hans Acha-Orbea,
Hans Pircher and Hans Hengartner

Scripps Clinic and Research Foundation
La Jolla, California 92037
University of Zurich
Zurich, Switzerland

I. Introduction

Murine, cloned cytolytic NK- and TK-cells may be classified

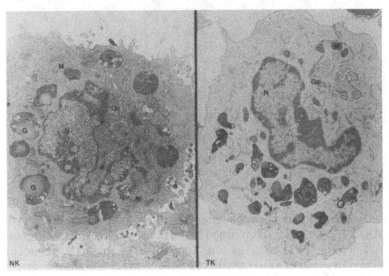

Fig. 1: Ultrastructural comparison of a cytolytic NK and
T-cell. Note the dense cytoplasmatic granules (G) and the
prominent Golgi complex (Go). M - Mitochondria; N - Nucleus

*Present address: New York Medical College, Department of
Microbiology/Immunology, Valhalla, New York 10595

as large, granular lymphocytes possessing a prominent Golgi complex and active ergastoplasma (Fig. 1). The granules are characterized by a dense homogeneous core surrounded by an area of vesicular structures and delimited by a bilayer membrane. Ultrastructural studies showed the positioning of granules towards the conjugation site of killer-target conjugates and the apparent release (secretion) of granule contents into the interstitial space (1-5). Subsequently, two types of membrane lesions poly P1 (160 Å diameter) and poly P2 (~70 Å diameter) became detectable on target membranes and on vesicular bodies (4,5,6) (Fig. 2). These studies led to the hypothesis that the granules contain the factors responsible for membrane lesion assembly and that they represent the cytolytic principle of cloned cytolytic NK and TK cells (7). Similar conclusions were reached by Henkart et al in the antibody dependent cytotoxicity system and with a rat lymphoma line that expressed NK-like cytotoxicity.

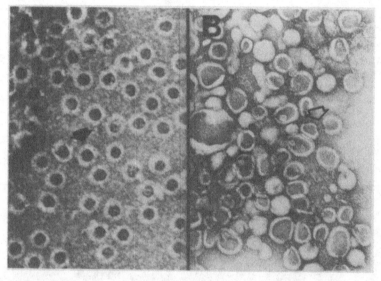

Fig. 2: Ultrastructural membrane lesions assembled by cytolytic lymphocytes. Panel A: High magnification of membrane bound poly perforin 1 (poly P1) complex in top view. Subunit structure is detectable in several complexes (arrow). Panel B: Lower magnification of poly P1 in side view (arrow) attached to single bilayer vesicles. Note the top-to-top aggregation of poly P1 on adjacent vesicles (arrow). Scale: the inner diameter of poly P1 corresponds to 160 Å.

In addition, this hypothesis is fully compatible with other studies analzying the kinetics, temperature dependence and drug inhibition of cell mediated cytolysis (for review see e.g. 9).

II. Isolation and characterization of T-cell granules

Granules have been isolated to date from four cytolytic T-cell clones and one long-term cytolytic T-cell line. The clones used were chosen because they allowed a comparison of the cytolytic activity of the intact cell with that of the isolated granules (Table I).

Table I

Name of clone or cell line	Haplotype of Effector Cell	Original Target Specificity	Present Target Specificity	Reference
CTLL-2	H2b	H2d	None (lost cytolytic activity)	10
HY3AG3	H2b (female)	H2b (male)	NK-like	11
3A2	H2d	H2b	H2b	
8/10	H2b	H2b + Hapten (AED)	H2b + Hapten	12
B6	H2b	H2d	H2d	13

CTLL-2, isolated in 1978, is a cloned cell line containing typical granules as defined by their azurophilic staining with Giemsa stain (12). CTLL-2 originally has been an H2d restricted cytolytic T-cell. During the many years in culture, this cell line has lost its cytolytic activity, yet retained its dependence on Il2 and its azurophilic granules. CTLL-2 can be stimulated to assemble poly P1 and poly P2 by concanavalin A (5). HY3AG3 has been isolated in 1978 as H2^b restricted male antigen specific and H2D^d specific cytotoxic T-cell (14). This clone has lost its original specificity and, instead, acquired NK-like killing activity, the most sensitive target being YAC-1, followed by El-4 (11). 3A2 is an alloreactive cytolytic T-cell clone restricted to H2b targets. 3A2 has retained its allospecificity throughout the culture period and requires regular antigen stimulation in addition to Il2 for continuous proliferation. Similarly clone 8/10 has retained its H2b restricted hapten (N-iodo-acetyl-N-[5-sulfonic-1-naphtyl]ethyl ene diamine) specificity (12). B6 is an uncloned long-term cytolytic T-cell line specific for H2d targets that has been in culture for five months and requires antigen stimulation and Il2.

a. CTLL-2 and B6 granules

10^9 cells are grown in 15 cm Petri dishes in the presence of 10-15 percent rat concanavalin A supernatant. The cells are harvested, disrupted by N_2-cavitation, and separated by Percoll gradient centrifugation. The details of the procedure have been described (13).

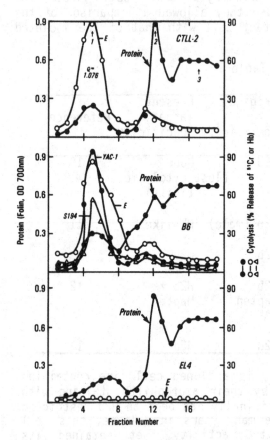

Fig.3: Percoll gradient fractionation of N_2-disrupted CTLL-2 (upper panel) B6 (middle panel) and E14 (lower panel). Sedimentations to the left. Upper panel Hemolytic activity of CTLL-2 fractions against sheep erythrocytes (E) and protein. Middle panel: Cytolytic activity of B6 fractions to sheep erythrocytes (E) and to tumor lines YAC-1 (H2a) and S194 (H2d) is plotted in addition to protein Lower panel: E14 shows no hemolytic activity toward sheep erythrocytes (E).

Fig. 3 (upper panel) shows the Percoll gradient profile of protein and of hemolytic activity of CTLL-2 after fractionation. Cytolytic activity is located in the high density area of the gradient containing the dense granules. The apparent density of granules from CTLL-2 (Fig. 3, upper panel) and from B6 (Fig. 3, middle panel) is the same as indicated by the same position of cytolytic activity in the gradient. As control in Fig. 3 (lower panel) is included a non-cytolytic cell line, E14. Although a protein peak sediments to a somewhat lower density than that of CTLL-2 or B6-granules, no cytolytic activity is detectable. This results suggests that cytolytic granules do not occur in EL4 cells.

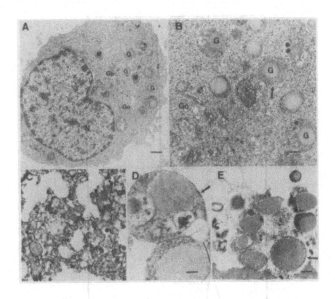

Fig. 4: Ultrastructure of intracellular granules of CTLL-2 (panel A,B) and of isolated granules (panel D,E). Panel C shows the composition of the low density material of Fig. 3 (arrow 2).

Fig. 4 summarizes the morphological characterization of intracellular CTLL-2 granules (panel A,B) isolated CTLL-2 granules from the high density area of the Percoll gradient (panel D,E) and, for comparison, the low density peak of the Percoll gradient (panel C).

b) HY3AG3, 3A2 and 8/10 granules

Granules from these cloned cell lines were prepared exactly as described above (13). Fig. 5 shows the Percoll density gradient profile of the cytolytic activity of HY3AG3 (lower panel) in comparison to CTLL-2 (upper panel). Cytolytic activity, as measured by red cell lysis, is located exclusively in the high density area of the gradient. 3A2 and 8/10 granules showed activity only in one out of three fractionations. The peptide composition of Percoll gradient fractions of HY3AG3 is shown in Fig. 6. Track 1-3 shows fractions across the high density granule and cytolytic activity containing peak. Track 4-6 shows the pattern of the lower density area of the Percoll gradient and of soluble proteins (track 6). Cytolytic granules have a unique peptide composition. The most abundant proteins are a cluster of three protein bands labeled K2,3,4 with molecular

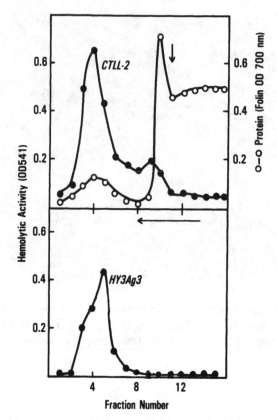

Fig. 5: Percoll gradient fractionation of clone HY3Ag3. Upper panel: CTLL-2 (same as in Fig. 3). Lower panel: Hemolytic activity of the fractionated T-cell clone. Sedimentation is to the left. The arrow in the upper panel shows the beginning of the Percoll gradient. Granules from clone 8/10 and 3A2 were prepared by the same procedure and used for SDS polyacrylamide gel electrophoresis (Fig. 8).

weights between 32-40,000. Lower molecular weight proteins, labeled K5 and K6, are somewhat variable. The highest molecular weight band, K1, migrates with about 58 kDa and 75 kDa under non-reducing and reducing condtions, respectively. A protein doublet of Mr 45-50 KDa (not labeled in Fig. 6) is usually detectable between K1 and K2 and probably also is a granule specific protein. However, further analysis is required to further clarify the precise peptide composition of cytolytic granules. CTLL-2 granules show a similar composition of K1-K6 compared to HY3AG3 granules (Fig. 7). In Fig. 8, the peptide pattern of granules derived HY3AG3, 3A2, 8/10 is compared. It is apparent that the peptide composition of granules derived from T-cell clones with completely different killing specificity is very similar, if not identical. This result may suggest that the killing step, mediated by granules, is identical in each of these clones, and that their specificity is provided by other cellular compartments.

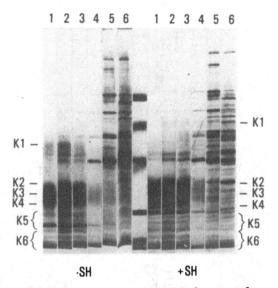

Fig. 6: Peptide composition of HY3Ag3 granules. A 7.5-15 SDS polyacrylamide gradient slab was used. Track 1-3: Samples from granule containing fractions. Track 4 and 5, samples from the low density area of Percoll gradients. Track 6 soluble proteins. K1 to K6 refer to granule proteins in track 1-3. The center track contains marker proteins (94 kDa, 68 kDa, 45 kDa, 32 kDa, 21 kDa, 14 kDa).

Granule mediated cytolytic activity appears to be restricted to granules obtained from cytolytic lymphocytes. As shown in Fig. 3 (lower panel), E14 granules do not effect any cytolytic activity. In addition, anti sera raised against CTLL-2 granules detect granules from other cytolytic T-cell clones but not granules from other non-cytolytic T-cells (Fig. 9). CTLL-2, B6 and the H2d- T-cell lymphoma S194 were cytocentrifuged onto microscope slides, fixed, permeabilized and exposed to anti CTLL-2 granules antiserum (raised in rabbits). After washing, binding of the first antibody was detected with a fluorescein labeled second antibody (goat anti-rabbit IgG). Anti CTLL-2-granule antibody stains granules of CTLL-2 and of B6 but fails to stain granules of S194 even though S194 is a T-cell lymphoma and contains numerous cytoplasmic granules. No staining of cytolytic granules was detected with non-immune rabbit IgG, excluding non-specific affinity of cytolytic granules for rabbit IgG (Fig. 9).

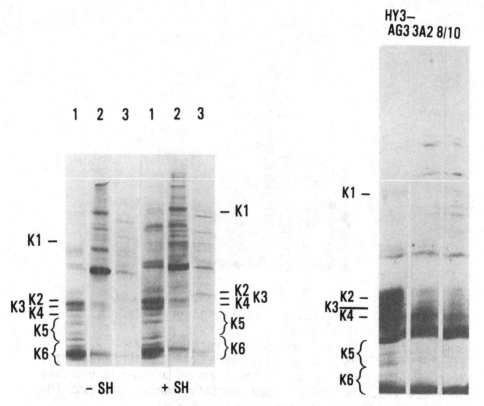

Fig. 7: Peptide composition of CTLL-2 granules on 7.5-15% SDS polyacrylimide slabs. Track 1: Granules, track 2: low density material, track 3: soluble proteins above gradient. K1 to K6 are labeled as in Fig. 6 and refer to peptides in track 1.

Fig. 8: Peptide composition of granules obtained from three T-cell clones after SDS PAGE under reducing conditions. Only the granules containing fractions are shown.

In summary, then, these studies suggest that cytolytic granules from various T-cell clones have a specific set of proteins with identical molecular weights and antigenic determinants that seem to be responsible for cytolytic activity. Non-cytolytic T-cells do not express granule mediated cytolysis and do not contain these antigenic determinants.

III. Target specificity of isolated T-cell granules

Although studies directed towards determining the specificity of cytolytic granules from the five T-cell lines described above are not complete, the pattern emerging from results to date suggests that T-cell granules are not H2-restricted. Different susceptibilities of various tumor cells to granule mediated cytolysis seems to be determined by certain properties of the target cell.

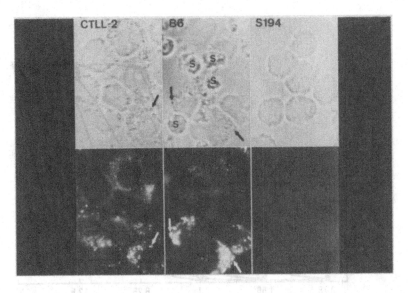

Fig. 9: Immunofluorescence of various T-cells treated with rabbit anti-CTLL-2 granule antibody. Upper panels: Phase contrast, lower panel: fluorescence. CTLL-2, B6 and S194 were fixed, permeabilized and then reacted with the first antibody. After washing, antibody binding was detected with a fluorescein labeled goat anti rabbit IgG.

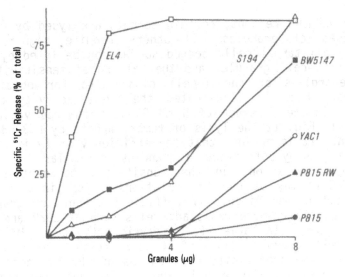

Fig. 10 legend next page

Fig. 10: Target sensitivity to CTLL-2 granules. 2×10^4 ^{51}Cr labeled target cells were incubated for 30 min with the amount of granules indicated. Non-specific release was less than 5% in controls incubated with Percoll-containing buffer.

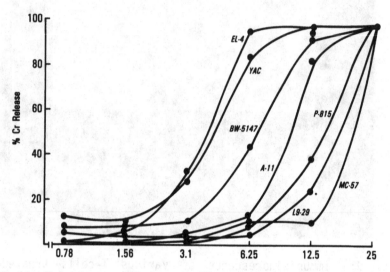

Fig. 11: Target sensitivity to HY granules. Assay was for 10 min at 37°. Note the logarithmic scale of the abscissa given in μl granule fractions from Percoll.

For unknown reasons, certain targets are lysed by relatively low doses of granules and others require higher amounts. However, all target cells tested so far can be lysed by isolated cytolytic T-cell granules and the pattern of sensitivity is the same regardless of the T-cell clone used for obtaining the granules. Fig. 10 illustrates the lytic activity of CTLL-2 granules in the presence of 5 mM Ca ions towards various tumor cells. In Fig. 11 the lysis of tumor targets by HY3AG3 granules is shown. It is obvious that the efficiency of lysis of various tumor targets by both types of granules is similar.

Slight variations in the sensitivity to certain targets (e.g. YAC-1) may be due to variations of sublines cultured in Zurich and in San Diego. If sufficient amounts of granules are added, relatively more resistant cells such as L929 and MC57 are readily lysed. In Table II, the lytic activity of HY3AG3 cells and HY3AG3 granules and of CTLL-2 cells and granules is compared. The specificity of granules of the two cell types is similar; however, the granule specificity does not reflect the specificty of the intact cell. For instance, the susceptibility

Table II. Comparison of cytolytic activity of intact cells and isolated granules

| Target | HY3AG3 | | CTLL-2 | |
	Cells*	Granules	Cells	Granules
YAC-1	++++	++	-	++
EL4	++	++++	-	++++
BW5147	ND	+++	-	+++
P815	+	+	-	+

*From reference 11

of EL4 and YAC1 to lysis by HY3AG3 cells is the reverse of their susceptibility to lysis by HY3AG3 granules. Similarly, CTLL-2 granules show high cytolytic activity whereas the intact cell has no cytolytic activity.

In Table III the cytolytic activity of B6 cells is compared to that of B6 granules with two target cells. B6 is an H2d restricted cytolytic T-cell and lyses the lymphoma line S194 (H2d) but not the NK-target YAC-1 (H2a).
In contrast, B6 granules lyse YAC-1 targets even better than S194 targets (see also Fig. 3) suggesting that H2-restriction is conferred by plasma membrane receptors and not by the granules. The cytolytic step itself appears to be nonspecific supporting the notion that NK- and TK-cell mediated killing employs the same molecular mechanism (4,5).

Table III. Lack of H2-restriction of B6 granules as opposed to H2-restriction of B6 cells

| Target | Lysis by B6 | |
	Cells	Granules
S194 (H2d)	++++	+++
YAC-1 (H2a)	-	++++

IV. Mechanism of killing

The experiments outlined in the previous chapters and in previous publications (7,8) showed that isolated granules are endowed with strong cytolytic activity. Quantitative titrations indicate that the amount of granules corresponding to a killer-target ratio of 1:1 to 3:1 is sufficient to cause 100 percent ^{51}Cr release from target cells within 5–10 min.
This result suggests that cytolytic granules represent the major, if not the entire, cytolytic principle of cytotoxic lymphocytes. In this context, the function of the cell is to provide for specific killer target contact and to mediate the release of granules.

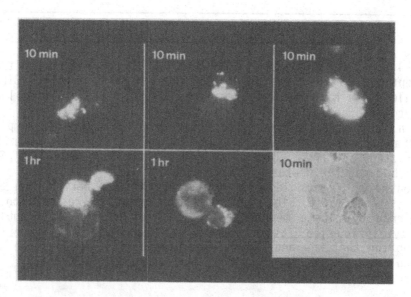

Fig. 12: Orientation of granules to the contact area of killer target conjugates. S194 targets were mixed with B6 killers at 1:1 ratio, centrifuged for 5 min at 400 rpm and incubated for the times indicated. Samples were then carefully resuspended and cytocentrifuged onto microscope slides. After fixing with paraformaldehyde and permeabilization with NP40, cytolytic granules were detected by immunofluorescence using rabbit anti CTLL-2 granule IgG and FITC goat anti rabbit IgG. Immunofluorescence micrographs are shown (left and middle panel). The right panels show fluorescence and phase contrast images of the same killer-target conjugate. Note the apparent transfer of cytolytic granules from killer to target cell.

Immunofluoresce studies in Fig. 12 (see also Fig. 9) directly
support the role of granules in the cytolytic reaction. B6
cytolytic T-cells were incubated with appropriate targets cells
(S194) for various time periods and the conjugates analyzed by
the immunofluorescent technique described in Fig. 12 using
anti-granule antibodies. It is evident from Fig. 12 that already
after 10 min the cytolytic T-cell granules are oriented towards
the conjugation area. The right panels in Fig. 12 are suggestive
of the release of granules from the killer cell and of their
transfer onto target membranes. After 1 hr the target cells have
assumed a diffuse fluorescent staining. These studies show a
very early involvement of cytolytic granules in the cytolytic
reaction mediated by intact killer cells. It is suggested that
the reorientation of cytoskeletal elements of killer cells
observed during the the early phase of killer-target contact (
15,16) brings the cytoplasmic granules to the conjugation site
and causes their release. The essential role of granules for
cytolysis is further substantiated by the finding that granules
during the cytolytic reaction give rise to target membrane bound
poly P1 and poly P2 complexes. Fig. 14 shows rabbit erythrocyte
membranes lysed by CTLL-2 granules. The typical membrane lesions
of poly P1 (left panel) and poly P2 are apparent (right panel).

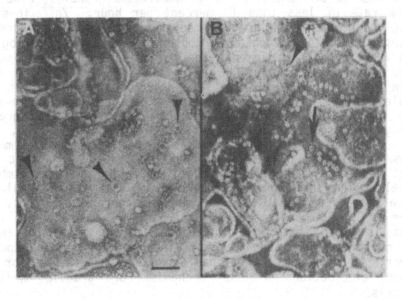

Fig. 13: Membrane lesions assembled by isolated granules on
rabbit erythrocyte membranes. Rabbit erythrocytes were
incubated for 1 hr at 37° with CTLL-2 granules corresponding
to 50 Z. After washing, the ghost membranes were trypsinized
and mounted for negative staining electron microscopy. Panel
A: Poly P1, Panel B: Poly P2. Same magnification in both
panels. Scale bar: A.

Poly perforin complexes may be extracted from membranes with deoxycholate and purified by gel filtration on Sepharose CL4B (7,13). Without reduction, poly P1 remains on top of a 2.5 percent stacking gel indicating disulfide-linked subunits exceeding 2.5 to 3×10^6 molecular weight. After reduction, protein bands of similar, but not identical, molecular weights (migrating as K2,3,4) are detectable. Since granules do not contain preassembled poly P complexes, this result suggests that, during cytolysis, perforins polymerize to disulfide linked poly perforin complexes. The poly P1 complex, as evident from the association pattern in Fig. 2 is endowed with hydrophobic domains on both ends of the tubular complex. In solution these domains give rise to stacked tail-tail, head-head, or head-tail aggregates. If bound to membrane vesicles, the second hydrophobic domains of poly P1 may either fuse with adjacent membrane or aggregate head-head with other membrane bound poly P1's (Fig. 2). It is probable that the second hydrophobic domain of poly P1 has important functions during target membrane insertion of poly perforin complexes.

Cytolysis by isolated granules is strongly temperature dependent and absolutely Ca^{++} dependent (Fig. 14). The dose response curve is sigmoidal. Granule mediated lysis of targets in the presence of Ca^{++} is extremely rapid (<2 min at 37°C) and strongly inhibited by low concentrations of serum. Ca^{++} alone in the absence of targets at 37°C inactivates granules, albeit at a slow rate of less than 10 percent per hour. Zn^{++} ions are strongly inhibitory for granule mediated cytolysis at micromolar concentrations. Based on these observations and by analogy to known reactions in complement, the following hypothetical scheme may be constructed (Fig. 15).

In the presence of Ca^{++}, contact between target and granules causes granule activation. The inhibitory effect of serum may be due to interference or competition with granule binding to targets. In the absence of granule binding, Ca^{++} alone activates only slowly. Granule activation sets into motion the polymerization of perforins that simultaneously insert into target membranes and cause lysis by formation of transmembrane channels. The inhibitory effect of Zn^{++} ions may be explained by the possibility that Zn^{++} polymerizes perforins in a similar manner as C9 of human complement (17).

It is clear that this hypothetical chain of events leaves many questions open and may be incorrect in some aspects. However, it provides a reasonable working hypothesis for the further elucidation of the mechanism of granule mediated cytolysis.

V. Analogies between poly P of lymphocytes and poly C9 of complement

The discovery of C9 polymerization in the complement cascade has greatly enhanced our understanding of the molecular mechanism of the formation of complement lesions. Poly C9 has been studied in some detail, and the results are briefly summarized here and compared to poly P1 in Table IV. Isolated C9 polymerizes spontaneously in a very slow reaction. The rate of C9

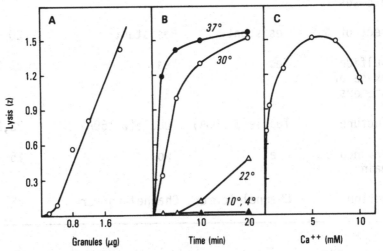

Fig. 14: Dose response, temperature, time, and Ca-dependence of granule mediated hemolysis of sheep erythrocytes.

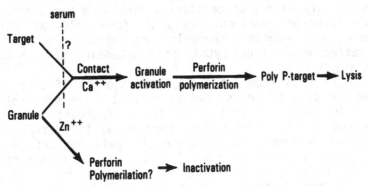

Fig. 15: Hypothetical scheme for granule mediated cytolysis and control.

Table IV. Similarities between poly C9 and Poly P1

	Poly C9	Poly Perforin 1	Reference
Physiological Polymerase	C5b-8	?	18,19
Effect of Zn	Polymerization	Polymerization	17
Effect of Proteases	Resistant	Resistant	20
Effect of SDS	Resistant	Resistant	20
Disulfide linkage of protomers	Yes	Yes	21,22
Structure	Tubule(ϕ 100Å)	Tubule(ϕ 160Å)	23,24
Hydrophobic domain	One	Two	25
Function	Channel-former	Channel-former	25

polymerization is drastically increased by Zn ions or by the C5b-8 complex (physiological polymerase). Even in the presence of C5b-8, C9 polymerization is strongly temperature dependent and ceases below 20°C. Poly C9 is a tubular complex of 160 Å length and 100 Å internal diameter which is resistant to dissociation by SDS and to degradation by proteases. C9 subunits in poly C9 may be covalently linked to one another by disulfide exchange reaction. Poly C9 forms ~70-100 Å wide functional transmembrane channels and appears to be the primary effector unit of cytolytic complement (see Young et al, this volume).

As can be seen from Table IV, the majority of properties described for poly C9 are shared by poly P1. The most notable exception is poly P1's content of two hydrophobic domains on opposite ends of its tubule. The question as to whether there is a complex analogous to C5b-8 in the poly perforin system remains open at the present time. The ultrastructural examination of poly P1 revealed no indication for a similar complex. It may, therefore, be assumed that the physiological mechanism of perforin polymerization is different from that of poly C9.

The accumulated evidence outlined in this chapter strongly supports the concept that cytotoxicity of NK and T-killer cells is mediated by their cytoplasmic granules. The cytolytic granules appear to be released into the killer-target conjugation site subsequent to specific contact

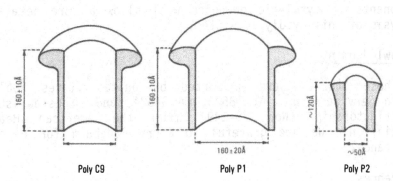

Fig. 16: Size comparison of poly P1 and poly P2 (murine) with poly C9 (human).

between the plasma membranes of the reacting cells. The killing step itself appears to be unspecific because isolated granules do not express the H2 restriction and the specificity of the parent cell. Furthermore, granules isolated from different H2 restricted T-clones and from clones with NK-like specificity have similar cytolytic activity towards various tumor targets and erythrocytes.

Cytolytic lymphocyte granules contain a characteristic set of proteins that is not detectable in cells lacking cytolytic activity. The same granule proteins are found in cytolytic cells of different clonal origin and of different specificity. The presence of cytolytic granule proteins in cell lines that have lost their cytolytic activity (e.g. CTLL-2) suggests a functional deficiency of these cells at a step required for granule release. The continued Il2 dependence of these cells could suggest a role of this interleukin in the regulation of cytolytic granule protein synthesis. Antigen, in contrast, does not seem to be required for granule synthesis. The cytolytic step itself appears to involve polymerization of granule perforins to tubular poly perforins forming transmembrane channels upon insertion into target membranes. Thus, the killing mechanism may be quite analogous to transmembrane channel formation by C9 polymerization in complement. The steps occurring prior to perforin polymerization have not been elucidated on a molecular level. The absolute requirement for Ca might suggest a Ca-dependent proteolytic or conformational activation during the early phase of granule activation. Although many questions of granule mediated cytolysis remain open at the present time, it is clear that a dissection of the components of cytolytic granules will allow a more detailed analysis of this cytolytic system.

Acknowledgement

These studies were supported by United States Public Health Service Grants AI 18525, CA 34524, and an Established Investigatorship (No. 79-149) from the American Heart Association. We are grateful to Kerry Pangburn for expert assistance.

References

1. Carpen, O, Virtanen, I., and Saksela, E., 1981, Cell. Immunol. 58: 97.
2. Carpen, O., Virtanen, I. and Saksela, E., 1982, J. Immunol. 128: 2691.
3. Henkart, M., Henkart, P., 1982, in: Mechanisms of Cell Mediated Cytotoxicity, p. 227, W. Clark, P. Golstein, ed., Plenum, New York.
4. Podack, E. R. and Dennert, G., 1983, Nature 302: 442.
5. Dennert, G. and Podack, E.R., 1983, J. Exp. Med. 157: 1483.
6. Dourmashkin, R.R., Deteix, P., Simone, C.B. and Henkart, P.A., 1980, Clin. Exp. Immunol. 42: 554.
7. Podack, E.R., 1984, in: Natural Killer Activity and its Regulation, p. 101, T. Hoshino, H.S. Koren, A. Uchida, ed. Excerpta Medica, Tokyo.
8. Henkart, P., Henkart, M., Millard, P. and Reynolds, C.W. in: Natural Killer Activity and its Regulation, p. 150, T. Hoshino, H.S. Koren, A. Uchida, ed., Excerpta Medica, Tokyo.
9. Green, W.R. and Henney, C.S., 1981, Critical Rev. in Immunology 1: 259.
10. Gillis, S., Baker, P.E., Ruscetti, F.W. and Smith, K.A., 1978, J. Exp. Med. 148: 1093.
11. Acha-Orbea, H., Groscurth, P., Lang, R., Stitz, L., and Hengartner, H., 1983, J. Immunol. 130: 2952.
12. Pircher, H., Hammerling, G. and Hengartner, H., 1984, Eur. J. Immunol., in press.

13. Podack, E.R. and Konigsberg, P.J., 1984, J. Exp. Med., submitted.
14. Von Bohmer, H., Hengartner, H., Nabholz, M., Lernhardt, W., Schreier, M.H. and Haas, W., Eur. J. Immunol. 9: 952.
15. Carpen, O., Virtanen, I., Lehto, V. and Saksela, E., 1983, J. Immunol. 131: 2695.
16. Kupfer, A., Dennert, G. and Singer, S.J., 1983, Proc. Natl. Acad. Sci. 80: 7224.
17. Tschopp, J., 1984, J. Biol. Chem., in press.
18. Podack, E.R., Tschopp, J., and Muller-Eberhard, H.J., 1982, J. Exp. Med. 156: 268.
19. Tschopp, J., Podack, E.R. and Muller-Eberhard, H.J., 1982, Proc. Natl. Acad. Sci. 79: 7474.
20. Podack, E.R. and Tschopp, J., 1982, J. Biol. Chem. 257: 15204.
21. Yamamoto, K., Kawashima, T. and Migita, S., 1982, J. Biol. Chem. 257: 8573.
22. Yamamoto, K., Migita, S., 1983, J. Biol. Chem. 258: 7887.
23. Podack, E.R., Tschopp, J., 1982, Proc. Natl. Acad. Sci. 79: 574.
24. Tschopp, J., Engel, A. and Podack, E.R., 1984, J. Biol. Chem. 259: 1922.
25. Tschopp, J., Muller-Eberhard, H.J. and Podack, E.R., 1982, Nature 298: 534.

DISCUSSION

Mescher: Are there any differences in granule morphology in the absence and presence of calcium?

Podack: If you incubate granules in calcium you form poly-perforins, but looking at the granules directly you don't see them.

Mescher: Do you see the polymerized form within the limiting membrane?

Podack: No.

Cohen: When you look at granules from non-cytotoxic cells, do you get the same protein bands as you see in granules from killer cells?

Podack: I have only analyzed EL-4 cells, and these granules have a different pattern, although it is difficult to say that there are no common proteins. Based on the fluorescence, the EL-4 granules do not have the antigens found in CTL granules, and the antibodies do react with all the major CTL granule proteins in western blots.

Hiserodt: Have you looked at your gels with silver stains to see how many minor proteins are present?

Podack: The gels I showed were overloaded and stained with Coomassie Blue, and you can see a number of minor bands. However I don't really know their relationship to the granules. But the granules seem to be complex system, and while these membrane lesions I have described are undoubtedly important, they may not be the only means of killing target cells. The granules may contain other factors contributing to this.

Nathan: To get granule staining with your antiserum, did you permeabilize the cells?

Podack: The best way to do this is to cytocentrifuge the cells onto the slides, air dry them, fix the paraformaldehyde, permeabilize them with NP-40, then treat with the primary antibody, wash and treat with the fluoresceinated antibody.

Nathan: Does your antiserum block CTL function?

Podack: Yes, but so do control sera and preimmune serum.

Kaufmann: Have you ever looked for these granules in helper T cells which are devoid of killing activity?

Podack: The one helper T cell clone I have examined did have granules, but they looked quite different morphologically from the CTL granules. I have looked at suppressor cells, and they have granules which are very similar morphologically to CTL granules.

Kaufmann: Did you test the granules from these other lymphocyte types for killing activity?

Podack: No, we haven't done that.

THE ROLE OF CYTOPLASMIC GRANULES IN CYTOTOXICITY

BY LARGE GRANULAR LYMPHOCYTES AND CYTOTOXIC T LYMPHOCYTES

Pierre Henkart, Maryanna Henkart, Paul Millard, Peter
Frederikse, Jeff Bluestone, Robert Blumenthal, Cho Yue
and Craig Reynolds

Immunology Branch and Laboratory of Theoretical Biology
NCI, Bethesda, Md., 20205, and Biological Therapeutics
Biological Therapeutics Branch, NCI
Frederick, Md. 21701

Three years ago, at the First Workshop on Mechanisms of
Cell-Mediated Cytotoxicity, we presented a summary of the evidence developed in our lab that the ADCC and NK cytotoxic
functions of large granular lymphocytes (LGL) operated via a secretory process (1). We showed by EM that for both NK and ADCC,
target contact induces a rearrangement of the LGL cytoplasmic
granules suggesting exocytosis. This secretion was evidenced by
deposition of material which had been in the granules into the
intracellular space, where 15 nm pore-like ring structures formed
from this material. These structures were identical to those
previously reported in a collaborative study with Dourmashkin
(2), where they were seen on target membranes after ADCC. The
pore-like structures were similar in appearance to those made by
complement but had a larger diameter; these findings correlated
nicely with molecular sieving experiments of markers released
from red cell ghosts attacked by complement and by LGL in ADCC
(3). Similar pore-like structures were reported to be associated
with cytotoxicity by a cloned cell line with NK activity (4).

Several groups studying cytototoxic T lymphocyte killing
have also produced evidence in support of an exocytosis of effector cell cytoplasmic granules during the post-binding stage of
the cytotoxic process. Zagury and collaborators presented evidence at the first Workshop (5) that granules containing
lysosomal enzymes moved towards the bound target and later

released their contents into the intracellular space. Somewhat similar observations have been made by Bykovskyva, et al (6). Further analogy of the CTL secretory process to that of LGL was provided by Dennert and Podack (7) who showed pore-like structures associated with CTL killing.

The above morphological evidence of a secretory process involving cytoplasmic granules is compatible with evidence for a secretion mechanism based on the role of calcium (8,9), and the action of various drugs (10-13) on both CTL and LGL cytotoxicity. We felt that the most direct test of hypotheses invoking granule exocytosis in lymphocyte cytotoxicity required a detailed study of the relevant granules and their properties, and I will describe here the results of our studies of the properties of isolated cytoplasmic granules of LGL tumors and CTL.

The first problem we faced was to find a source of adequate amounts of granules to allow a rigorous purification which could be monitored biochemically. LGL tumors having NK and/or ADCC activity (14,15) proved to be a convenient source of material for this, and we devoted a considerable effort into developing a procedure for the purification of these granules (16). Since histochemical studies had indicated that the granules contained lysosomal enzymes (5,14,17), we monitored such activities, along with morphology, to guide our purification. Fig. 1 shows the results of a Percoll gradient, which is the final step in the

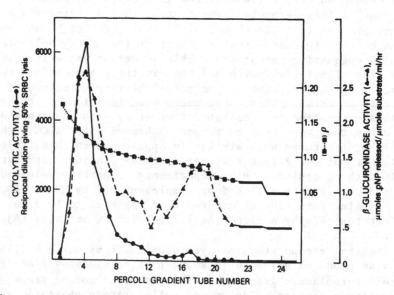

Fig. 1. Percoll gradient purification of LGL tumor homogenate. Fraction 1 is at the bottom, and fractions 23 and 24 contain 4X more sample than the others. This is not an equilibrium gradient. From ref. 16.

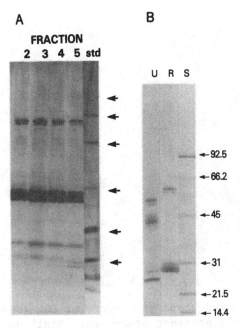

Fig. 2. SDS gel of proteins from Percoll gradient fractions. A.
Silver stain of sequential fractions in the granule region,
showing purity of granules. Arrows point to molecular weight
standards shown in B. B. Coomassie stained gells run under
reduced (R) and unreduced (U) conditions. Reduced standards are
shown in lane S. From ref. 16.

purification of LGL tumor granules, and the association of the
lysosomal enzymes B-glucuronidase with the characteristic lytic
activity of the granules. Other enzymatic activities in this
gradient provide evidence that this gradient yields pure
lysosomal granules devoid of other cellular components (3). Fig.
2 shows SDS gels of the proteins in those tubes where cytolytic
activity is found, showing a unique set of bands of 60, 58, 30,
28 and 27 kd associated with the lytic activity. This figure
also demonstrates the biochemical purity of the granules, since
proteins from other parts of the gradient are not found in the
granule pool. The major LGL tumor granule protein components do
not appear to coincide with known proteins from other granules,
and overall consideration of the biochemical and enzymatic
contents of these granules has led to the conclusion that they
are distinct from the cytoplasmic granules of mast cells or PMN
(16). Fig. 3 shows that a pool of the lytically active material
consists of a pure population of granules which are morphologically indistinguishable from those in the intact LGL tumor
cells.

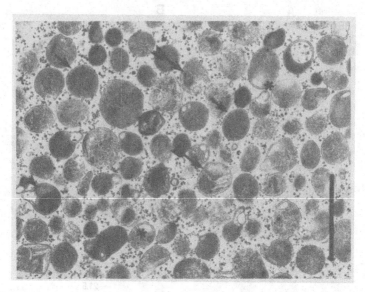

Fig. 3. Electron microscope appearance of LGL tumor granules purified by Percoll gradient procedure. Small dots are residual Percoll. Bar, 1 micron. From ref. 16.

The most striking property of the granules is their potent lytic activity (18), which was not initially easy to detect because of its peculiar properties. As shown in Fig. 4, small amounts of granules are lytic to a variety of cells, with red cells being the most sensitive. It can readily be seen that the target cell selectivity in granule-mediated killing is very different from NK cells or NK tumor cells, which do not lyse red cells or normal lymphocytes. However, among the lymphoid tumor cells tested there is a general correlation of susceptibility to NK cells and to the lytic effects of the granules.

This cytolytic effect is so fast that it is not easy to get a good time course at 37° with conventional sampling techniques. Fig. 5 shows the lysis of red cells and YAC tumor cells at room temperature. The speed of this lysis very clearly distinguishes it from the lymphotoxin type of supernatant factors such as NKCF.

The lytic activity of LGL tumor granules is highly dependent on divalent ions, as shown in Fig. 6. These curves are strikingly similar to those for the programming for lysis stage of CTL killing (19). The granule mediated lytic activity is unstable in the presence of calcium, however, decaying with a half life of 10 minutes at room temperature in 2mM $CaCl_2$. This dual effect of calcium probably explains why the lytic potential of the granule cytolysin was not previously detected.

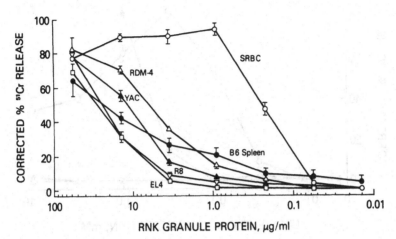

Fig. 4. Lytic activity of LGL tumor granules on various cells.
Granules were diluted in calcium-free PBS, followed by addition
of an equal volume of target cells in balanced salt solution containing a physiological calcium concentration. After 20 min at
37°, supernatants were harvested and counted. RDM-4, YAC, R-8
and EL-4 are murine lymphoid tumor lines. From ref. 18.

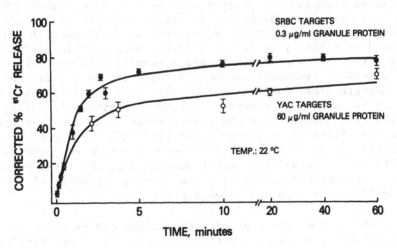

Fig. 5. Kinetics of granule mediated lysis of red cells and YAC
tumor cells. The temperature of this experiment was 22°. From
ref. 18.

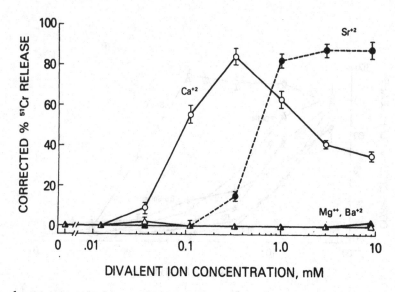

Fig. 6. Divalent ion dependence of LGL tumor granule cytolytic
activity on YAC cells. From ref. 18.

The granule lytic activity described has been reproducibly
found in each of six independent cytotoxic rat LGL tumors. When
we use our Percoll gradient purification technique to prepare
granules from non-cytotoxic lymphoid cells, they generally do not
possess detectable lytic activity (e.g. blood T cells, spleen,
thymus, EL-4 and most other lymphoid tumors). In most of these
cases a peak of lysosomal enzymes is found at the position of the
LGL tumor granules, indicating that some sort of equivalent granules are isolated. In contrast to these non-cytotoxic cells, LGL
purified from normal rat blood give granules with the same level
of lytic activity (on a per cell basis) as LGL tumor granules.
This activity has similar divalent ion dependence and rapid kinetics to that obtained from LGL tumors. Thus, the lytic property
of the cytoplasmic granules is not a peculiar property of the LGL
tumor cells we have chosen to work with.

When granules are treated with calcium and examined in the
electron microscope using negative staining, the characteristic
pore-like structures described above can be seen. The apearance
of these structures on the granule membranes correlated with the
cytolytic effects of granules in that they were apparent within a
few minutes and were completely dependent on calcium. When
erythrocytes were lysed by the granules, these structures could
be seen associated with the ghost membranes (18).

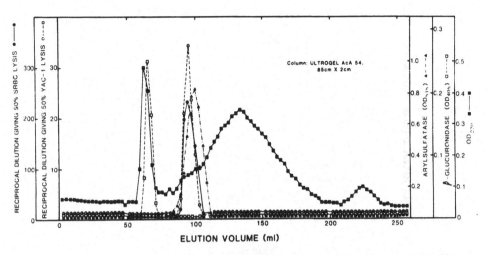

Fig. 7. Gel filtration of LGL tumor granule cytolysin on ACA 54.
The elution buffer contains 2M NaCl. On this column, BSA elutes
at about 80ml. (●) Lytic activity on SRBC; (○) Lytic activity
on YAC; (▲) Arylsulfatase; (□) B-glucuronidase; (■) OD_{220}.

The lytic activity associated with granules can be
solubilized, and we have termed the active material a cytolysin
in view of its lytic properties. The cytolysin is heat-labile
and Pronase sensitive, suggesting a protein. The activity can be
solubilized by high ionic strength, and Fig. 7 shows the gel filtration behavior of this material which suggests a molecular
weight of the native material of about 60kd. At this stage there
are still three major protein bands (of 60, 58, and 29 kd), and
we have no strong evidence as to which of these is responsible
for the activity. Obviously, further purification and characterization of the cytolysin is currently underway in our lab.

Because of the previous data suggesting that the cytolysin
acts by a membrane pore insertion mechanism, we tested the cytolysin on liposomes, using the carboxyfluorescein (CF) release
assay (20). As shown in Fig. 8, these studies revealed a rapid
release of CF from small and large liposomes of all compositions
in the presence of calcium (21). The divalent ion dependence of
this process was virtually identical to the cytolytic activity.
Finally, the characteristic pore-like structures appeared to be
inserted into the liposomes, as shown in Fig. 9. As was found
with complement (22), penetration of the negative stain into the
liposomes correlated nicely with the presence of these pore

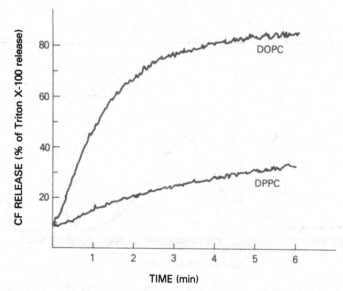

Fig. 8. Carboxyfluroescein release from small unilamillar liposomes induced by partially purified LGL tumor granule cytolysin. DOPC, dioleoyl phosphatidyl choline, which is in a "fluid" phase; DPPC, dipalmitoyl phatidylcholine, which is in a "solid" phase at 22°, where these measurements were made. From ref. 21.

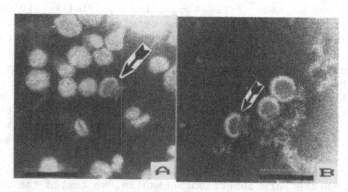

Fig. 9. Appearance of liposomes after carboxyfluorescein release by partially purified LGL granule cytolysin. Electron micrograph after negative stain with phosphotungstate. Arrows show clear examples of inserted pore structures. Two other liposomes in panel B have inserted pore structures, while the majority of liposomes in A have neither pore structures nor penetration of the negative stain. From ref. 21.

structures. These experiments provide strong support for the model of pore insertion into the lipid bilayer via creation of an amphipathic complex as the mechanism of cytolysin activity.

The potent lytic activity of the cytolysin in LGL granules clearly adds strong support for the previously described model (1) for lymphocyte cytotoxicity involving granule exocytosis after target cell recognition by a membrane receptor. However, it is not easy to design critical experiments to test the question of whether granule cytolysins are responsible for the lethal damage inflicted by cytotoxic lymphocytes. One approach we have taken is the use of rabbit antibodies against the purified LGL tumor granules. By fluorescence microscopy, such antibodies stain cytoplasmic granules in LGL tumor cells, LGL, and CTL, but not normal splenocytes, thymocytes, or peripheral T cells. The antibodies do not stain the membranes of any of these cells, but require a permeabilization of the membrane in order for the granule staining to be detectable. These results are compatible with the demonstrated purity of the granules used as the immunogen. By Western blots, anti-granule antibodies react with 4 of the 5 major granule proteins. IgG from the anti-granule sera specifically block granule cytolysin activity, an effect which is demonstrable by overlaying an Ouchterlony gel diffusion with a layer of red cells in agarose, as in the Jerne plaque assay. More importantly, F(ab')$_2$ fragments of these antibodies specifically block the lytic activity of LGL in NK and ADCC assays in addition to the cytolysin activity. Some of this data is presented in Table I, along with the demonstration that the antibodies do not interfere with LGL-target binding, as would be expected for specific anti-granule antibodies. We regard these experiments with anti-granule antibodies as strong direct evidence for a role of granule components in the LGL-mediated killing process. Since the antibodies are made against most of the granule componments, we cannot conclude that the anti-

Table 1

EFFECT OF ANTI-GRANULE ANTIBODIES ON ADCC AND NK CYTOTOXICITY AND CONJUGATE FORMATION[1]

Treatment	[51]Cr Release[2]		%Conjugates[3]	
	YAC-1	P815+Ab	YAC-1	P815+Ab
PBS control	34±3	37±3	20±2	33±2
Anti-TNP[4]	30±6	38±2	17±4	26±0
Anti-LGL granules[3]	3±1	14±1	18±4	35±2

1. Percoll purified rat LGL.
2. E/T=25, 4 hour assay.
3. E/T=2, scored after 5 min at 37°.
4. F(ab')$_2$, 300 ug/ml in the assay.

cytolysin antibodies block the cell mediated process, but this is clearly the simplest and most appealing hypothesis. More definitive statements should be possible as our purification improves and more defined anti-cytolysin antibodies become available.

All the studies I have described so far have been with LGL tumor cytoplasmic granules and LGL-mediated cytotoxicity. We have begun to extend these findings to CTL, but have had to make do with more limited amounts of granules simply because one cannot grow as many CTL as LGL tumor cells. While we have not been able to establish the biochemical purity of these CTL granules, it is clear that granules having a lytic activity which is generally similar to that in the LGL can be isolated from cloned CTL using the same procedure we developed for LGL tumor cells. These granules are also associated with lysosomal enzyme activity and thus appear to be the ones described by Zagury (5). Fig. 10 shows the cytolytic activity of these granules on a number of different target cells. In general, the pattern of sensitivity correlates well with the LGL granules, and it is clearly not related to the very strong H-2K^b specificity of the cloned CTL from which the granules were derived. Both the kinetics and the divalent ion dependence of the lytic activity of CTL granules are generally similar to that of LGL granules, although subtle differences are reproducibly found. The addition of calcium to the granules from cloned CTL gives rise to

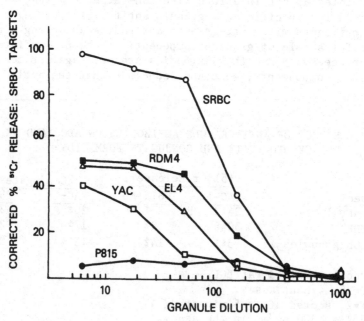

Fig. 10. Lytic activity of cytoplasmic granules from cloned CTL. Conditions similar to Fig. 4.

130

pore-like cylindrical structures in the EM, as seen in Fig. 10. These structures are decidedly smaller than those we observe from the LGL tumor granules, and they appear to correspond to the smaller of the two sizes reported by Dennert and Podack to be associated with cytotoxicity by cloned CTL (7).

The use of cloned CTL for such experiments was open to the criticism that the granule cytolytic activity was really a reflection of an NK-like cytotoxic mechanism (23,24) which was present in these cells, and that it had nothing to do with the CTL-mediated target cell damage. While one can point to the strict H-2k[b] specificity of killing by the cloned CTL used in these experiments, and to the anti-Lyt-2 blocking of the cytotoxicity, the question remains as to whether the cytolytic granules may represent a latent LGL-like characteristic of these cells. As one approach to this question, we have looked for lytic granules in primary and secondary allo-MLR cultures having good CTL activity, since in the mouse such cultured lymphocytes have no detectable NK activity under these conditions. As can be seen in Table 2, such granules contain detectable cytolytic activity while control preparations from normal spleen cells do not. By comparison with cloned CTL preparations the levels of activity observed seem reasonable. The lytic properties of these granules with regard to kinetics, divalent ion dependence, and target cell selectivity appear similar to the granules from cloned CTL.

We have looked at a number of functionally different T cell lines growing in vitro with the expectation that only those with cytotoxic activity would produce granules which are cytolytic. We have found that life is not as simple as we had imagined. Some cytotoxic lines have failed to give detectable cytolytic activity in their granules, e.g., Yael Kaufman's CTL hybridoma cells, the TB-1 tumor, and human LGL and CTL clones. One might view the failure to detect lytic granules in these cytotoxic cells as evidence against the model of granule exocytosis.

Table 2

CYTOLYTIC ACTIVITY OF GRANULES FROM CTL

Cell source	Granule lytic activity, Lytic units/10[8] cell-equiv.*
Normal spleen	<10
Spleen, 5 day 1° allo cult.	23-260
Spleen, 5 day 2° allo cult.	200-600
Cloned CTL, H-2 K[b] specific	1600-4200
LGL tumor, normal LGL	1000-4000

*See ref. 18 for definition of these units.

However, we believe that this can be explained by the potent potent inhibitory ability of many cellular components, especially those comprised of membranes. We have shown that liposomes are very potent inhibitors of cytolysin activity, as might be expected by a membrane insertion mechanism for the active species. We have detected similar inhibitory material in the Percoll gradient in the granule region from some cells, and we believe that this explains our failures to find active cytolysin in some granule preparations. These results underline the need for rigorous purification of the granules as we have done only for the LGL tumor cells.

Perhaps more surprising has been our finding of lytic activity in granules from several lines of non-cytotoxic cultured lymphocytes, which indicates that the presence of cytolysin containing granules is not restricted to CTL. Two cell lines which gave 800-4000 lytic U/10^8 cell-equivalents (in the range of LGL and cloned CTL) are Line 53, a line which arose spontaneously from spleen cells cultured in IL-2, and line 3310, a proliferative line responding to the Mls locus. Both of these were obtained from the laboratory of Dr. Steven Rosenberg, of NIH. When tested for their ability to lyse tumor target cells presence of Con A under conditions where CTL will non-specifically kill inappropriate targets, both Line 53 cells and 3310 cells were negative. Thus these two separate cell lines which had never shown cytotoxic activity give granules which are potently lytic, and they share the calcium dependence and rapid kinetics of the cytolysins from LGL and CTL. While we do not have a full interpretation of these results at present, we would speculate that these cells lack other components required for lytic activity. We clearly have a long way to go before we fully understand the complex control of the secretory process in lymphocytes.

Overall, the results of our study of granules from cytotoxic lymphocytes have strongly supported the granule exocytosis model which we (1) and Zagury (5) proposed three years ago on the basis of morphology. According to this model, the cytoplasmic granules of cytotoxic lymphocytes are differentiated organelles specialized to inflict damage on target cells. If so, it is possible that other granule components in addition to the cytolysin may participate to provide several avenues of destruction of the target cell. To speculate further, it could be that these other components can gain access to the target cell only via the large pores created by the cytolysin. The characterization of the various granule components is currently underway in our lab, and should provide some evidence as to the validity of these ideas.

REFERENCES

1. Henkart, M. P., and P. A. Henkart. 1982. Lymphocyte mediated cytolysis as a secretory process. In: Clark, W.R., and Golstein, P (Eds) Mechanisms in Cell Mediated Cytotoxicity. New York, Plenum Press. p. 227.

2. Dourmashkin, R. R., P. Deteix, C. B. Simone, and P. A. Henkart. 1980. Electron microscopic demonstration of lesions on target cell membranes associated with antibody-dependent cytotoxicity. Clin. Exp. Immunol. 43:554.

3. Simone, C. B., and P. Henkart. 1980. Permeability changes induced in erythrocyte ghost targets by antibody-dependent cytotoxic effector cells: evidence for membrane pores. J. Immunol. 124:954.

4. Podack, E. R., and G. Dennert. 1983. Assembly of two types of tubules with putative cytolytic function by cloned natural killer cells. Nature (Lond.). 302:442.

5. Zagury, D. 1982. Direct analysis of individual killer T cells: Susceptibility of target cells to lysis and secretion of hydrolytic enzymes by CTL. Adv. Exp. Med. Biol. 146:149.

6. Bykovskaja, S. N., A. N. Rytenko, M. O. Rauschenbach, and A. F. Bykovsky. 1978. Ultrastructural alteration of cytolytic T lymphocytes following their interaction with target cells. II. Morphogenesis of secretory granules and intracellular vacuoles. Cell. Immunol. 40:175.

7. Dennert, G., and E. R. Podack. 1983. Cytolysis by H-2 specific T killer cells. Assembly of tubular complexes on target membranes. J. Exp. Med. 157:1483.

8. Henney, C. S. 1973. On the mechanism of T-cell mediated cytolysis. Transplant. Rev. 17:37.

9. Martz, E., W. L. Parker, M. K. Gately, and C. D. Tsoukas. 1982. The role of calcium in the lethal hit of T lymphocyte-mediated cytolysis. Adv. Exp. Med. Biol. 146:121.

10. Carpen, O., I. Virtanen, and E. Saksela. 1981. The cytotoxic activity of human natural killer cells requires an intact secretory apparatus. Cell. Immunol. 58:97.

11. Neighbour, P. A., and H. S. Huberman. 1982. Sr+2-induced inhibition of human natural killer (NK) cell-mediated cytotoxicity. J. Immunol. 128:1236.

12. Quan, P. C., T. Ishizake, and B. Bloom. 1982. Studies on the mechanism of NK cell lysis. J. Immunol. 128:1786.

13. Brondz, B. D., A. E. Snegirova, Y. A. Rassulin, and O. G. Shamborant. 1973. Modification of in vitro immune lymphocyte-target cell interaction by some biologically active drugs. Immunochemistry. 10:175.

14. Ward, J. M., and C. W. Reynolds. 1983. Large granular lymphocyte leukemia. A heterogeneous lymphocytic leukemia of F344 rats. Am. J. Path. 111:1.

15. Reynolds, C. W., E. W. Bere, and J. M. Ward. 1984. Natural killer activity in the rat. III. Characterization of transplantable large granular lymphocyte leukemias in the F344 rat. J. Immunol. 132:534.

16. Millard, P. J., M. P. Henkart, C. W. Reynolds, and P. A. Henkart. 1984. Purification and properties of cytoplasmic granules from cytotoxic rat LGL tumors. J. Immunol. 132:3197.

17. Grossi, C. E., A. Cadoni, A. Zicca, A. Leprini, and M. Ferrarini. 1982. Large granular lymphocytes in human peripheral blood: Ultrastructural and cytochemical characterization of the granules. Blood. 59:277.

18. Henkart, P. A., P. J. Millard, C. W. Reynolds, and M. P. Henkart. 1984. Cytolytic activity of purified cytoplasmic granules from cytotoxic rat LGL tumors. J. Exp. Med. 160:75.

19. Gately, M. K., and E. Martz. 1979. Early steps in specific tumor cell lysis by sensitized mouse T lymphocytes.III Resolution of two distinct roles for calcium in the cytolytic process. J. Immunol. 122:482.

20. Weinstein, J. N., S. Yoshikami, P. Henkart, R. Blumenthal, and W. A. Hagins. 1977. Liposome-cell interaction: Transfer and intracellular release of a trapped fluorescent marker. Science (Wash. D. C.). 195:489.

21. Blumenthal, R., P. J. Millard, M. P. Henkart, C. W. Reynolds, and P. A. Henkart. 1984. Liposomes as targets for granule cytolysin from cytotoxic LGL tumors. Proc. Natl. Acad. Sci. U. S. A. 81:5551.

22. Bhakdi, S., and J. Tranum-Jensen. 1983. Membrane damage by complement. Biochim. Biophys. Acta. 737:343.

23. Brooks, C. G., D. L. Urdal, and C. S. Henney. 1983. Lymphokine-driven "differentiation" of cytotoxic T cell clones into cells with NK-like specificity: Correlations with display of membrane macromolecules. Immunological Rev. 72:43.

24. Acha-Orbea, H., P. Groscurth, R. Lang, L. Stitz, and H. Hengartner. 1983. Characterization of cloned cytotoxic lymphocytes with NK-like activity. J. Immunol. 130:1952.

134

DISCUSSION

Dennert: For the TB-1 tumor what effector:target ratio do you have to use to get killing?

Henkart: As I remember, at about 20:1 we got reasonable lysis, like 20%. It is not a potent cytotoxic cell.

Dennert: In our hands tumor cells such as TB-1 and BW-5147 and a number of other thymic lymphomas required very long incubations and very high E:T ratios to give any target lysis. During the incubation, the medium became very acidic, and I have real doubts as to whether the target cell lysis was physiologic.

Henkart: I can say that in our hands in a four hour incubation with a 20:1 E:T ratio, TB-1 gave a 20% ^{51}Cr release.

Springer: What kind of pharmacologic agents induce degranulation, and have you looked at the effect of lectins?

Henkart: Depending on the type of cell, many agents can cause degranulation. For example, in NK cells, strontium works well, as shown in very nice published experiments by Neighbour and Huberman. But the problem with these lymphocyte systems is that you don't have a real assay for degranulation per se. When we have more refined antibodies we hope to work out a radioimmunoassay for granule components, but at present we have no quantitative means of looking at degranulation.

M. Henkart: Morphologically, degranulation does occur with lectins.

Henney: Do you need degranulation to get lysis?

Henkart: We really haven't been able to address this question directly. The EM evidence certainly suggests that granule exocytosis does occur.

Henney: CTL-L2 doesn't kill, but seems to have perfectly good granules. Does strontium induce lysis with these cells?

Henkart: We have not tried this.

Podack: CTL-L2 does not kill, but you can induce formation of the complexes if you add PMA and Con A. However, we have not been able to detect killing under these conditions.

Nathan: Does the antibody whose F(ab')$_2$ inhibited NK cells, inhibit CTL killing?

Henkart: Good question, and I wish I could tell you the answer is yet, but it is no. We tried hard to do this. In fact, the antibody nicely inhibits killing by CTL granules, but just does not inhibit intact CTL killing. We would speculate that the CTL-target junction is tighter and makes a better barrier to antibody penetration, as Wright and Silverstein have recently shown can occur in the macrophage system.

Targan: If this cytolysin is secreted in an active form, why doesn't it kill the effector cell?

Henkart: The issue of why the effector cell is not killed is a paramount one, and we are currently designing experiments to look at this. The granule exocytosis model requires that the effector cell have a period of resistance to the cytolysin. If you take purified LGL and label them with chromium, the granules kill them in a way which is typical of other lymphocytes, so they are not inherently resistant.

Targan: There seems to be a small difference in the kinetics of NK cell induced killer cell independent lysis versus the very rapid kinetics that you have seen. Is it possible that the secreted form of the cytolysin is less active than the isolated form?

Henkart: The lysis mediated by these cytolysins is rapid, potentially more rapid than one sees in the killer cell independent lytic phase. Such rapid lysis would be expected by the very large target cell membrane pores seen in the EM, and in fact we showed by sieving experiments that such large pores are created in red cell ghosts in an ADCC. There are many potential differences between the situation where we add purified granules in the presence of calcium and the delivery of granule contents by a degranulation.

Hudig: Have you recovered proteins from the phospholipid vesicles?

Henkart: What preliminary experiments we did indicated that all the granule proteins had affinity for lipid, so we have not pursued this approach. That may be more like the sort of thing that Eckhard has been doing.

Podack: We have created the complexes in the absence of target cells, extracted with detergent and isolated them, as I showed in the EM.

Nathan: Is there any formal evidence that C9 is not involved in the granule lytic effects?

Henkart: No, but I would say that the major granule proteins are too small to be C9.

Tirosh: In cell mediated cytolysis there are cases where the lysis is independent of calcium. Have you found similar effects using the granules?

Henkart: We have studied a number of different types of nucleated cells and red cells; all have shown a rather similar calcium requirement for lysis by granules. We have not seen your data showing calcium independent CTL lysis.

Unknown: When you tested macrophages, were they differentiated so that they were cytotoxic?

Henkart: At least one preparation what we have tested was activated by C. parvum. However, I want to caution you that we are hesitant to make a strong interpretation of a negative result for granule mediated cytotoxicity. In some of these cases we have not rigorously established the purity of the granules, there may be interfering membrane components in the granule region of the gradient; these may mask a cytolytic activity, so a negative result has to be interpreted cautiously.

Young: If I could add a comment, when we acid extract granules from macrophages activated by C. parvum or BCG, we can recover hemolytic agents. This correlates very well with the macrophages being resident or activated.

Berke: Because such granule material can be extracted from a wide range of cells, and since such different cell types can mediate ADCC, it seems to me that we are dealing with a genuine lytic mechanism which may be operational in non-specific killing like ADCC and NK. The experiment which needs to be done is to freeze-etch killer-target conjugates and demonstrate those ring-like structures in the intercellular space. We have attempted such experiments with negative results, but this is technically difficult. Perhaps we should collaborate with Bhakdi and Tranum-Jensen.

Bhakdi: I'm afraid both Tranum-Jensen and I are a bit overloaded just now.

Hiserodt: When you treat your targets with cytolysin in the absence of calcium and get no killing, do you know for sure that you do not get ring structures?

M. Henkart: When we have looked, we haven't seen them. The cleanest example is where we have used isolated granules in the absence of added membranes. Here in the absence of calcium there are only smooth membranes, but if you add calcium you get ring structures as soon as you can make the negative stain preparation.

A UNIFIED THEORY FOR THE MECHANISM OF THE LETHAL HIT BY CYTOTOXIC
T LYMPHOCYTES (CTL) AND NATURAL KILLER (NK) CELLS AS DEFINED BY
ANTISERA CAPABLE OF BLOCKING THE LETHAL HIT STAGE OF CYTOTOXICITY

John C. Hiserodt

Department of Pathology
University of Michigan
Ann Arbor, Michigan 48109

INTRODUCTION

Understanding the mechanisms in which cytotoxic lymphocytes
(particularly cytotoxic T lymphocytes (CTL) and natural killer
(NK) cells) mediate the lysis of target cells has been a fundamental problem in molecular immunology. While these reactions
involve complex biochemical and physiological processes the mechanism of cytotoxicity has been resolved into several operationally
identifiable stages (1-4). In the most simplistic scheme, the
effector lymphocyte must recognize and bind to the appropriate
target. Subsequent to binding, the killer cell undergoes of
series of physiological responses collectively termed activation.
It is during this activation phase that the killer cell initiates
infliction of the lethal hit on the target. Once the lethal hit
has been completed the killer cell can detach and recycle to other
targets. Target cells having received the lethal hit are "programmed to lyse" and will rapidly do so during the final stage of
the lytic reaction known as the killer cell independent stage.

Resolution of the various stages outlined above has been
achieved in most studies by their dependency on the divalent
cations Ca^{++} and Mg^{++} or by various pharmacologic interventions
(2-6). Recently, however, antibodies have been developed which
appear to react with structures employed by the killer cell at
each of the above mentioned stages. Monoclonal antibodies against
Lyt 2 (7) or LFA-1 (8,9) appear to inhibit the binding of CTL to
the specific target. Triggering of the cytolytic response can be
inhibited by antibodies reactive with other T cell structures such
as T-200 (10,11). Inhibition of the lethal hit has been more
difficult to achieve using serologic probes. Hiserodt and

Bonavida were the first to demonstrate inhibition of the CTL lethal hit by antibodies generated against purified CTL cells (this antiserum was termed RAT*) (12). Subsequently, similar heterologous antibodies were generated which were capable of blocking the lethal hit stage of human CTL (13,14) murine NK cells (15,16) and human NK cells (17). Thus, the ability to reverse the lethal hit by the appropriate antibodies appears to represent a general phenomenon indicating transfer of some form of killer cell derived material to the target must be a requisite step for infliction of the lethal hit.

During studies with the RAT* antibody we found that cell free cytosolic extracts from CTL could neutralize its ability to inhibit the CTL lethal hit. With this information we decided to generate a new antibody raised against the cytosolic fraction of a CTL clone. In addition, because this CTL clone does not possess standard NK surface markers the resultant antibody could be used to address questions regarding the relationship of the lethal hit between CTL and NK lymphocytes.

MATERIALS AND METHODS

Animals and Cell Lines: Mice were obtained from Jackson Laboratories and were 6-10 weeks of age. Strains included C57Bl/6, CBA/J, DBA/2 and Balb/c. Target cells included the P815 mastocytoma ($H-2^d$), EL4 lymphoma ($H-2^b$) maintained in ascites in DBA/2 and C57Bl/6 mice, respectively and the S-194 myeloma ($H-2^d$) and YAC-1 lymphoma ($H-2^a$) maintained in vitro in RPMI 1640 10% FCS. The CTL clone B6.1.SF.1 was a generous gift of Dr. Markus Nabholz and has been described previously (18). This is an IL-2 dependent CTL clone (Thy 1^+, lyt2$^+$) from a C57Bl/6 mouse with specificity for the H-Y antigen and cross reacts with $H-2D^d$. The helper T cell clone A-11 was a gift from Dr. Eli Sercarz. This clone is of Balb/c origin with specificity for hen egg lysozyme.

Production and Use of Antisera: Rat anti CTL-lysate antisera (αCTLL) were produced in Lewis rats by the following protocol: 2 x 10^8 B6.1.SF.1 CTL cells were harvested, washed with PBS, and suspended to a density of 5 x 10^7/ml in PBS. The cells were completely lysed by freezing and thawing by transferring 4 times from an ethanol/dry ice bath to a 37°C water bath. The samples were then centrifuged at 20,000 xg for 30 min at 4°C. The supernatants were collected, filtered through 0.22 μ millipore filters and 0.5 ml aliquots stored in liquid nitrogen. Antisera was generated by emulsifying equal volumes of the CTL extract with Freunds complete adjuvant and injecting intradermally in six sites over the back of anesthetized rats. This procedure was repeated in 2 weeks using the frozen aliquots. The third immunization was given after 3 additional weeks with antigen suspended in Freunds incomplete adjuvant. Control serum consisted of preimmune serum or pooled Lewis rat serum from normal animals. All animals were bled from the tail, the serum was collected, heat inactivated (56°C, 45 minutes), diluted 1:4 in PBS and absorbed on the following cell populations for 30 min. at 4°C: (1) Three consecutive absorptions on washed P815 mastocytoma cells at 1×10^8 cells/ml of 1:4 diluted antiserum; (2) 2 consecutive absorptions on washed Balb/c spleen cells at 1×10^8 lymphoid cells/ml of antiserum; (3) 2 consecutive absorptions on washed Balb/c Thymocytes at 1×10^8 cells/ml of antiserum. All experiments performed in this study were done using antisera absorbed in this way. IgG and Fab'$_2$ fractions were also obtained from the same absorbed antiserum by standard methodology employing column chromatography on Sephacryl S-300 and pepsin digestion. Anti Lyt 2 and anti H-2D were obtained from the Salk Institute Cell Distribution Center.

Rat α NK Serum: This antiserum was prepared similar to αCTLL except cell free cytosolic extracts of Balb/c Nu/Nu spleen cells were used as the immunogen. Briefly, Balb/c Nu/Nu splenic lymphocytes were collected from Ficoll hypaque gradients and passed over nylon wool columns. The nonadherent cells were then used to make cell free cytosolic extracts identical to the procedure described for the αCTLL. Immunization procedures and preparations of RαNK IgG was similar to that for αCTLL.

Murine Effector Cells: Alloimmune peritoneal exudate lymphocytes (PEL) or splenic T cells were obtained from day 9 (PEL) or day 12 (spleen) P815 immune mice by incubating the cell suspension on nylon wool columns (Leukopak) and eluting off the nonadherent T lymphocytes. The viability of all cell preparations was determined by suspension in 0.1% trypan blue and were routinely >98%.

Cytotoxicity Assays: The ^{51}Cr-release microcytotoxicity was employed using 96-well, round bottom microplates (Lindbro). Briefly 1×10^4 chromium labeled (Na$_2$^{51}CrO$_4$, New England Nuclear) target cells (in 50 µl) were mixed with various numbers of CTL (in 50 µl) to give E:T ratios between 2 to 20:1 in a final volume of 200 µl. These cells were allowed to interact at 37°C for three to four hours after which the percentage of ^{51}Cr release was calculated using standard formulas.

Mixed Lymphocyte Reaction (MLR): Spleen cells from 60 to 90 day memory C57Bl/6 anti P815 mice were obtained and stimulated in a one way mixed lymphocyte reaction by mixing 50×10^6 memory spleen cells with 10×10^6 irradiated (2000 R) DBA/2 spleen cells in a total volume of 20 ml of RPMI 1640 with 10% FCS and 5×10^{-5}M mercaptoethanol and incubated at 37°C in a 5% CO$_2$ incubator. Cells were harvested by centrifugation on Ficol-Hypaque (p = 1.090) prior to use for testing.

<u>Enumeration of CTL-target Cell Conjugate Frequency</u>: 5×10^5 C57 anti-P815 effector PEL in 0.1 ml were mixed with 5×10^5 P815 target cells in 0.1 ml in the presence of various amounts of αCTLL, RαNK, or NRS antibody. The cells were pelleted (400 xg for 3-5 minutes) and allowed a further incubation for five minutes at 37°C. The cells were then suspended by ten suspensions through a Gilston pipetteman set at 100 µl. CTL-target cell conjugate frequency was enumerated immediately after suspension. Binding frequency was calculated by the following formula:

$$\% \text{ Binding} = \frac{\text{Number of lymphocytes bound to 1 or more targets}}{\text{Total Number of lymphocytes}} \times 100$$

For determination of binding frequency, 200 lymphocytes were routinely counted.

<u>Preparation of Cell Free Cytosolic Extracts (CFE)</u>: Cells were washed twice in PBS at 4°C. They were suspended in PBS at 10^8 cell/ml and lysed by freezing and thawing by transferring four times from an ethanol/dry ice bath to a 37°C water bath. The samples were then centrifuged at 20,000 xg for 30 minutes at 4°C and the supernatant was harvested, filtered through an 0.2 µ millipore filter, and stored at -70°C. Protein concentration was determined by the method of Lowry.

RESULTS

<u>Anti CTLL IgG Inhibits Cytotoxicity in a Variety of CTL Effector and Target Cell Combinations</u>. Table 1 shows the results of blocking experiments using highly absorbed αCTLL IgG and different effector and target cell combinations. Inhibition of cytolysis was observed irregardless of the source or strain of effector CTL or target cell used. Inhibition was also observed when normal CBA/J spleen cells were tested for NK activity against the standard NK target YAC-1. In contrast, cytolysis of P815 cells by thioglycollate elicited peritoneal macrophages or by human K cells (ADCC) was not affected by αCTLL antibody.

<u>Analysis of the Mechanism of αCTLL Inhibition of CTL Mediated Cytotoxicity</u>. Figure 1 shows the results of experiments in which the IgG or Fab'_2 fragments of highly absorbed αCTLL antibody were tested for their effects on CTL-target cell binding and cytolysis. Clearly, αCTLL IgG and/or Fab'_2 is a potent inhibitor of cytolysis (measured by ^{51}Cr-release) with virtually 100% inhibition obtained at 20-40 µg of IgG or Fab'_2. In contrast, no inhibition in the frequency of CTL target conjugates was observed even when performed in up to 100 µg of αCTLL IgG or Fab'_2. αCTLL IgG did not dissociate the CTL-P815 conjugates since the percentage of conjugates remained unchanged even after 1 hour at 37°C. In addition, preincubation of the CTL at 4°C in αCTLL IgG for up to 1 hour prior to addition of targets also did not reduce the

frequency of CTL-target conjugates and removal of the antibody by washing reversed its inhibitory effect. Delayed addition of αCTLL IgG (in Ca^{++} pulse experiments) demonstrated that inhibition of cytolysis occurred during and beyond that of EDTA and thus beyond the latest Ca^{++} dependent step of cytolysis (Figure 2).

Table I

αCTLL IgG Inhibits CTL Activity Irregardless of
Target Cell Haplotype or Source of CTL

Group	Effector cell	Source	Target	NRS IgG	αCTLL IgG
1	B6.1.SF.1 ($H2^b$)	Clone	S194 ($H2^d$)	72	10
	B6.1.SF.1	Clone	P815 ($H2^d$)	43	3
2	C57B1/6 ($H2^b$)	PEL	P815	43	9
	C57B1/6	Spleen	P815	31	5
	C57B1/6	2° MLC	P815	55	6
3	Balb/c ($H2^d$)	PEL	EL4 ($H2^b$)	40	10
4	CBA/J ($H2^k$)	PEL	P815	59	12
5	Normal CBA/J	Spleen	YAC ($H2^a$)	38	14
6	CBA/J	Peri-toneal macro-phages	P815	48	51

Effector CTL and ^{51}Cr labeled targets were obtained as described in methods. All cytotoxicity assays were performed at E:T ratios of 5:1 except the alloimmune spleen cells which were at 20:1. Group 5 measured the effect of αCTLL on NK activity (E:T 50:1, 4 hrs). Group 6 employed thioglycollate elicited CBA/J peritoneal macrophages in an 18 hr cytotoxicity assay aginst P815 targets (E:T = 30:1).

Cell Free Cytosolic Extracts (CFE) Obtained from CTL or CTL Clones Neutralize the Blocking Activity of αCTLL IgG and Fab'$_2$:
Figure 3 shows the results of experiments in which cell free cytosolic extracts (CFE) derived from alloimmune CTL inhibited the blocking activity of αCTLL antibody. As little as 10-30 μg of cytosolic protein extracted from in vivo elicited CTL (PEL) (Fig. 3A) or the CTL clone B6.1.SF.1 (Fig. 3B) significantly neutralized

the blocking activity of 20 µg of αCTLL IgG or Fab'$_2$. Higher amounts of CFE protein yielded virtually 100% neutralization. Cytotoxicity in the presence of only the CTL-CFE was unaffected. However, it must be noted that if unstable cytolysins were present in these preparations they may not have been detected since the CFE and antibody were preincubated for 30' in Ca^{++} containing medium prior to addition of effectors and targets.

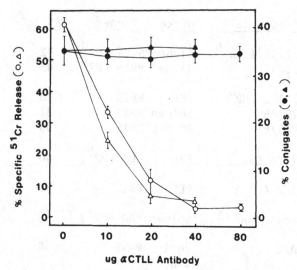

Figure 1. αCTLL inhibits CTL mediated cytotoxicity without affecting target cell binding. αCTLL IgG or Fab'$_2$ were added into a standard ^{51}Cr release cytotoxicity assay using day 10 C57B1/6 anti P815 PEL (5:1 E:T ratio) as effector cells and ^{51}Cr labeled P815 targets. αCTLL antibody was also assessed for its effects on CTL-P815 binding in the standard binding assay described in Methods. o, o IgG: Δ, (Fab')$_2$.

Effects of CTL Extracts on the Blocking Activity of Other CTL Inhibitory Antibodies Such as anti-Lyt 2 and Anti-target Cell (anti H-2^d) Antisera. Experiments were preformed to determine whether material(s) present in the CTL extracts could inhibit other antisera capable of blocking CTL mediated cytotoxicity. Figure 4 shows that when CTL-CFE were mixed with inhibitory doses of monoclonal rat anti-Lyt 2 or H-2^b anti H-2^d antisera (anti target antisera) no inhibition of the ability of these antibodies to block cytolysis was observed. In other experiments (not shown) CTL-CFE prepared from human CTL (PBL αIM-9) also did not affect the blocking effects of αCTLL IgG. Finally CTL-CFE from murine CTL did not contain proteases which degraded the αCTLL IgG.

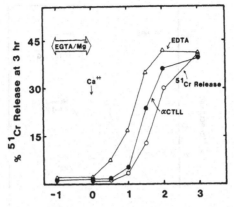

Figure 2. αCTLL IgG inhibits CTL mediated cytotoxicity during and beyond the Ca^{++} dependent stage of cytolysis. Day 10 C57Bl/6 anti P815 PEL were mixed with P815 targets (E:T 5:1) in the presence of 2.5 mM EGTA/Mg^{++}. After 60 minutes at 37°C 5 mM Ca^{++} was added to each well. At various times EDTA or αCTLL IgG (30 μg) were added and the entire assay was left to incubate for 3 hours when all wells were harvested. Kinetics of Cr^{51} release were also determined at each time point indicated.

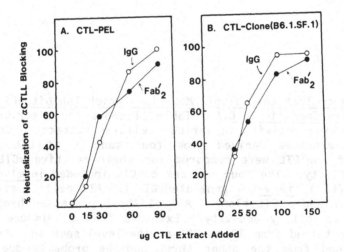

Figure 3. Neutralization of αCTLL IgG or Fab'$_2$ blocking of CTL activity with cell free cytosolic extracts (CFE) obtained from CTL (PEL) or the CTL clone B6.1.SF.1. CFE protein was preincu-bated with 20 μg of αCTLL IgG or Fab'$_2$ and the mixture was tested for blocking of cytotoxicity in a standard 3 hour ^{51}Cr release assay. The percent cytotoxicity in the experiment shown was 58% (5:1 PEL:Tg ratio) in the presence of 20 μg NRS IgG and 12% and 10% respectively in 20 μg of αCTLL IgG or Fab'$_2$.

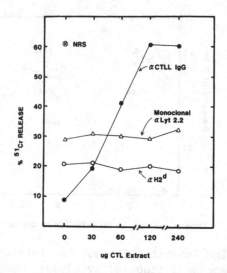

Figure 4. Inhibition of CTL activity by Anti Lyt 2 or anti target (H-2^d) antibodies is not affected by CTL-CFE. CFE prepared from day 10 alloimmune PEL was mixed with 20 µg αCTLL IgG, monoclonal anti-Lyt 2, or H-2^b anti H-2^d serum. The mixture was then tested for blocking activity in a standard cytotoxicity assay (5:1 PEL:Tg ratio).

Evidence That the Soluble Materials Which Inhibit αCTLL Blocking Are Specific to CTL.

Table II shows the distribution of αCTLL blocking activity in various cellular extracts. Cell free cytosolic extracts derived from four sources of CTL and six sources of non-CTL were compared for their relative αCTLL inhibitory activity. The four sources of CTL included in vivo generated CTL (PEL), in vitro generated CTL (2° MLR cells), alloimmune splenic CTL and a CTL clone. All of these possessed high levels of αCTLL inhibitory activity. Extracts from alloimmune spleen, however contained from 10 to 30% of the level seen in extracts of CTL obtained from the other three sources probably due to the relatively low frequency of CTL in an alloimmune spleen. None of the various sources of non-CTL (i.e., normal C57B1/6 spleen, thymocyte, macrophage, two tumor cell lines, EL4 and P815, and a helper T cell clone) contained materials which could significantly neutralize αCTLL blocking.

Table II

Distribution of αCTLL Inhibitory Activity In
Cell Free Cytosolic Extracts from Various Cell Populations

Cell Population[a]	(Protein)[b] mg/ml/10[8] cells	αCTLL Inhibitory Activity (Units/ ml of CFE)[c]
CTL clone (B61.SF.1)	2-4	200-500
CTL (PEL	2-4	200-500
CTL (2° MLC)	2-4	200-500
CTL splenic T cells	1-3	50-100
Normal C57B1/6 spleen	1-3	10-20
Helper T cell clone (A-11)	3-4	<10
B6 thymocytes	1-3	<10
B6 macrophages (thioglycollate)	8-10	<10
EL4 tumor	9-12	<10
P815 tumor	9-12	<10

[a]Cell free extract (CFE) for each population were obtained as described in Methods. The 2° MLC was generated using spleen cells from 60-90 day memory C57B1/6 anti P815 mice. These cells were cultured (10:1 R:S ratio) with irradiated DBA/2 spleen cells for 4 days prior to use.

[b]As determined by the Lowry method.

[c]αCTLL inhibitory activity is defined in units/ml of CFE as follows: 1 unit of CFE is that volume of CFE which will inhibit 50% of the blocking activity of 20 μg of αCTLL IgG. Thus, if 10 μl of CFE inhibits 50% of αCTLL blocking there would be 100 units/ml of inhibitory activity in that CFE. All extracts were prepared using 10[8] lymphoid cells/ml.

Kinetics of Appearance of αCTLL Inhibitory Activity in Secondary MLC Generated CTL. To determine the kinetics of appearance of αCTLL inhibitory activity, memory cells present in the spleens of P815 immune mice (90 days post immunization) were cultured in secondary MLC. Specific CTL cytotoxicity and αCTLL inhibitory activity present in CFE were determined at various times after initiation of the cultures. As can be seen in Table III, CFE from memory spleen cells had undetectable levels of specific CTL or αCTLL neutralizing activity. As early as day 1 after initiation of the MLC, cytotoxic and αCTLL neutralizing activity begin to appear. By day 4 of MLC, very high levels of

Table III

Kinetics of Appearance of αCTLL Inhibitory
Activity and Alloimmune Cytotoxicity During 2° MLC

Days in 2° MLC Culture[a]	CTL Activity LU(30)/10^7 cells	αCTLL Inhibitory Activity (Units/ml of CFE)[b]
Day 0 (memory CTL)	<20	<20
Day 1	560	110
Day 4	3880	750
Day 14	840	240
Day 4 (controls)[c]	<20	<10

[a]The MLC cultures were prepared as described in methods.

[b]Units/ml are calculated as described in Table II.

[c]Control cultures did not receive DBA/2 stimulator cells.

CTL cytotoxic activity and αCTLL neutralizing activity are present. These activities persist through day 14, but drop off subsequently. Memory spleen cells cultured without stimulator cells failed to develop cytotoxicity or αCTLL neutralizing activity.

Physical-chemical and Biochemical Properties of Cell Free Cytosolic Extracts of CTL. Preliminary physical-chemical analysis of cytosolic extracts from CTL (PEL) or the CTL clone showed that the antigenic structure(s) (reactivity with αCTLL IgG) were rapidly lost when heated to 50°C or when incubated at 4°C for extended periods of time (>48 hrs) (Table IV). The material was also destroyed at low pH. While treatment with trypsin or neuraminidase had no effect on antigenic activity, treatment with pronase completely abrogated reactivity with αCTLL IgG.

Gel filtration chromatography (Sephacryl S-300) of CTL-CFE showed peaks of antigenic activity eluting in several areas of the column (Fig. 5). While the major peak of activity eluted around 60 kd consistent peaks were also seen in the void volume (>300 kd), 120 kd, and 20 kd. The relative amount of the material eluting in the void volume varied in different experiments and appeared to be due to the time elapsed between extraction and application to the column. In addition, when extracted in the presence of the reducing agent 2-ME or protease inhibitors (including benzamidine, EACA and PMSF) the size of the 60 kd peak was reduced and the size of the 20 kd peak was greatly enhanced (Fig. 6, compare to Fig. 5).

Table IV
Physical-chemical Properties of αCTLL
Inhibitory Material(s) Present in Cell Free
Cytosolic Extracts (CFE) of CTL

Treatment	% Inactivation of CFE
4°C (24 hr)	20
37°C (1 hr)	30
50°C (30 min)	100
pH2	100
Trypsin	5
Neuraminidase	10
Pronase	80

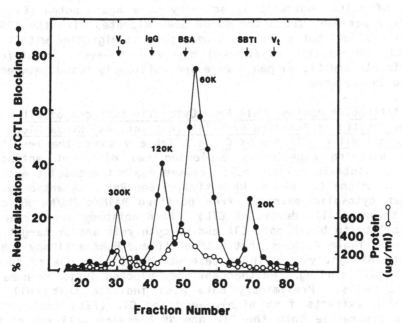

Figure 5. Gel filtration chromatography (Sephacryl S-300) of cell free cytosolic extract from alloimmune CTL (PEL). 1 ml of CFE (10^8 PEL) was applied to a 1.5 x 50 cm column. Fractions were mixed with 20 μg αCTLL IgG and tested for CTL blocking activity. Control lysis (5:1 PEL:Tg ratio) was 66% and 14% in 20 μg αCTLL IgG alone.

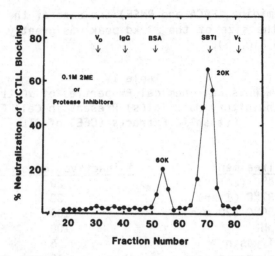

Figure 6. Gel filtration chromatography (S-300) of cell free cytosolic material from alloimmune CTL (PEL) extracted in the presence of 0.1M mercaptoethanol or protease inhibitors. (Compare to elution profile of Figure 5).

When analyzed by sucrose density centrifugation multiple peaks of αCTLL neutralizing activity were again noted (Fig. 7). In the experiment shown the major peak migrated with the 19S IgM marker (∿10^6 mw) but other peaks were present migrating with the 3S (60 kd) and smaller mw (20 kd) markers. However, in different experiments additional peaks were inconsistently noted between the 3S and 19S markers.

Antibodies Against Cell Free Cytosolic Extracts of CTL
Clones (αCTLL) or Purified NK Cells (Rat anti NK) Cross Block
the Lethal Hit of CTL and NK Cells. Table V shows the results of cross blocking experiments employing two different antibodies against cytotoxic cells. αCTLL raised against cytosolic extracts of a CTL clone (devoid of NK activity) and Rat α NK antibody made against cytosolic extracts from purified Balb/c Nu/Nu NK cells (and theoretically devoid of CTL). Each antibody was tested for its ability to block both CTL and NK cytolysis and/or target cell binding. Table V shows that both αCTLL and RαNK antibody inhibit CTL and NK cytolysis. In no case was inhibition due to reduced target cell binding. Neither antibody blocked lysis by human NK or CTL cells. Preliminary data also indicate that cell free cytosolic extracts from highly purified CTL (PEL) could effectively neutralize both the CTL and NK blocking activity of both antibodies (Data not shown).

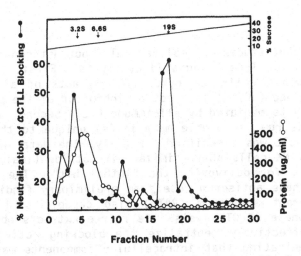

Figure 7. Sucrose density sedimentation of cell free cytosolic extracts from alloimmune CTL (PEL). 0.5 ml of CFE (10^8 PEL) was applied to a 10 to 40% linear sucrose gradient. After ultracentrifugation fractions were dialyzed against PBS and mixed with 20 µg of αCTLL IgG for neutralizing activity. Control lysis (5:1 PEL:Tg ratio) was 52% and 17% in 20 µg αCTLL IgG alone.

Table V

Inhibition of CTL and NK Cytolysis by
αCTLL or Rat α NK Antibodies

Cytotoxic Cells	% Inhibition of Cytotoxic Activity[a]		% Inhibition of Target cell Binding[b]	
	αCTLL	RαNK	αCTLL	RαNK
CTL (PEL)	>90	>70	<10	<10
CBA/J NK (YAC)	>60	>70	<10	<10
Human NK (K562)	<10	<10	<10	<10

[a]Antibodies (20 µg IgG) were added to Standard CRA using C57Bl/6 anti P815 PEL (E:T - 5:1), CBA/J spleen cells with YAC-1 targets (E:T - 50:1) or Human PBL and K562 targets (E:T 30:1).

[b]Target binding at 1:1 E:T ratio employing 20 µg of antibody.

151

DISCUSSION

The present studies reveal several important contributions to the mechanism of T-cell mediated cytolysis. First, rat antibody directed against cell-free cytosolic extracts of a cytotoxic T lymphocyte clone (αCTLL) is a potent inhibitor of the post-binding cytolytic events mediated by alloimmune CTL. Second, with the use of this antiserum, a soluble material(s) unique to the cytolytic function of CTL was identified. Finally, the data indicate that both CTL and NK cells share similar (if not identical) mechanisms and materials for delivering the "lethal hit". The concept for generating these antiserum rose from preliminary findings employing a different antiserum (RAT) also capable of blocking the lethal hit phase of CTL lysis. Cell free extracts obtained from CTL could effectively neutralize the blocking activity of that antiserum indicating that intracellular components may be important in the CTL lytic process. In order to make a more "purified" antibody we used cell free extracts derived from a CTL clone and absorbed the antiserum extensively to eliminate irrelevant antibodies.

Preliminary studies demonstrated that the mechanism of inhibition of cytolysis by αCTLL was not due to trivial processes such as toxicity, lymphocyte or target cell agglutination, or precipitation of ^{51}Cr labeled proteins released from dead targets. Inhibition was obtained using purified Fab'_2 molecules ruling out a mechanism(s) in which antigen-antibody complexes or antibody F_c regions were responsible for the blocking effects. Inhibition by αCTLL appeared to be restricted to the post-binding cytolytic phase of killing since αCTLL antibodies did not affect the capacity of CTL to recognize and bind to specific target cells and even once bound the CTL did not prematurely detach from the targets. Even after preincubation in high levels of αCTLL IgG, CTL could still bind target cells and removal of the antisera prior to addition of targets removed the blockade. Indeed, it was demonstrated that the αCTLL IgG could inhibit CTL activity during and beyond the Ca^{++} dependent step(s) in the lytic reaction. These data indicate that αCTLL appears to recognize material(s) which are expressed during CTL cytotoxicity only subsequent to target binding and would therefore be independent of the target cell recognition mechanisms. The ability of αCTLL to inhibit killing irregardless of the H-2 haplotype of the CTL or target supports this concept. These observations are in contrast to previous studies employing other antibodies capable of blocking cytotoxicity. Monoclonal antibodies directed against Lyt 2 (7), LFA-1 (8) or gp 180,95 (9), all of which inhibit CTL activity in the absence of C', appear to inhibit cytolysis by preventing target binding. By direct analysis Fan et al. (7) showed that anti-Lyt 2 does not affect the post-binding stage of CTL cytolysis.

Soluble material(s) present in cell free cytosolic extracts of cytotoxic T cells inhibits αCTLL blocking activity. This αCTLL inhibitory activity was found to be present in several sources of alloimmune CTL (whether in vivo or in vitro derived) as well as the CTL clone used to make the αCTLL antibody and other CTL clones (with different specificities) (data not shown). This activity was not found in cell-free cytosolic extracts of resident or activated macrophages, thymocytes, normal C57Bl/6 spleen cells, P815 cells, a non-cytotoxic T cell tumor (EL4) or a noncytotoxic helper T cell clone. This suggested that the αCTLL neutralizing activity may represent a material(s) intrinsic to and specific for the functional activity of CTL and not just unique to different-iated T cells per se. This was supported by the observation that splenic memory CTL were devoid of αCTLL inhibitory material but rapidly developed this material during secondary MLC precisely parallel to the development of CTL activity. In addition, cells of T cell origin but devoid of cytolytic function (i.e., EL4, thymocytes, normal splenic T cells) were also devoid of blocking activity. Thus, differentiation into immunocompetent T cells per se is insufficient for the expression of this material. Finally, positive evidence that αCTLL blocking activity was derived from CTL and not other forms of antigen activated T cells present in a whole population was obtained from the finding that a CTL clone but not a helper T cell clone contained αCTLL blocking activity.

It is noteworthy that while normal C57Bl/6 spleen cells were without detectable blocking activity, spleen cells from certain strains such as CBA or BALB/C nude did contain low but detectable levels of αCTLL inhibitory activity (unpublished results). This suggests that similar material(s) may also be present in NK cells and that the inability to detect this material in the spleens of normal mice may reflect the relatively low frequency of active NK killer cells in the strain tested (i.e., B6 vs. CBA). Indeed, the ability of αCTLL and RαNK antibody to cross block both CTL and NK cytolysis without inhibiting target binding strongly supports this possibility.

By the use of a soluble phase immunoabsorbent assay the physical-chemical and biochemical properties of the CTL derived cytosolic material reactive with αCTLL IgG was determined. The antigenicity of this material was unstable to brief heating or extended storage at 4°C. It was also lost at low pH. Treatment with trypsin or neuraminidase did not alter antigenic reactivity with αCTLL IgG but treatment with pronase dramatically lowered reactivity. These findings suggest the material to be protein in nature.

When analyzed by gel filtration chromatography (S-300) material reactive with αCTLL IgG was heterogenous in size. While the major peak of reactivity eluted in the 60 kd range consistent peaks were also noted in the void volume (>300 kd), at 120 kd, and around 20 kd. In different experiments the percentage of material eluting in the void volume appeared to be due to the time which elapsed between extraction of the material and application to the column. In some experiments when application occurred several hours after extraction, the majority of αCTLL neutralizing material eluted in the void volume (only a small 60 kd peak was seen). This is best exemplified in the sucrose density gradient shown in Fig. 7. Here, the majority of αCTLL blocking activity migrates with the 19S IgM marker (∿900 kd), with smaller peaks eluting with the 3S (60 kd) and smaller (20 kd) markers. However, it must be noted that other sucrose gradients showed different elution patterns with several peaks of activity migrating between the 3S and 19S markers. Thus, one can conclude this material can spontaneously polymerize through a series of high MW intermediates to form very high MW (∿10^6d) complexes.

Interestingly, extraction of CTL cytosolic material in the presence of 2 mercaptoethanol or protease inhibitors caused a dramatic shift in the gel filtration elution profile in which the 60 kd peak was greatly reduced and the 20 kd peak greatly enhanced. This is interpreted as meaning the 60 kd peak is derived from disulfide bonding of 20 kd monomers. The fact that protease inhibitors (in the absence of a reducing agent) also prevented formation of the 60 kd structure suggests that some form of protease activity is also required to allow polymerization of the 20 kd subunits. Whether the 60 kd structure represents a trimer of three 20 kd subunits or a 20 kd subunit complexed to another molecule(s) will require further study.

It is clear from this and other studies that transfer of protein like materials from the killer cell to the target is requisite for target cell lysis. The ability to block the lethal hit with antibody probes (first done with RAT[*] in the murine CTL system and followed by similar antibodies capable of blocking the lethal hit of human CTL, murine NK cells and human NK cells) indicates this process is at least initially a reversible one. Further support for this comes from the observation that the NK lethal hit is blocked by trypsinization of the lethally hit target (19). Furthermore, reduction of the temperature to 4°C also blocks the lethal hit by CTL or NK cells and this can be reversed by raising the temperature back to 37°C indicating the lethal hit remains affixed to the target for sometime. It is important to note, however, that the sensitivity of the lethal hit to antibody or trypsin blockade is transient and only present during the early stages of killer cell independent lysis.

The capability to inhibit the CTL lethal hit using αCTLL antibody together with biochemical analysis of CTL derived cytosolic materials involved in cytolysis allows us to hypothesize the following theory regarding the mechanism of the CTL (and NK cell) lethal hit. Subsequent to target cell binding the CTL is triggered to initiate directed secretion of the cytolytic mediators. It is possible these cytolytic mediators are derived from the intracellular granules identified in LGL and CTL clones as has been suggested by Henkart et al. (20). The lack of "granules" in some cytolytic clones, however, indicate other mechanisms for delivery of cytolytic mediators may also exist (21). We propose these cytolytic mediators are carried as inactive or only weakly active subunits and once released are polymerized into high MW complexes in the membrane of the target, a theory originally proposed by Hiserodt and Granger analyzing the mechanism of action of lymphotoxin molecules (22). Polymerization will require the formation of stabilizing disulfide bonds and may be initiated by target cell derived or effector cell derived proteolytic "polymerases". The idea of a target cell associated polymerase is especially attractive as this could explain the spectrum of target cell sensitivities to these cytolytic mediators. The "NK sensitive" targets are those targets possessing a surface enzymes which can mimic or partially mimic the "polymerase" derived from the killer cells. In this regard it has been demonstrated that pretreatment of target cells with certain protease inhibitors renders these cells resistant to lysis by purified lymphotoxin molecules (23).

Completion of the polymerization reaction will result in the development of a transmembrane pore as has been already observed in targets lysed by human K cells (24) or murine NK (25) and CTL (26). The ability of an antibody directed against the cytolytic mediators to inhibit target lysis will necessarily depend upon the relative stage of completion of such "pores" during the polymerization process.

Intrinsic to this model is the possibility that at various stages of cytolysin polymerization the target cell may undergo dramatic physiologic consequences. This model does not preclude the possibility that prior to completion of the final "pores" the target cell membrane may depolarize perhaps by Ca^{++} gates created by intermediate "pores" or by other ion fluxes. Thus, it is possible that irreversible target cell damage may even occur before completion of a visible "pore". However, in either case target cell death was affected directly by materials derived from the killer and transferred to the target most likely via a secretory mechanism. Certainly future studies on the biochemistry of killer cell derived cytolytic mediators and the physiologic mechanisms of target cell death will be exciting.

REFERENCES

1. Mechanisms of Cell-Mediated Cytotoxicity. in Adv. Expt. Medicine and Biology, Vol. 146 (Ed. W.R. Clark and P. Golstein), Plenum Press, New York, 1982.
2. Martz, E. Mechanism of specific tumor cell lysis by allo-immune T lymphocytes: Resolution and characterization of discrete steps in the cellular interaction. In: Contemporary Topics in Immunobiology. (ed. O. Stutman) Plenum Press, N.Y. 7:301, 1977.
3. Golstein, P., and Smith, E.T. The lethal hit stage of mouse T and non T cell mediated cytolysis. Differences in cation requirements and characterization of an analytical "cation pulse" method. Eur. J. Immunol. 6:31, 1976.
4. Berke, G. Cytotoxic T-lymphocytes: Ho do they function. Immunological Rev. 72:5, 1983.
5. Gately, M.K., Wechter, W.J., and E. Martz. Early steps in specific tumor cell lysis by sensitized mouse T lymphocytes. IV. Inhibition of Programming for lysis by pharmacologic agents. J. Immunol. 125:783, 1980.
6. Hiserodt, J.C., Britvan, L.J., and S.R. Targan. Characterization of the cytolytic reaction mechanism of the human natural killer (NK) lymphocyte: Resolution into binding, programming and killer cell-independent steps. J. Immunol. 129:1782, 1982.
7. Fan, J., Ahmed, A., and Bonavida, B. Studies on the induction and expression of T cell mediated immunity. X. Inhibition by Lyt 2,3 antisera of cytotoxic T lymphocyte-mediated antigen-specific and nonspecific cytotoxicity: Evidence for the blocking of the binding between T lymphocytes and target cells and not the post-binding cytolytic steps. J. Immunol. 125:2444, 1980.
8. Davignon, E., Martz, E., Reynolds, T., Kurzinger, K., and Springer, T.A. Lymphocyte function associated antigens one (LFA-1): a surface antigen distinct from Lyt 2,3 that participates in T lymphocyte-mediated killing. Proc. Natl. Acad. Sci. USA 78:4535, 1981.
9. Pierres, M., Goridis, C., and Golstein, P. Inhibition of murine T cell cytolysis and T cell proliferation by a rat monoclonal antibody immunoprecipitation two polypeptides of 94,000 and 180,000 molecular weight. Eur. J. Immunology 12:60, 1982.
10. Pasternak, M.S., Sitkowski, M.V., and H.N. Eisen. The site of action of TLCK on cloned cytotoxic T lymphocytes. J. Immunol. 131:2477, 1983.
11. Targan, S. and W. Newman. Definition of a "trigger" stage in the NK cytolytic reaction sequence by a monclonal antibody to the glycoprotein T-200. J. Immunol. 131:1149, 1983.

12. Hiserodt, J.C., and Bonavida, B. Studies on the induction and expression of T cell-mediated immunity. XI. Inhibition of the "lethal hit" on T cell mediated cytotoxicity by heterologous rat antiserum made against alloimmune cytotoxic T lymphocytes. J. Immunol. 126:256, 1981.

13. Neville, M.E., and J.C. Hiserodt. Inhibition of human antibody dependent cellular cytotoxicity, T cell mediated cytotoxicity, and natural killing by heterologous rat antiserum made against alloimmune human cytotoxic lymphocytes. J. Immunol. 128:1246, 1982.

14. Ware, C.F., and Granger, G.A. Mechanisms of lymphocyte-mediated cytotoxicity I. The effect of anti-human lymphotoxin antisera on the cytolysis of allogeneic B cell lines by MLC-sensitized human lymphocytes in vitro. J. Immunol. 126:1919, 1981.

15. Lawlor, D.A., Saunders, P.H., and Ware, C.F. Rat antisera directed against alloimmune cytotoxic T lymphocytes inhibit cytotoxic T lymphocyte and natural killer activity: Strain specificity of inhibition. Cellular Immunol. 62:128, 1982.

16. Kahle, R., Hiserodt, J. and B. Bonavida. Characterization of antibody mediated inhibition of natural killer (NK) cytotoxicity: Evidence for blocking of both recognition and lethal hit stages of cytolysis. Cell. Immunol. 80:97, 1983.

17. Hiserodt, J.C., Britvan, L.J. and S.R. Targan. Inhibition of human natural killing by heterologous and monoclonal antibodies. J. Immunol. 129:2248, 1982.

18. Bohmer, V., Hengartner, H., Nabholz, M., Lernhardt, W., Schrier, M.H., and Haas, W. Fine specificity of a continuously growing killer cell clone specific for H-Y antigen. Eur. J. Immunol. 9:592, 1979.

19. Hiserodt, J.C., Britvan, L.J., and S.R. Targan. Studies on the mechanism of the human natural killer cell lethal hit: Evidence for transfer of protease-sensitive structures requisite for target cell lysis. J. Immunol. 131:2710, 1983.

20. Henkart, M., Blumenthal, R., Millard, P., Reynolds, C., and P. Henkart. Correlation of ring structures and activity of the calcium dependent cytolysin from LGL granules. Fed. Proc. 43:1756, 1984.

21. Schneider, E.M., G.P. Pawelec, S. Uangru, and P. Wernet. A novel type of human T cell clone with highly potent natural killer-like cytotoxicity divorced from large granular lymphocyte morphology. J. Immunol. 133:173, 1984.

22. Hiserodt, J.C. and G.A. Granger. The human lymphotoxin system. J. Reticuloendothelial Soc. 24:427, 1978.

23. Weirtzen, M. and G.A. Granger. The Human LT System. VIII. A target cell-dependent enzymatic activation step required for the expression of cytotoxic activity of human lymphotoxin. J. Immunol. 125:719, 1980.

24. Doumashkin, R.R., P. Deteix, C.B. Simone, and P. Henkart. Electron microscope demonstration of lesions on target cell membranes associated with antibody dependent cellular cyto-toxicity. Clin. Exp. Immunol. 43:554, 1980.

25. Podack, E.R., and G. Dennert. Assembly of two types of tubules with putative cytolytic function in cloned natural killer cells. Nature (Lond.) 302:442, 1983.

26. Dennert, G. and E.R. Podack. Cytolysis by H-2 specific T killer cells. Assembly of tubular complexes on target membranes. J. Exp. Med. 157:1483, 1983.

DISCUSSION

Dennert: Do any of your antibodies react with granules or with NKCF?

Hiserodt: I haven't tested either, but this is in the works.

Podack: Have you done Western blots against whole cell extracts rather than looking at gel filtration?

Hiserodt: No.

M. Henkart: Have you tried immunocytochemistry to see what part of the cells stain?

Hiserodt: I haven't had time yet.

Young: (inaudible)

Hiserodt: What I have done is to take the CTL extract and neutralize the anti-NK antibody. The anti-NK neutralizing activity comes out on the columns at very similar positions as the anti-CTL neutralizing activity.

Young: Do thiols break down the polymers to lower molecular weights?

Hiserodt: No, but I have preliminary data that high salt (2M KCl) can break these materials into smaller forms.

Springer: Regarding your sucrose sedimantation profile, polymerization while the gradient is running would give you a smear. Since you get a sharp peak, the polymerization must have occurred prior to running the gradient.

Hiserodt: Well, I showed you one of my best gradients, and I have seen smears and chatter in other gradients. If you put the material right away onto the gradient, you tend to eliminate the high molecular weight form. Letting it sit for a few hours tends to generate the aggregate. I see intermediate forms in many gradients.

Ware: Your work is somewhat similar to experiments we did in Granger's lab in 1981, looking at antibodies made against supernatants of activated CTL. Those antibodies would block killing, and we would do a fluid phase immunoabsorption to identify the molecular weight range of the antigen. We found it was mainly in the void volume peakof greater than 200kd, which would be consistent with what you are finding if the material is allowed to incubate for awhile. In our experiments we were correlating this activity with lymphotoxin.

Hiserodt: The relationship between this material and lymphotoxin or NKCF is currently unclear.

Mescher: Have you looked for this blocking activity in pellets of your homogenates?

Hiserodt: When I take the pellet and resolubilize it, I get a lot more activity--but not as much as the original soluble material.

Bonavida: We have found that different batches of serum from animals immunized by the same protocol show different types of blocking activity. Some block at conjugate formation, and others at later stages, so that each batch must be carefully characterized. How many rats have you immunized with your extracts, and how many of those have shown the activity you have described?

Hiserodt: We have used CTL clones to get around that kind of problem. We immunized 5 rats with the CTL extracts, and all 5 inhibited CTL lytic activity without affecting binding. This may be due to the immunogen in these experiments.

Brooks: Do the antibodies inhibit the activity of cytotoxic factors?

Hiserodt: We are going to do that shortly.

Berke: I am surprised that your antibody didn't prevent conjugation. Did you add antibody to the cells prior to mixing them together, or did you test its ability to reverse pre-formed conjugates?

Hiserodt: I have done this in a variety of ways. I have pretreated the effectors for an hour, and left the antibody in, and conjugation still occurs at normal levels. These antibodies also do not dissociate conjugates, as otherantobodies do.

Berke: This behaves like your rat* antibody in the sense of its acting on something which is generated after effector-target binding. Would not you expect that the extract itself to be cytolytic to the target?

Hiserodt: The extract probably is cytotoxic, but since it has been incubated in calcium containing medium, it probably has lost lytic activity as was shown for the granule cytolysin.

HUMAN NK RESISTANT TUMOR CELL LYSIS IS EFFECTED BY IL-2 ACTIVATED KILLER CELLS

Elizabeth A. Grimm, Anthony A. Rayner[1] and Debra J. Wilson

Surgical Neurology Branch
Natl. Inst. of Neurological and Communicative Disorders and
Stroke, National Institutes of Health
Bethesda, MD 20205
[1]Current Address: 585 HSE, UCSF Medical Center
Parnasus Avenue, San Francisco, CA 94143

INTRODUCTION

In experimental animal systems, transfer of cell populations immune to solid tumors has been successful in mediating the regression of such tumors. In human systems, much conflicting and confusing data has been reported attempting to define the analogous effector cells. Our approach to define human anti-tumor effectors cells was to avoid as many in vitro induced artifacts as possible, and to employ fresh (or cyropreserved, uncultured) surgical biopsy specimens of tumors as target cells, and to generate effectors in human serum with naturally occurring immune stimulants. We have found that normal or cancer patients' PBL incubated for 2-3 days in preparations of IL-2, including purified recombinant IL-2 (RIL-2) acquires the unique capacity to kill human tumors in 4 hour chromium release assays (1-6). These lymphokine-activated killer cells (LAK) kill NK resistant fresh tumors with an efficiency and polyspecificity that has not been found reproducible in any other anti-tumor lytic system, and therefore provides yet another interesting and potentially biologically relevant system in which to examine the mechanism of cell mediated cytotoxicity. This report addresses some of the basic aspects of LAK killing, such as the killing efficiency of whole populations versus clones, kinetics of lysis as measured by the chromium release assay, correlation of chromium release with the expression of LAK effector cell markers, and morphology and phenotype of LAK effector cells, thereby setting the groundwork for further detailed studies of the mechanism of tumor killing by LAK.

FRESH TUMORS, CULTERED CELLS, AND TNP-MODIFIED PBL ARE LYSED BY
LAK

LAK populations generated from both normal persons and
cancer patients' PBL were found to kill fresh and cultured tumor
targets tested (> 100 fresh tumors tested currently), as well
as, TNP-modified PBL (for review, see 6). Usually, little or no
lysis of unmodified PBL, Con A blasts, LAK or normal tissue
cells has been found (Table I). Initially it was tempting to
speculate that the mechanism of LAK lysis was specific for
rapidly dividing cells only, but the efficient lysis of TNP-PBL,
and lack of lysis directed toward Con A blasts now provides
evidence to the contrary.

TABLE I

SUMMARY OF TARGET CELLS SUSCEPTIBLE TO LYSIS BY HUMAN LAK

LYSED	NOT LYSED
FRESH TUMORS:	NORMAL LUNG (6)
SARCOMA (1-3,6)	NORMAL LIVER (6)
ADENOCARCINOMA (1)	NORMAL KIDNEY (6)
MELANOMA (1)	PBL[1] (1-3,7)
LYMPHOMA (8)	CON A BLASTS[2] (2)
OVARIAN CA ASCITIES (1)	LAK[2,3]
NEURILEMOMA (6)	
CULTURED CELLS: (2,6,7)	
K562, DAUDI, 3T3	
MOUSE TUMORS:	
MCA 105, P815, EL4	
EBV TRANSFORMED B CELL LINES	
FETAL CELLS (6)	
PLACENTAL CELLS (6)	
TNP - PBL[3]	

[1]FEW EXCEPTIONS NOTED IN <u>CANCER RESEARCH</u>
[2]LOW AND ERRATIC LYSIS
[3]NOT PUBLISHED

DISTINCTIONS BETWEEN NK CELLS, LAK, AND CTL

While terminology should be utilized carefully and
specifically in order to clarify distinctions in new results, new
names are often given to findings prior to full analysis and
establishment of unique characteristics. Therefore, we felt it
was of utmost importance to justify the new name, LAK, given to
these IL-2 activated killer cells and have presented six criteria
below that establish human LAK as a unique lytic phenomenon.

Table II

LAK MEDIATED ANTI-SOLID TUMOR KILLING REPRESENTS SYSTEM DISTINCT FROM HUMAN NK AND CTL

	NK	LAK	CTL
DEVELOPMENT KINETICS	PRESENT IN FRESH PBL	DAY 2,3	DAY 5,6
STIMULUS	IFN AUGMENTS	IL-2, (NOT IFN)	SPECIFIC ANTIGENS
SPECIFICITY OF CYTOTOXICITY	BONE MARROW, LEUKEMIA, SOME CULTURED CELLS K562	FRESH SOLID TUMORS ALL NK TARGETS	SPECIFIC ANTIGEN EX-PRESSING CELLS
PRECURSOR LOCATION	TDL- PBL+	TDL+ SPLEEN+ PBL+ TUMOR+ BM +	PBL+
SEROLOGIC PHENOTYPE OF EFFECTOR	OKM1 + LEU7 + OKT11 + OKT3 - LEU 1 -	OKT3 + OKT8 + 4F2 + OKM1 -	OKT3 + OKT8 + 4F2 + OKM1 -
SEROLOGIC PHENOTYPE OF PRECURSOR	NOT KNOWN	OKM1 - OKT3 - LEU-1 - OKT10 - TAC - OKT11 -	OKT3 + LEU-1 + OKT11 + OKM1 -

Previously, Henny presented the distinctions between NK cells and CTL in the mouse (8) and Rosenstein's results (studying murine LAK) established it as distinct as well (9).

KILLING OF FRESH TUMOR CELLS BY LAK CAUSES OPTIMUM CHROMIUM
RELEASE IN 3-4 HOURS

Some previous reports suggested that solid tumor cells
required 18 hours of interaction with effector populations for
substantial lysis to occur, while others have consistently used
shorter term assays. Because CTL are known to kill in 3-4
hours, we analyzed the kinetics of solid tumor lysis by LAK.
Our results confirm that 3-4 hours is optimal for LAK lysis of
tumors, especially because of the heightened spontaneous
chromium release in the longer term assays.

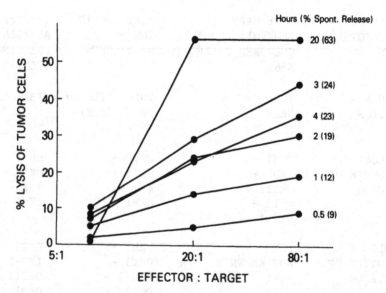

Figure 1. Kinetics of tumor lysis by LAK; spontaneous release at
each time point is given in the parenthesis.

LAK POPULATIONS AND LAK CLONES KILL AUTOLOGOUS AND ALLOGENEIC TUMORS WITH POLYSPECIFICITY

In order to ascertain whether LAK represented a population of effectors each with unique specificity, or whether all LAK killed multiple targets, LAK clones and subclones were generated. While the details of these experiments are to be published elsewhere (10-12) the main findings indicate that individual LAK are polyspecific.

An unseparated LAK cell population produce substantial lysis (67 $\pm$ 3% chromium release at 40:1) of the patient's autologous sarcoma, and a panel of six allogeneic tumors (5 sarcomas and a colon cancer, (33 $\pm$ 2% to 66 $\pm$ 1% lysis at 40:1 effector target ratio). Clones derived from 1 and 3 cell/well limiting dilution cultures and were observed to significantly kill the same panel of tumor targets in 58/61 combinations. The autologous sarcoma was lysed by clones from 33-53%, and six allogeneic tumors up to 68% at an effector target ratio of 40:1. In all experiments, autologous PBL were included as target cells and were not lysed.

Polyspecificity of LAK was also confirmed at the population level in cold target inhibition experiments in which HLA typed allogeneic individuals' tumors totally inhibited the lysis of autologous tumor cells (Grimm, to be reported elsewhere). Taken together, these results imply that the initial recognition unit and subsequent mechanism of lysis of fresh tumors is common on all tumor cells as well as specificity expressed by all LAK effectors.

CLONING OF LAK DOES NOT INCREASE THE PERCENTAGE OF KILLERS AS DETERMINED IN THE SINGLE CELL LYSIS ASSAY.

Because preliminary single-cell lysis experiments indicated that only 10-30% of the cells in any LAK population were killer cells, we tested whether an increase in killer cells would be evident in LAK clones. An enriched homogeneous population of LAK would be a useful to studying the mechanism of cytotoxicity; however, as indicated in Table III the % killer cells was not increased.

Table III

SINGLE TUMOR CELL LYSIS BY LAK CLONES

Exp.	Clone[1]	Predominant Phenotype	% Binders[2]	% Dead Target[3]	% Killers
1.	1AA1	LEU 3	56	38	21
	1AE12	LEU 3	37	69	26
	1BB5	NT	39	71	28
	Whole LAK	NT	45	45	30
2.	1AE12	LEU 3	18	34	7
	1BH10	LEU 2	13	88	11
	1BA6	LEU 2	40	86	34
	Whole LAK	NT	33	45	15

[1] Clones were the same as those expressing polyspecificity and details of their selection and growth are published elsewhere (12). For this assay, the clones were grown for 3 days in the absence of feeders and aliquots used for FACS analysis of phenotype and single cell lysis to the fresh autologous sarcoma, containing 93% tumor cells.

[2] The % binding LAK cells was determined by visually examining the conjugates in the LAK-target mixture prior to incubation. A minimum of 100 cells was counted.

[3] The % dead conjugating sarcoma was counted after the 4 hour incubation of conjugates in agarose, followed by staining with trypan blue as reported previously (13).

Our lack of enrichment of effector cells after cloning confirms the report by Zagury who cloned by micromanipulation and analyzed the subsequent CTL clones in single cell lysis assays (14). In both Zagury's and our studies, there was little doubt as to the clonality of the effectors. Therefore, we hypothesize that either we are cloning a precursor, which continually differentiates into terminal lytic cells while replicating itself; or that lytic ability is a function of the effector cells stage in the cell cycle (analogous to activation). These and other models are now being tested. It is curious that some clones express the Leu 2 and others express the Leu 3 phenotype and in data not shown, these clones did lyse with identical polyspecificity.

LAK AND LAK CLONES GROWN FOR GREATER THAN 33 DAYS REQUIRE PHA FOR EXPRESSION OF CYTOLYTIC ACTIVITY

In previously reported studies with long term in vitro expanded LAK, cytolytic activity was maintained as long as the cells were replicating, which was documented for up to 70 days (6). Partially purified, lectin free IL-2 was utilized as the source of growth factor for those previous studies. Preliminary results employing purified IL-2 from recombinant DNA technology (5) have indicated that the lytic activity is lost after approximately 2-3 weeks. Addition of PHA and pooled allogeneic feeder cells to the cultures (or clones) resulted in re-expression of lytic activity. In order to determine whether PHA was serving merely as a bridge to induce lectin dependent cellular cytotoxicity (LDCC) or whether the PHA was needed to "activate" a lytic mechanism within the effete LAK clones, PHA was preincubated with the 3 clones shown in Table IV for 3 days, 8 hours, 1/2 hour all followed by three washes, or PHA included in the cytotoxicity assay as a control for LDCC.

TABLE IV

ROLE OF PHA IN LAK CLONE LYSIS[1]

CULTURE SUPPLEMENT	1BA6[2]	1BH10	1AE12
RIL-2	1 + 2	7 + 2	2 + 1
RIL-2 + 1/2 HR PHA[3]	24 + 2	NT	-2 + 3
RIL-2 + 8 HR PHA	49 + 1	50 + 4	25 + 3
RIL-2 + PHA 3 DAYS	45 + 3	33 + 1	8 + 2
RIL-2 + PHA IN ASSAY (LDCC)	63 + 4	46 + 5	35 + 7

[1] Lysis was performed in a 4 hour assay to autologous sarcoma tumor at E:T = 40:1.

[2] Clone 1BA6 was 33 days in vitro, 1BH10 and 1AE12 were 35 days.

[3] PHA (Burroughs-Wellcome) was used at 0.1 µg/ml final concentration.

167

Clearly both roles suggested for PHA were found to be possible depending on the conditions in which it was used. When PHA was added to the assay only, the clones grown only in RIL-2 expressed the highest lysis. However, incubation of clones for 30 minutes prior to assay stimulated some activity, and 8 hours preincubation was as effective as 3 days. This induction of cytolytic activity is reminiscent of the induction of cytolytic activity in CTL hybridomas by Kaufmann (15).

MORPHOLOGY OF LAK EFFECTOR CELLS

LAK effector cells were enriched by continuous growth in IL-2. A photograph of a cytocentrifuge preparation of LAK cells is shown in Figure 2. These cells were highly enriched for LAK and displayed lysis of 30% at an E:T = 0.6:1. These cells appear similar to large T cell blasts. They have cytoplasmic granules, and a large round nuclei. The cells have an average diameter of 20 μm.

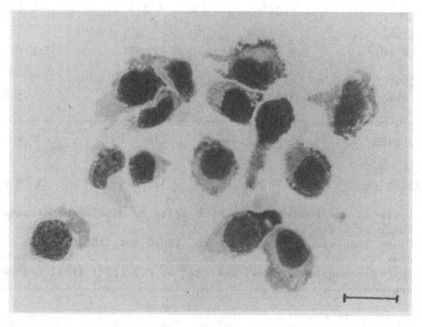

Figure 2. Photograph of LAK effector cells. The bar is 20 μm.

RELATIVE SENSITIVITY OF NK vs LAK EFFECTORS TO NH₄Cl

It has long been realized that NK mediated lysis was sensitive to short treatments with NH_4Cl, while CTL mediated lysis was insensitive. Therefore, we tested whether LAK lysis of autologous tumor was inhibited by treatment of the LAK cells with 0.83% NH_4Cl, (buffered with Phosphate). Table V shows one of these experiments. While we could reproducibly eliminate the NK activity, the LAK activity was reduced approximately 4-fold, but never eliminated.

TABLE V

LAK EFFECTORS ARE PARTIALLY SENSITIVE TO NH₄Cl

EFFECTOR	TARGET CELLS	% LYSIS AT EFFECTOR:TARGET RATIO		
		60:1	15:1	4:1
LAK	TUMOR	69 + 5	55 + 5	30 + 1
LAK - treated[1]	TUMOR	43 + 2	32 + 4	11 + 1
PBL	TUMOR	2 + 1	3 + 1	6 + 1
PBL - treated[1]	TUMOR	-1 + 2	2 + 1	4 + 4
LAK	K562	74 + 1	64 + 6	37 + 1
LAK - treated[1]	K562	32 + 1	12 + 1	1 + 1
PBL	K562	43 + 2	17 + 1	4 + 1
PBL - treated[1]	K562	1 + 1	-1 + 1	1 + 1

[1] These effector populations were incubated in phosphate buffered 0.83% NH_4Cl for 60 seconds, followed by two washes immediately prior to the chromium release assay.

LAK EFFECTORS DEVELOP EXPRESSION OF T CELL MARKERS

While LAK precursors do not express T, B, or NK cell markers, we have consistently observed that the LAK effectors express the phenotype of CTL (1-3). In order to examine the kinetics of appearance of CTL markers a series of kinetic studies have been performed (6). A most interesting finding is that LAK develop expression of Tac, the IL-2 receptor, as detected by FACS analysis, in correlation with the expression of lysis (Table VI).

It was also observed at the clonal level that non-lytic clones lost their expression of Tac, and regained it when cultured under conditions that restored the cytotoxicity (data not shown). Anti Tac does not inhibit the chromium release assay when the antibody was included for the 4 hours, though anti Tac does inhibit the activation when present in the culture medium (6).

TABLE VI

DEVELOPMENT OF LAK ACTIVITY CORRELATES WITH EXPRESSION OF TAC

% CELLS WITH PHENOTYPE	DAY					
	0	1	2	3	4	5
OKM1	15	18	10	12	NT	13
LEU 7	9	NT	10	11	NT	7
OKT 9	0	1	3	5	NT	11
TAC	0	0	10	31	47	58
LYTIC UNITS	0	7	20	NT	59	NT

CONCLUSION

The mechanism by which LAK effector cells mediate tumor cell destruction is unknown. Lysis occurs rapidly at 37°, and 4 hours of incubation is optimal. The mechanism is neither an antibody mediated cytotoxicity (ADCC) or merely lectin-dependent cytotoxicity (LDCC) as summarized previously (1-6). LAK kill tumors with an unexplained polyspecificity and is such killing partially sensitive to treatment with NH_4Cl. The report of successful adoptive therapy is mouse systems with LAK (16,17) provides the basis for proposing that LAK is a biologically relevant system in which to further examine the mechanism of cell-mediated cytotoxicity.

REFERENCES

1. Grimm, E.A., Mazumder, A., Zhang, H.Z, and Rosenberg, S.A. The lymphokine activated killer cell phenomenon: Lysis of NK resistant fresh solid tumor cells by IL-2 activated autologous human peripheral blood lymphocytes. J. Exp. Med. 155:1823-1841 (1982).

2. Grimm, E.A., Gorelik, E., Rosenstein, M.M., and Rosenberg, S.A. The lymphokine-activated killer cell phenomenon: In vitro and in vivo studies. Interluekins, Lymphokines, and Cytokines. S. Cohen and J. Oppenheim,(eds.). Academic Press, New York, pp. 739-746 (1983).

3. Grimm, E.A., Ramsey, K., Mazumder, A., Wilson, D.J., Djeu, J., and Rosenberg, S.A. Lymphokine-activated killer cell phenomenon: II. The precursor phenotype is serologically distinct from peripheral T lymphocytes, memory CTL, and NK cells. J. Exp. Med. 157:884-897 (1983).

4. Grimm, E.A., Robb, R.J., Roth, J.A., Neckers, L.M., Lachman, L., Wilson, D.J., and Rosenberg, S.A. The lymphokine-activated killer cell phenomenon. III. Evidence that IL-2 alone is sufficient for direct activation of PBL into LAK. J. Exp. Med. 158:1356-1361 (1983).

5. Rosenberg, S.A., Grimm, E.A., McGrogan, N., Doyle, M., Kawasaki, E., Koths, K., and Mark, D.F. Biologic activity of recombinant human interleukine-2 produced in E. Coli. Science. 223:1412-1415 (1984).

6. Grimm, E.A., and Rosenberg, S.A. The human lymphokine-activated killer cell phenomenon in Lymphokines. 9:Edgar Pick, (ed.) Academic Press, (in press).

7. Lotze, M.T., Grimm, E.A., Mazumder, A., Strausser, J.L., and Rosenberg, S.A. Lysis of human solid tumors by autologous cells sensitized in vitro to alloantigens. J. Immunol. 127:266-271 (1981).

8. Henney, C.S. Dintinction between NK cells and CTL in Advances in Exp. Med. Biol. 146:353-356 (1982).

9. Rosenstein, M., Yron, I., Kaufmann, Y., and Rosenberg S.A. Lymphokine-activated killer cells: Lysis of fresh syngeneic natural killer-resistant murine tumor cells by lymphocytes cultured in interleukin-2. Cancer Research. 44:1946 (1984).

10. Rayner, A.A., Grimm, E.A., Lotze, M.T., and Rosenberg, S.A. Demonstration of shared recognition and lysis of autologous and allogeneic fresh human tumors by cloned lymphokine-activated killer calls (LAK): Implications for immunotherapy. Surgical Forum (in press).

11. Rayner, A.A., Grimm, E.A., Lotze, M.T., Chu, E., and Rosenberg, S.A. Lymphokine-activated killer cells (LAK). Analysis of factors relevant to the immunotherapy of cancer. (submitted).

12. Rayner, A.A., Grimm, E.A., Wilson, D.J., and Rosenberg, S.A. Clonal and lytic analysis of IL-2 activated lymphocyte: Lymphokine-activated killer (LAK) cell clones lyse multiple fresh human targets. (submitted).

13. Grimm, E.A., and Bonavida, B. Mechanism of cell-mediated immunity at the single cell level. I. Estimation of cytotoxic T lymphocyte frequency and relative lytic efficiency in individual effector populations. J. Immunol. 123:2861-2869 (1979).

14. Zagury, D., Morgan, D., Lenoir, G., Fouchard, M., Feldman, M. Human normal CTL clones. Generatioin and properties. Int. J. Cancer. 31:427-432 (1983).

15. Kaufmann, Y. Lyt 2 negative and T cell growth factor independent cytotoxic T lymphocyte hybridomas. Adv. in Exp. Med. Biol. W.R. Clark and P. Goldstein (eds.) 146 (1982).

16. Mazumder, A., and Rosenberg, S.A. Successful immunotherapy of natural killer-resistant established pulmonary melanoma metastases by the intravenous adoptive transfer of syngeneic lymphocytes activated in vitro by interleukin-2 J. Exp Med. 159:495-507 (1984).

17. Mule, J.J., Shut, S., Schwarz, S., and Rosenberg, S.A. Successful adoptive immunotherapy of established pulmonary metastases of multiple sarcomas with lymphokine-activated killer cells and recombinant IL-2. Science. (in press)

DISCUSSION

A. Kimura: Is the expression of MHC products on these various tumors required for lysis?

E. Grimm: No. K562 is lysed, and has very little class I or class II.

W. Clark: Did you say that the peak of activity is at 2-3 days, or that you first see it at 2-3 days?

E. Grimm: You first see it at 2-3. It peaks at 3-5 days. If we wash and continue adding fresh factor and fresh medium, you actually grow out LAK to a very pure population.

W. Clark: Have you looked to see if there is this type of activation when you do what is generally considered to be a polyclonal activation with T cell mitogens?

E. Grimm: Yes. In fact, one of my coworkers, A. Mazumder, was studying PHA activation of lymphocyte fractions using the cells in clinical trials. For a long time, he was sure that these were the same as LAK. And so we did a number of side-by-side tests. What happens in the PHA system, for example, is that PHA stimulates every T cell that you find in culture, including suppressor cells, and so the vast majority of T cells start proliferating, and the culture conditions become very toxic very fast. Now, if he dilutes out the system, adds some fresh medium, and adds some IL2, LAK cells will grow out. Certainly IL2 is produced under those conditions, and if you look late enough, if the cells didn't deplete the nutrients resulting from the PHA, then you could find LAK. But, initially, the PHA stimulated killing is not sensitive to irradiation of precursors, whereas LAK is. The PHA activated killers peak between day 1 and day 2. By day 3, anything that survived had a good chance of being contaminated with LAK, whereas the other killers died early.

J. Hiserodt: Are the LAK precursors Fc receptor positive? And also, have you looked at histochemistry of your cultured cells for nonspecific esterase?

E. Grimm: We have looked, and they are nonspecific esterase negative. We have tried to block Fc receptors as a prelude to FACS work, and saw no Fc receptors, but we have not done classical Fc rosetting, so I can't answer with regard to that technique. These cells do not mediate an ADCC, and the killing is not blocked by staph A under conditions which do block ADCC.

D. Adams: Could it be that rather than expanding a subset, interleukin has really changed the specificity to which CTLs are directed? Though that may be semantic, frameworks like that shape the experiments we do.

My second point is directed at the specificity. I must say, I was not convinced that the killers were not reactive against rapidly dividing cells. At least in our hands, when we have modified tumor cells with TNP, we have frequently found that though background release is not raised, these cells become much more sensitive to injury. So I would have a hard time putting this in a meaningful frame until we know more about whether contact is required, what is being recognized, some of the kinetics of lysis and some of the things that other people have worked on. Perhaps these will tell us whether this is the same thing replayed in a somewhat different way or is very different.

E. Grimm: I agree completely, TNP is notorius. I tested some other modifications of lymphocytes, influenza infected lymphocytes, and some other biochemical modifications. None of them have resulted in being good LAK targets.

E. Podack: Do you see any increase in activity after cloning? And how do you determine that only 30% of the cloned cells are active?

E. Grimm: We were hoping that cloned cells would give us a continuous population with which to study cytotoxicity. Therefore, we did what we call a single cell cytotoxicity assay in which we form conjugates, isolate them in agarose, incubate the conjugates for several hours, and then stain with trypan blue to see how many of the bound tumor target cells are lysed. From this sort of assay, we have determined the percentage killer cells.

D. Redelman: Did you look at Tac [IL2 receptor] expression on the precursor?

E. Grimm: You would expect Tac to be there. Anti-Tac blocks the activation of LAK cells, and Tac is on the effector. But we have not been able to detect Tac by FACS analysis on day zero. However, we have been able to kill LAK precursors with very high concentrations of anti-Tac plus complement, 10 to 20-fold more concentrated than was used for FACS. So we're still trying to sort this out. There may be some very low levels of Tac there which are up-regulated by IL2.

D. Redelman: At the normal concentrations that one uses for [FACS] staining, 1:10,000 or 1:30,000 dilution of the standard prep, I see that anywhere from 5 to 25% of resting peripheral blood cells have very little evidence of Tac on them.

You said that after a couple of months or so, your cells

tended to die out. Have you attempted to put in some lectin along with purified growth factors?

E. Grimm: Absolutely. Neither lectin nor feeders help.

D. Redelman: Does the interleukin 2 that you're using induce interferon production?

E. Grimm: We have tested supernatants from various stages of LAK activation and have not found any interferon.

G. Berke: Do you need interleukin 2 present during the killing assay?

E. Grimm: No.

SECTION 3. NK CELL MEDIATED CYTOTOXICITY

INTRODUCTION

The finding that large granular lymphocytes can be purified and are the effector cells responsible for NK cell mediated cytotoxicity in all mammalian species studied has allowed rapid progress in the study of mechanisms of NK cytotoxicity. The finding by Wright and Bonavida that NK cells secrete NKCF, a soluble factor which shows cytotoxic activity on NK targets (Mechanisms in Cell-Mediated Cytotoxicity, p. 379), has been followed up by several groups, and comprises the first group of chapters in this section. As the reader will see, there is not yet full agreement on some aspects of NKCF among different laboratories, but the chapters by Wright and Bonavida, Ortaldo, et al., and Deem and Targan support the hypothesis that NKCF is involved in the NK cell-mediated lethal damage. The chapter by Wayner and Brooks argues against this hypothesis as well as the proposed role of reactive oxygen intermediates.

The biochemical pathways which operate between target cell recognition by NK cell surface receptors and the target cell lethal damage remain largely obscure. The chapters by Jondal and collaborators and by Hudig, et al., represent current efforts to elucidate two such pathways, largely through the use of pharmacological agents.

The final chapter in this section is again concerned with the interactions of lymphokines and cytotoxic lymphocytes, but in a new and different way. Ransom, et al. provide evidence that the lymphokine they have termed leukoregulin can act on the target cell and thus enhance the efficiency of NK cytotoxicity.

BIOCHEMICAL CHARACTERIZATION OF NATURAL KILLER CYTOTOXIC FACTORS

Susan C. Wright, Stanley M. Wilbur[*]
and Benjamin Bonavida

Department of Microbiology and Immunology
UCLA School of Medicine
Los Angeles, CA

[*]Department of Microbiology
University of Southern California
Los Angeles, CA

INTRODUCTION

Earlier studies of the NK lytic mechanism produced evidence for the stimulus secretion model and led to the postulation that lytic mediators are transferred from the effector to the target cell (1). Subsequent work in our laboratory demonstrated that soluble natural killer cytotoxic factors (NKCF) can be detected in the supernatants of effector cells stimulated with NK targets or with lectin (2,3). Further experiments were performed to analyze the functional characteristics of these factors. It was found that NKCF are released from human PBL (4) or murine spleen cells (2) that bear the phenotypic characteristics of NK cells. Release of NKCF is inhibited by some of the same protease inhibitors (5) shown previously to inhibit NK CMC (6). Pretreatment of effector cells with interferon enhances the release of NKCF (7) whereas interferon pretreatment of YAC-1 cells impairs their ability to stimulate release of the factors (8), thus accounting for the dual effects of interferon on NK CMC (9). NKCF lyse only NK sensitive targets (2,4) and YAC-1 variants selected for resistance to NKCF are also resistant to NK CMC (10).

Based on the above evidence we have proposed a model for NK CMC (8,10) in which, following effector-target cell binding, the target stimulates the effector to release NKCF. These factors then bind to and lyse the target cell.

179

More recent work in our laboratory has concentrated on the purification and biochemical characterization of NKCF produced by murine, rat, and human effector cells. Our initial results are presented in this report.

MATERIALS AND METHODS

Cell lines

All cell lines used in this study were maintained in suspension culture in RPMI-1640 supplemented with 10% FCS, 1% L-glutamine, 1% sodium pyruvate, and 1% non-essential amino acids (all from GIBCO). Cell lines cultured in the absence of antibiotics were screened at least twice a month for the presence of mycoplasmas according to Chen's (11) technique using the Hoeschst stain and fibroblast indicator cells. All cell lines were found to be mycoplasma-free and this result was confirmed using the adenosine phosphorylase-mediated nucleoside toxicity test as described by McGarrity and Carson (12).

Production of NCKF

Plastic non-adherent spleen cells or human PBL were cultured in the absence of FCS in RPMI-1640 supplemented with 1% L-glutamine, 1% sodium pyruvate, 1% non-essential amino acids, and 1% penicillin-streptomycin. Effector cells were mixed with YAC-1 or U937 stimulator cells to obtain a 25:1 effector to stimulator ratio. The final density of effector cells in all cultures was 5×10^6 cells/ml. Cultures were started in a total of 1 to 3 ml in 17x100 mm tissue culture tubes (Falcon #2057). In experiments where NKCF was induced by Con A, the lectin was added to the effector cell cultures at 2.5 µg/ml. Con A at 2.5 µg/ml added to media alone was not cytotoxic in the NKCF assay. After 24 h incubation at 37°C in 5% CO_2 and 95% air, the cell free supernatants were harvested and stored in either 4°C or -20°C until assaying for NKCF activity.

NKCF Assay

Murine and rat NKCF were assessed by measuring cytotoxicity against YAC-1 target cells. YAC-1 cells were labeled with ^{51}Cr (Amersham, 1 mCi/ml) that was always used prior to the date of calibration. 0.2 ml of ^{51}Cr was added to 4×10^6 YAC-1 cells in 10 ml of media in a 25 cm^2 tissue culture flask. The flask was incubated vertically at 37°C in 5% CO_2, 95% air for 20-24 h. Target cells were then washed 3 times and suspended at a final density of 2×10^5/ml in RPMI-1640 supplmented with 1% penicillin-streptomycin and 10% FCS. The assay was set up in triplicate in 96-well U bottom sterile microtiter plates. 50 µl of target cell suspension was added to each well. Different volumes of cell free supernatant containing NKCF (100 μl, 50 μl, and 25 μl) were added to each well, and the final volume was adjusted to 0.2 ml by adding RPMI + 1% penicillin-streptomycin. The final concentration of FCS in all wells was 2.5%. Wells for spontaneous and total ^{51}Cr release contained target cells plus 150 μl RPMI + 1% penicillin-streptomycin. After 20 h incubation at 37°C in 5% CO_2, the amount of ^{51}Cr released into 0.1 ml of supernatant from each well was determined. Total counts per minute was determined by resuspending the target cells and counting the radioactivity in 0.1 ml of cell suspension. In all experiments, the percentage of spontaneous release was less than 35%. The percent cytotoxicity was calculated as follows:

$$\% \text{ cytotoxicity} = \frac{\text{test cpm} - \text{spontaneous cpm}}{\text{total cpm} - \text{spontaneous cpm}} \times 100$$

The assay for human NKCF was similar to that for the rodent, except that U937 was used as the target cell. U937 targets were labeled with ^{51}Cr using either the overnight labeling procedure as for YAC-1, or using a short term procedure in which $1-10 \times 10^6$ cells are labeled with 0.1 ml ^{51}Cr in a total of 0.3 ml for 1-2 h at 37°C. All subsequent steps of the human NKCF assay were identical to those of the rodent assay except that the test was incubated for 24 h instead of 20 h.

Adsorption of NKCF

One ml of supernatant containing NKCF was mixed with 5×10^6 YAC-1 cells and incubated at 37°C for 20 h in one well of a 24-well plate. In some adsorptions, α-methyl-D-mannoside or fructose-6-phosphate was added to the NKCF-YAC-1 mixture. The adsorbed supernatants were dialyzed for 24 h and then tested for residual NKCF activity.

HPLC

Two ml of supernatant was injected into a Perkin Elmer series 3B high pressure liquid chromatograph (Tustin, CA). The column was a TSK SW 3000 (Altex Assoc., CA) and was run in RPMI-1640 at a flow rate of 1 ml/min.

RESULTS

Biochemical Characterization of Whole Rodent Supernatants

Whole supernatants containing NKCF produced by either murine or rat spleen cells were subjected to a number of tests and then assayed for residual NKCF activity. The biochemical characteristics of rodent NKCF produced using Con A or YAC-1 or U937 stimulator cells are listed in Table 1. These results indicate that NKCF are heat-sensitive proteins in which sialic acid residues are not essential for lytic activity. The factors are inactivated by incubating at pH 2 for 20 h. The observation that reduction and alkylation of these supernatants abrogates lytic activity suggests that disulfide bonding is essential for NKCF activity. The possibility that NKCF may be proteolytic enzymes was investigated using various protease inhibitors that have been found by other investigators to inhibit NK CMC (6,13). These agents were added directly to the NKCF assay at their highest nontoxic concentrations. The following agents were found to have no effect on NKCF lytic activity: human α-1-antitrypsin (0.5 mg/ml), soybean trypsin inhibitor (0.5 mg/ml), lima bean trypsin inhibitor (0.5 mg/ml), tosyl-phenyl-chloromethylketone (TPCK, 1×10^{-6}M), tosyllysylchloromethylketone (TLCK, 1×10^{-5}M), and acetyl-tyrosine-ethyl ester (ATEE, 5×10^{-4}M).

Table 1. Biochemical Characteristics of Murine or Rat NKCF Produced By Stimulation With Tumor Cells or Con A

Treatment	Effect on NKCF Lytic Activity
56°C 2 h	partial inhibition
63°C 2 h	complete inhibition
trypsin	complete inhibition
neuraminidase	no effect
pH 2	complete inhibition
reduction & alkylation	complete inhibition
protease inhibitors	no effect
Na periodate 0.01M	complete inhibition

Table 2.   Inhibition of NKCF Adsorption to YAC-1 by
α-Methyl-D-Mannoside and Fructose-6-Phosphate

Supernatant[1]	Concentration α-methyl-D-mannoside	Concentration fructose-6-phosphate	% Cytotoxicity[2]		
			100 μl	50 μl	25 μl
not adsorbed	-	-	40±2.0	36±4.0	29±2.6
adsorbed with YAC-1	-	-	4±4.7	5±4.4	4±4.0
"	100mM	-	37±2.0	34±1.0	27±4.0
"	50mM	-	42±4.4	41±3.0	31±26
"	25mM	-	18±2.1	13±1.0	7±0.6
"	-	100mM	40±3.5	37±2.9	25±3.6
"	-	50mM	23±3.0	20±3.2	16±1.7
"	-	25mM	17±2.0	9±3.2	9±1.5

[1]Supernatants from cultures of rat spleen cells stimulated with
Con A were adsorbed with YAC-1 cells as described in Materials and
Methods in the presence of the various concentrations of the two
monosaccharides.

[2]NKCF activity was assessed against YAC-1 targets in a 20 h ^{51}Cr
release assay.

The finding that oxidation of supernatants with sodium
periodate abrogates lytic activity suggests that NKCF may be glycoproteins in which carbohydrate determinants are essential for
lytic activity. Additional evidence implicating the involvement
of carbohydrate determinants in target cell lysis by NKCF was
reported in an earlier study indicating that α-methyl-D-mannoside
could inhibit lysis of YAC-1 by NKCF (3). The mechanism of this
inhibition was further investigated in the present study. In preliminary experiments, it was found that pre-incubation of NKCF in
100 mM α-methyl-D-mannoside followed by dialysis resulted in no
inhibition of NKCF activity. These findings suggest that it is
not irreversible binding of the factors to the sugar that causes
their inactivation. Adsorption experiments were then performed in
the presence of α-methyl-D-mannoside or fructose-6-phosphate,
which we have also found to inhibit NKCF activity. The results
shown in Table 2 demonstrate that adsorption of the rat Con-A
induced supernatant with YAC-1 cells in the absence of any sugar
removed almost all lytic activity. However, adsorption in the
presence of 50 mM or 100 mM α-methyl-D-mannoside or 100 mM
fructose-6-phosphate resulted in no change in the cytotoxic
activity. NKCF activity was partially removed at lower concentrations of either sugar. These findings suggest that car-

bohydrate residues present either on the NKCF molecules or on the YAC-1 cell membrane are involved in the binding of the factors to the target cell.

Partial Purification of NKCF

Supernatants from cultures of human PBL stimulated either with U937 (Fig. 1) or Con A (Fig. 2) were fractionated by HPLC gel filtration. Each fraction was tested for cytotoxic activity against U937 target cells in a 24 h ^{51}Cr release assay. Peak cytotoxic activity was found in fractions corresponding to an apparent MW of 20,000 to 30,000. The lytic activity of these fractions was greater than that of the unfractionated supernatant, suggesting that whole supernatants may contain inhibitors of NKCF lytic activity. Similar results were obtained using supernatants produced by murine or rat spleen cells stimulated with either YAC-1 or Con A.

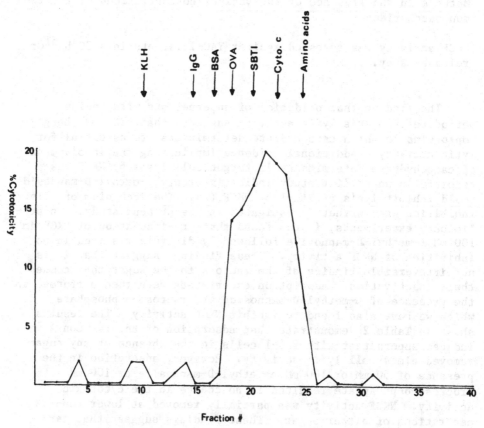

Fig. 1   Supernatants of PBL stimulated with U937 were frac-
         tionated and assayed for NKCF activity.

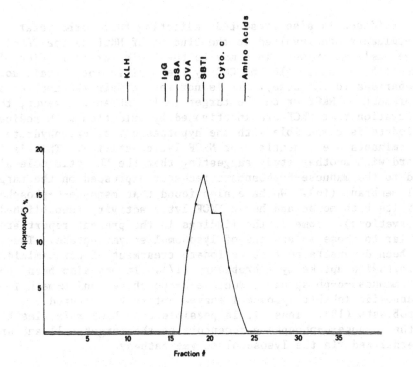

Fig. 2   Supernatants of PBL stimulated with Con A were fractionated by HPLC gel filtration and assayed for NKCF
activity.

DISCUSSION

This investigation examines the biochemical characteristics
of soluble cytotoxic factors produced by human, murine, or rat
effector cells stimulated with either tumor cells or Con A. The
data indicate that NKCF are glycoproteins with an apparent MW of
20,000-30,000 daltons. The gel filtration experiments suggest
that all NKCF lytic activity is mediated by molecules of a single
size. However, we cannot rule out the possibility that molecules
of a different MW that alone are not toxic may also participate in
target cell lysis by whole supernatants.

By all parameters tested thus far, we have not detected any
differences in NKCF produced by the three different species, nor
were there differences in factors generated by tumor cell or Con A
stimulation. We have also reported that Con A-induced supernatants exhibit the same target specificity as do tumor cell
induced factors (14). The biochemical and functional similarities
exhibited by these supernatants suggest that NKCF produced by
stimulation with tumor cells or Con A are identical. However,
further purification and characterization will be necessary to
determine if this is true.

Evidence is also presented indicating that carbohydrate determinants are involved in the binding of NKCF to the YAC-1 target cell membrane. This may be the basis for inhibition of mouse (15) or human (16) NK CMC by the addition of certain monosaccharides to the assay. It is not yet certain whether the sugar is present on NKCF or on the target cell membrane, however, the observation that NKCF are inactivated by oxidation with sodium periodate is compatible with the hypothesis that carbohydrate determinants are essential for NKCF lytic activity. This is in accord with another study suggesting that the NK lytic molecules bind to the mannose-6-phosphate receptor expressed on the target cell membrane (16). We have also found that mannose-6-phosphate inhibits both mouse and human NKCF lytic activity (unpublished observations). Some of the findings in the present report are similar to those in studies of lysosomal enzyme uptake. Thus, it has been demonstrated that periodate treatment of hexosaminidase inhibits its uptake by fibroblasts (17). It has also been shown that mannose-6-phosphate, fructose-6-phosphate, and α-methyl-D-mannoside inhibit lysosomal enzyme uptake by cultured fibroblasts (18). Thus, it is possible that NKCF molecules bind to the mannose-6-phosphate receptors on the target cell and are internalized via the lysosomal enzyme pathway.

An alternative interpretation of the data is that NKCF possess lectin-like receptors and bind to carbohydrate determinants on the target cell membrane. This interpretation is favored by Blanca et al. (19) who reported that K562 treated with tunicamycin were relatively resistant to lysis by NKCF. Further analysis of NKCF and their interaction with target cells will be necessary to distinguish between the two hypotheses.

Recent progress in the biochemical characterization of NKCF now allows comparison, on a molecular level, of NKCF factors to the well-studied cytotoxic lymphokine, lymphotoxin (LT). LT is released upon lectin stimulation of lymphocytes and the cytotoxic activity is most commonly measured using the L929 fibroblast target cell. A number of different investigators have proposed that LT may be involved in various types of CMC reactions (20-22). Whole supernatants containing human LT have been shown to contain four MW classes of LT: complex (>200,000), α (70 to 90,000), β (25-50,000), and γ (10-20,000) (23). Our results indicate that NKCF would correspond to γ or β LT, however, the comparison may not be valid since the MW of NKCF was determined by HPLC gel filtration as opposed to the conventional gel filtration techniques used for LT. Aggarwal et al. (24) have purified human LT and found that it exhibits an apparent MW of 60,000 on TSK-HPLC. However, the same molecule exhibited a MW of 20,000 on SDS-PAGE suggesting that a 60,000 MW oligomer may be dissociated under reducing conditions to a monomer. Recent work has indicated that certain forms of LT can lyse human NK sensitive targets, with Molt-4 being much more sensitive than K562 (25). We have reported a similar target sensitivity for human NKCF (4). Furthermore, adsorption experiments suggest that L929 targets are lysed by LT forms different from, or in addition to, those that lyse NK targets (25). As was observed in the NKCF system, lysis of NK targets by whole supernatants containing LT is inhibited by α—methyl-D-mannoside (20), although lysis of L929 cells is weakly or not at all inhibited by the same sugar (26). The MW of the LT form which lyses NK targets has not been determined.

Taken altogether, the data suggest that NKCF may be a subclass of conventional LT or else a related molecule. It appears that the conventional LT assay employing L929 targets will detect lytic molecules with differences in MW and functional characteristics from NKCF. Thus, to clarify the possible relationship between NKCF and LT will require the use of purified material and a standardized assay system.

Another mechanism which has been proposed for NK CMC involves the transfer of pore-forming molecules from the effector cell granules to the target cell. These perforins then polymerize and form pores in the target membrane resulting in cell lysis, analogous to the complement system (27-30). It is possible that there is more than one mechanism employed by NK cells to lyse targets. One subpopulation of NK cells may lyse the target by pore formation whereas another population may release NKCF to lyse the target. Alternatively, NKCF may be derived from the NK cytoplasmic granules and may be related to pore-forming molecules. One possibility is that NKCF are subunits which can polymerize and form ring structures on the target cell membrane. Both ring structures and soluble cytolysins have been recovered from purified cytoplasmic granules from the RNK tumor cell line (28,29). In agreement with this, we have demonstrated that RNK tumor cells produce NKCF (31). Both NKCF and ring structures can be induced under the same conditions, i.e, by mixing NK effector cells with NK targets or by stimulating with Con A (27). Although NKCF are much too small to consist of fully formed ring structures, these tubules have been isolated and SDS gel analysis has revealed several proteins (30) within the MW range of NKCF. It has also been reported that RNK granules contain several proteins with MW similar to NKCF (28). Furthermore, antisera prepared against RNK granules has been shown to inhibit the lytic activity of NKCF (29). One major difference between RNK granules and NKCF is that the granule cytolysin lyses targets much more rapidly (within 1h). This could be at least partly due to the fact that whole supernatants containing NKCF are too dilute and/or may contain inhibitors preventing rapid target lysis. Semi-purified preparations of NKCF exhibit more potent lytic activity and a faster rate of lysis than whole supernatants. The granule cytolysin and NKCF may also differ in that the cytolysin is not NK specific. However, it has been shown that, with the exception of red blood cells, the order of target sensitivity to the cytolysin is the same as that for NK sensitivity (29). Thus, it is possible that target specificity is dependent on NKCF concentration and we are currently investigating whether more highly concentrated NKCF will lyse NK resistant targets.

It has been reported that RNK granules in the presence of calcium rapidly lose cytotoxic activity (29). Since NKCF is produced in the presence of calcium, it could be that these factors are break-down products of the granule-derived cytolysins.

An alternative to the possibility that NKCF are either sub-units or break-down products of pore-forming molecules is that the NKCF act together with pore-forming molecules to lyse the target. Thus, it is possible that perforins produce a pore in the target membrane to facilitate the rapid entry of NKCF into the cytoplasm where it inflicts lethal damage.

Further work is necessary to analyze the possible relationships between NKCF, lymphotoxin, granule cytolysins, and ring structures. The initial results of our biochemical characterization of NKCF provide the basis to examine this question and to further analyze the role of NKCF in the NK lytic mechanism.

REFERENCES

1. J.C. Roder, R. Kiessling, P. Biberfield, and B. Anderson. Target-effector interaction in natural killer (NK) cell system. II. The isolation of NK cell and studies on the mechanism of killing. J. Immunol. 121:2509, 1978.

2. S.C. Wright, and B. Bonavida. Studies on the mechanism of natural killer (NK) cell-mediated cytotoxicity (CMC). I. Release of cytotoxic factors specific for NK-sensitive target cells (NKCF) during coculture of NK effector cells with NK target cells. J. Immunol. 129:433, 1982.

3. S.C. Wright, and B. Bonavida. Selective lysis of NK-sensitive target cells by a soluble mediator released from murine spleen cells and human peripheral blood lymphocytes. J. Immunol. 126:1516, 1981.

4. S.C. Wright, M.L. Weitzen, R. Kahle, G.A. Granger, and B. Bonavida. Studies on the mechanism of natural killer cell-mediated cytotoxicity. II. Coculture of human PBL with NK-sensitive or resistant cell lines stimulates release of natural

killer cytotoxic factors (NKCF) selectively cytotoxic to NK-sensitive target cells. J. Immunol. 130:2479, 1983.

5. S.C. Wright, and B. Bonavida. Evidence for the involvement of proteolytic enzymes in the production of natural killer cytotoxic factors, In: Natural Killer Activity and Its Regulation, T. Hoshino, H.S. Koren, A. Uchida, eds. Excerpta Medica, Amsterdam, p. 145, 1984.

6. D.C. Quan, T. Ishizaka, and B.R. Bloom. Studies on the mechanism of NK cell lysis. J. Immunol. 128:1786, 1982.

7. S.C. Wright, and B. Bonavida. Studies on the mechanism of natural killer cell-mediated cytoxicity. III. Activation of NK cells by interferon augments the lytic activity of released natural killer cytotoxic factors (NKCF). J. Immunol. 130:2960, 1983.

8. S.C. Wright, and B. Bonavida. Studies on the mechanism of natural killer cell-mediated cytotoxicity. IV. Interferon-induced inhibition of NK target cell susceptibility to lysis is due to a defect in their ability to stimulate release of natural killer cytotoxic factors (NKCF). J. Immunol. 130:2965, 1983.

9. G. Trinchieri, and D. Santoli. Anti-viral activity induced by culturing lymphocytes with tumor-derived or virus-transformed cells. Enhancement of human natural killer cell activity by interferon and antagonistic inhibition of suseptibility of target cells to lysis. J. Exp. Med. 147:1314, 1978.

10. S.C. Wright, and B. Bonavida. YAC-1 variant clones selected for resistance to natural killer cytotoxic factors (NKCF) are also resistant to natural killer cell-mediated cytotoxicity. Proc. Natl. Acad. Sci. 80:1688, 1983.

11. T.P. Chen. In situ detection of mycoplasma contamination in cell cultures by fluorescent Hoeschst 33258 stain. Exp. Cell. Res. 104:255, 1977.

12. G.J. McGarrity, and D.A. Carson. Adenosine phosphorylase-mediated nucleoside toxicity. Application towards the detection of mycoplasmal infection in mammalian cell cultures. Exp. Cell. Res. 139:199, 1982.

13. D. Hudig, T. Haverty, C. Fulcher, D. Redelman, and J. Mendelsohn. Inhibition of human natural cytotoxicity by macromolecular antiproteases. J. Immunol. 126:1569, 1981.

14. S.C. Wright, and B. Bonavida. Studies on the mechanism of natural killer cell-mediated cytotoxicity. V. Lack of NK specificity at the level of induction of natural killer cytotoxic factors in cultures of human, murine, or rat effector cells stimulated with mycoplasma free cell lines. J. Immunol., in press, 1984.

15. O. Stutman, P. Dien, R.E. Wisum, and E.C. Lattime. Natural cytotoxic cells against solid tumors in mice: Blocking of cytotoxicity by D-mannose. Proc. Natl. Acad. Sci: 77:2895, 1980.

16. J.T. Forbes, R.K. Bretthaer, and T.N. Oeltmann. Mannose 6-, fructose 1-, and fructose-6-phosphates inhibit human natural cell-mediated cytotoxicity. Proc. Natl. Acad. Sci. 78:5797, 1981.

17. S. Hickman, L.S. Shapiro, and E.F. Neufeld. A recognition marker required for uptake of a lysosomal enzyme by cultured fibroblasts. Biochem. Biophys. Res. Commun. 57:55, 1979.

18. A. Kaplan, D.T. Achord, and W.S. Sly. Phosphohexosyl components of a lysosomal enzyme are recognized by pinocytosis receptors on human fibroblasts. Proc. Natl. Acad. Sci. 74:2026, 1977.

19. I.R. Blanca, J.R. Ortaldo, and R.B. Herberman. Studies of soluble natural killer cytotoxic factor(s) released by human peripheral blood lymphocytes, In: Natural Killer Activity and Its Regulation, T. Hoshino, H.S. Koren, A. Uchida, eds., Excerpta Medica, Amsterdam, 1983.

20. M.L. Weitzen, E. Innis, R.S. Yamamoto, and G.A. Granger. Inhibition of human NK-induced cell lysis and soluble cell-lytic molecules with anti-human LT antisera and various saccharides. Cell. Immunol. 77:42, 1983.

21. S.M. Walker, and Z.J. Lucas. Role of soluble cytotoxins in cell-mediated immunity. Transpl. Proc. V:137, 1973.

22. L.L. Kondo, W. Rosenau, and D.W. Wara. Role of lymphotoxin in antibody dependent cell-mediated cytotoxicity (ADCC). J. Immunol. 126: 1131, 1981.

23. G.A. Granger, R.S. Yamamoto, D.S. Fair, and J.C. Hiserodt. The human LT system I: Physical-chemical heterogeneity of LT molecules released by mitogen activated human lymphocytes in vitro. Cell. Immunol. 38:338, 1978.

24. B.B. Aggarwal, B. Moffat, and R.N. Harkins. Human lymphotoxin. Production by a lymphoblastoid cell line, purification, and initial characterization. J. Biol. Chem. 259:686, 1984.

25. M.L. Weitzen, R.S. Yamamoto, and G.A. Granger. Identification of human lymphocyte-derived lymphotoxins with binding and cell-lytic activity on NK-sensitive cell lines in vitro. Cell. Immunol. 77:30, 1983.

26. M.K. Toth, and G.A. Granger. The human lymphotoxin system-IV. Identification of various saccharides on LT molecules and their contribution to cytotoxicity and charge heterogeneity. Molec. Immunol. 16:671, 1979.

27. E.R. Podack, and G. Dennert. Assembly of two types of tubules with putative cytolytic function by cloned natural killer cells. Nature 302:442, 1983.

28. P.J. Millard, M.P. Henkart, C.W. Reynolds, and P. Henkart. Purification and properties of cytoplasmic granules from cytotoxic rat LGL tumors. J. Immunol. 132:3197, 1984.

29. P. Henkart, M. Henkart, P. Millard, and C.W. Reynolds. Isolation and cytolytic activity of granules from natural occurring LGL tumors, In: Natural Killer Activity and Its Regulation, T. Hoshino, H.S. Koren, A. Uchida, eds. Excerpta Medica, Amsterdam, p. 156, 1984.

30. E.R. Podack. Assembly of transmembrane tubules (polyperforins) on target membranes by cloned NK and TK cells: Comparison to poly C9 of complement, In: Natural Killer Activity and Its Regulation, T. Hoshino, H.S. Koren, A. Uchida, eds., Excerpta Medica, Amsterdam, p. 101, 1984.

31. S.C. Wright, C.W. Reynolds, and B. Bonavida. Production of natural killer cytotoxic factors (NKCF) by the RNK rat tumor cell, In: Natural Killer Activity and Its Regulation, T. Hoshino, H.S. Koren, A. Uchida, eds., Excerpta Medica, p. 138, 1984.

BOTH NK SENSITIVE AND RESISTANT MYCOPLASMA FREE CELL LINES STIMULATE RELEASE OF NKCF

Susan C. Wright and Benjamin Bonavida

Department of Microbiology and Immunology
UCLA School of Medicine
Los Angeles, CA

INTRODUCTION

Studies on the NK lytic mechanism in our laboratory have produced evidence that natural killer cytotoxic factors (NKCF) may be the lytic mediators. Our model for the NK lytic mechanism proposes that after binding of the NK cell to the target, the target stimulates the effector to release NKCF (1,2). In support of this, we have found that effector cell populations enriched for NK cells in either human (3) or mouse (4) produce NKCF during coculture with NK sensitive tumor stimulator cells. The objective of this investigation was to determine if there is any NK specificity at the level of induction of NKCF release. Experiments were also carried out to determine if mycoplasma infection of tumor stimulator cells had any effect on the production of cytotoxic supernatants by murine or rat spleen cells. It was found that both NK sensitive and resistant mycoplasma free cell lines could stimulate release of NKCF. Some mycoplasma infected cell lines could generate cytotoxic supernatants, however, it is not clear whether the lytic activity is due to NKCF or some other agent.

MATERIALS AND METHODS

Mycoplasma Test

To test for mycoplasma infection of cell lines, we routinely used the technique developed by Chen (5). Cell lines were cultured for at least 1 week in the absence of antibiotics before mycoplasma testing began. Both culture supernatants and the cells from each line were tested by adding to monolayers of indicator cells. For most tests, we used the human fibroblast, LR'62, as indicators. In some tests, fetal C57Bl/6 fibroblasts were employed as indicator cells and produced identical results. After 3 days of culture, mycoplasma was visualized by the Hoechst 33258 stain. A positive and negative control was included in every test. Criteria for a cell line to be declared mycoplasma free were that they must produce 4 negative test results and no positive results over a 1 month test period. After meeting these criteria, cells were continually tested on a weekly basis throughout the duration of this study. The mycoplasma status of all cell lines was confirmed using a second type of test based on adenosine phosphorylase-mediated nucleoside toxicity (6). This test employed the mycoplasma detection system purchased from Bethesda Research Laboratory and for all cell lines yielded results identical to that obtained with the Chen technique. Cell lines that were found to be infected with mycoplasma are marked with an asterisk.

Cell Lines

YAC-1, YAC-A*, K562, and K562* were all obtained from different laboratories. U937 was obtained from E. Ades (Eli Lilly), and in addition to our routine mycoplasma screening procedures it has also been found to be mycoplasma free by anaerobic culturing techniques (E. Ades, personal communication). Both K562 and U937 are human NK sensitive target cells that are not lysed by rodent NK cells in our laboratory. The cloned NK like A'5Al cell line was obtained from C. Brooks (Fred Hutchinson Cancer Research Center) and methods to produce such lines have been described previously (7). Culture media for the propogation of A'5Al and production of NKCF was RPMl 1640 supplemented with 20% murine ConA supernatant, 10% FCS, 1% L-glutamine, 1% nonessential amino acids, 1% sodium pyruvate, and 1% penicillin-streptomycin. A'5Al cells were also found to be mycoplasma-free by the Chen technique (5).

Production and Assay of NKCF

See "Biochemical characterization of natural killer cytotoxic factors," this volume.

RESULTS

Stimulation of Release of NKCF by Mycoplasma Free Cell Lines

The results of two representative experiments are shown in Table 1. On some occasions, spleen cells spontaneously release NKCF in the absence of any stimulating agent, as shown in experiment #1. However, U937 and ConA induced the production of significantly higher levels of NKCF, although YAC-1 did not stimulate. In the second experiment, U937 and YAC-1 were equally effective in stimulating NKCF

Table 1. Stimulation of Release of NKCF by Mycoplasma-Free Cell Lines

Effector Cells	Stimulator	% Cytotoxicity[a]		
		100ul	50ul	25ul
Exp. 1				
Rat spleen	-	17±1.5	13±2.0	12±1.0
	YAC-1	15±2.1	13±1.7	12±0.6
	U937	36±3.8	19±2.0	18±1.2
	ConA	44±4.0	39±3.5	30±2.0
Exp. 2				
Rat spleen	-	12±2.1	5±1.5	4±1.0
	YAC-1	22±4.0	13±0.6	7±3.5
	U937	21±1.0	10±4.0	5±1.5
	ConA	33±3.1	33±1.2	30±3.5
Mouse spleen	-	9±1.5	3±1.5	0±0
	YAC-1	22±1.5	16±4.0	5±3.8
	U937	22±2.0	19±1.5	10±2.0
	ConA	35±1.7	32±4.4	23±3.5

[a]Supernatants were assayed for cytotoxicity against YAC-1 targets in a 20h ^{51}Cr release assay.

production by mouse or rat spleen cells. The data also indicates that ConA induces higher levels of NKCF production than either stimulator cell.

Whereas murine or rat spleen cells occasionally release NKCF in the absence of any stimulating agent, we found that the cloned NK-like A'5Al cell line consistently releases NKCF into the culture supernatant (unpublished observations). It was essential to dialyze the supernatant to detect lytic activity that was significantly higher than that mediated by the growth media containing 20% ConA-induced supernatant. Unlike rodent spleen cells, the addition of YAC-1 stimulator cells did not increase NKCF production by the A'5Al cell line.

Relative Ability of Mycoplasma Free and Infected Cell Lines to Stimulate Release of NKCF

The results of four representative experiments are shown in

Table 2. Effects of Mycoplasma Infection of Stimulator Cells

Effector Cells	Stimulator	% Cytotoxicity[a]		
		100ul	50ul	25ul
Exp. 1				
Mouse spleen	-	10±1.0	6±4.4	5±3.6
	YAC-1	23±3.5	21±3.5	10±2.1
	YAC-A*	25±1.0	17±3.2	15±2.4
	ConA	38±3.0	32±3.4	21±1.0
Exp. 2				
Mouse spleen	-	22±4.2	12±2.3	4±1.0
	YAC-1	32±3.5	28±2.6	20±1.7
	YAC-A*	30±5.1	24±2.5	24±2.5
Exp. 3				
Rat spleen	-	0±0	4±1.2	3±2.1
	K5621	28±2.9	24±1.2	15±0.6
	K562*	22±3.0	21±0.6	18±1.7
	ConA	21±0.6	17±1.7	12±1.0
Exp. 4				
Rat spleen	-	7±4.5	4±5.5	9±4.2
	YAC-1	21±0.6	16±4.0	14±2.6
	YAC-A*	41±4.4	39±7.6	34±3.5

[a]Supernatants were assayed for cytotoxicity against YAC-1 in a 20h ^{51}Cr release assay.

Table 2. It can be seen that mycoplasma infected stimulator cells induced the production of supernatants with equivalent or higher levels of cytotoxicity than uninfected stimulator cells. In other experiments we have also observed that some mycoplasma infected lines did not generate cytotoxic supernatants (data not shown).

DISCUSSION

This study has investigated some of the conditions under which rodent spleen cells or the NK-like cell line, A'5Al will release NKCF. Murine or rat spleen cells release NKCF in response to stimulation with mycoplasma-free tumor cells or ConA. Although U937 and K562 are sensitive to human NK cells, they are not lysed by mouse or rat NK cells. Thus, there is no NK or species specificity at the level of induction of factor release. We have obtained similar results in the human NKCF system (8).

We have also observed a certain degree of variability in the ability of a tumor cell line to stimulate NKCF production. Thus, in some experiments, effector cells may not respond to any stimulator cell or else they may respond to some but not to others. This is in contrast to the observation that high levels of NKCF can be produced with greater consistency using ConA. The cell type that produces NKCF in response to ConA is currently being investigated.

Several mycoplasma-infected lines tested as stimulator cells were found to generate cytotoxic supernatants that in some cases were more highly cytotoxic than supernatants produced using uninfected cells. The observations that some species of mycoplasma are mitogenic (9) and some may induce interferon (IFN) production (10) provide possible reasons why some infected lines may stimulate higher levels of NKCF production than mycoplasma-free cell lines. Thus, we have demonstrated that mitogenic lectins induce NKCF production (8,11) and that IFN pretreatment of effector cells augments the production of these factors (12).

An alternative interpretation of the data is that supernatants generated using mycoplasma infected stimulator cells do not contain high levels of NKCF, but instead are toxic due to an artifact of the culture conditions. This would be compatible with the findings of Wayner and Brooks (13) who were able to generate cytotoxic supernatants by culturing murine spleen cells with various types of mycoplasma infected cell lines. However, they concluded that the cytotoxic activity was not mediated by NKCF but instead was due to the presence of mycoplasma organisms in the supernatant. This was based on the observation that they could remove most of the cytotoxic activity by filtration or centrifugation. Thus, to avoid the possibility of introducing such artifacts, one should use only mycoplasma free stimulator cells or lectin to generate NKCF.

In contrast to the conditions for stimulation of NKCF release from spleen cells are the results obtained with the cloned A'5Al NK-like cell line. Under normal culture conditions, this cell line spontaneously releases NKCF into the supernatant in the absence of stimulator cells. We did not observe NKCF production in the absence of 20% ConA supernatant used to propagate the line. This suggests that residual ConA or other factors in the ConA supernatant may be stimulating the A'5Al cells to release NKCF. Unlike spleen cell supernatants, A'5Al supernatants must be dialyzed in order to detect significant levels of cytotoxic activity. This suggests that low MW inhibitors of NKCF activity may be produced by A'5Al cells. Failure to dialyze the supernatant may at least partially account for why Brooks et al. (7) were unable to detect cytotoxic activity in the supernatants of NK-like cell lines. The finding that a cloned cell line that mediates high levels of NK activity also produces NKCF provides further support for the role of NKCF in the NK lytic mechanism.

ACKNOWLEDGEMENT

The authors wish to thank Doctor Colin Brooks for the NK clone used in this study. This work is supported by grant CA35791 from the National Cancer Institute.

REFERENCES

1. S. C. Wright and B. Bonavida, YAC-1 variant clones selected for resistance to natural killer cytotoxic factors (NKCF) are also resistant to natural killer cell-mediated cytotoxicity. Proc. Natl. Acad. Sci. 80:1688 (1983).

2. S. C. Wright and B. Bonavida, Studies on the mechanism of natural killer cell-mediated cytotoxicity. IV. Interferon-induced inhibition of NK target cell susceptibility to lysis is due to a defect in their ability to stimulate release of natural killer cytotoxic factors (NKCF). J. Immunol. 130: 2965 (1983).

3. S. C. Wright, M. L. Weitzen, R. Kahle, G. A. Granger, and B. Bonavida, Studies on the mechanism of natural killer cell mediated cytotoxicity. II. Coculture of human PBL with NK-sensitive or resistant cell lines stimulates release of natural killer cytotoxic factors (NKCF) selectively cytotoxic to NK-sensitive target cells. J. Immunol. 130:2479 (1983).

4. S. C. Wright and B. Bonavida, Studies on the mechanism of natural killer (NK) cell-mediated cytotoxicity (CMC). I. Release of cytotoxic factors specific for NK-sensitive target cells (NKCF) during coculture of NK effector cells with NK target cells. J. Immunol. 129:433 (1982).

5. T. P. Chen, In situ detection of mycoplasma contamination in cell cultures by fluorescent Hoeschst 33258 stain. Exp. Cell Res. 104:255 (1977).

6. G. J. McGarrity and D. A. Carson, Adenosine phosphorylase-mediated nucleoside toxicity. Application towards the detection of mycoplasmal infection in mammalian cell cultures. Exp. Cell. Res. 139:199 (1982).

7. C. G. Brooks, K. Kuribayashi, G. E. Sale, and C. S. Henney, Characterization of five cloned murine cell lines showing high cytolytic activity against YAC-1 cells. J. Immunol. 128:2326 (1982).

8. S. C. Wright and B. Bonavida, Studies on the mechanism of natural killer cell mediated cytotoxicity. V. Lack of NK specificity at the level of induction of natural killer cytotoxic factors in cultures of human, murine, or rat effector cells stimulated with mycoplasma free cell lines. J. Immunol., in press (1984).

9. Y. Nast, In vitro studies on the mitogenic activity of mycoplasmal species toward lymphocytes. Rev. Infec. Dis. 4:5205 (1982).

10. B. C. Cole, J. C. Overall, Jr., P. S. Lombardi, and L. A. Glasgow, Induction of interferon in bovine and human lymphocyte cultures by mycoplasmas. Inf. and Immun. 14:88 (1976).

11. S. C. Wright and B. Bonavida, Selective lysis of NK-sensitive target cells by a soluble mediator released from murine spleen cells and human peripheral blood lymphocytes. J. Immunol. 126:1516 (1981).

12. S. C. Wright and B. Bonavida, Studies on the mechanism of natural killer cell-mediated cytotoxicity. III. Activation of NK cells by interferon augments the lytic activity of released natural killer cytotoxic factors (NKCF). J. Immunol. 130:2960 (1983).

13. E. A. Wayner and C. G. Brooks, Induction of NKCF-like activity in mixed lymphocyte-tumor cell culture: Direct involvement of mycoplasma infection of tumor cells. J. Immunol. 132:2135 (1984).

DISCUSSION

Bhakdi: Is the NKCF consumed during the process of killing? For example, after a typical experiment where 20% of the target cells are killed, if you add fresh factor, are another 20% killed?

Wright: I haven't done that experiment. But you do remove NKCF activity if you add YAC cells.

Herberman: Can you distinguish between absorption and inactivation of the factor?

Wright: No.

Hiserodt: If you saturate the NKCF binding sites with factor, are the cells still sensitive to NK cell mediated lysis? One might expect a reduction in the cell mediated lysis if it is operating via this pathway.

Wright: If you add NKCF to the cell medIAted cytotoxicity assay, you get about the same levels of killing. But I don't know if I saturated the binding sites.

Ortaldo: In our experiments with human NKCF, we see a consistent but small increase in cell mediated lysis if we add NKCF. This may not be significant. I interpret that as either a lack of saturation or to difficulties in reducing the rapid cell mediated lysis.

Adams: I am a bit concerned about the TLCK experiment because of the toxicity of this reagent due to its reaction with things other than proteases. It doesn't take much to shut down protein synthesis. Related to this type of problem, how much of the inhibitors did you use to treat the supernatants? In our supernatant system it often takes very large amounts to see inhibition, and we generally dialyze out the excess reagent prior to assay for inhibition.

Wright: I first did preliminary experiments to test for toxicity against YAC cells. The TPCK was at 10^{-6}M. I haven't used higher concentrations and then dialyzed.

Podack: Do you know what the charge properties of this molecule are, say by binding to ion exchange columns or electrophoretic experiments?

Wright: Those experiments are in progress.

Young: Do you know if the factor has any ionic requirements?

Wright: I haven't been able to establish any calcium requirement because of the long term incubation required by the NKCF assay. The target cells are not healthy if there is no calcium.

Berke: The kinetics of NKCF lysis seem to offer a fundamental problem for the interpretation that this is the lytic agent. If it is a problem of low concentrations of factor in your assays, you should see enhanced kinetics when you concentrate it. This slow kinetics of ^{51}Cr release also brings up the question of whether you are really measuring target cell death or if the label is being released by non-lethal events like cell division.

Wright: On the last point there is no cell division during the assay, because the cells stop dividing after chromium labelling. With regard to the concentration question, if you concentrate the factors by various techniques you will get increased levels of killing and faster kinetics.

Bhakdi: On that point, from the dose response you showed, it looked like you had no difference between 25, 50 or 100 ul.

Wright: With some supernatants you do see a plateau, this is not unusual.

Seaman: When you vary your stimulator/responder ratio during NKCF generation, which population do you hold constant?

Wright: I hold the responder number constant and add varying numbers of stimulators. The optimum ratio varies according to the population of responder cells.

Nathan: Getting back to the question of whether the ^{51}Cr release during the NKCF assay is due to cell death, have you used other criteria for death?

Wright: Yes, all my early experiments were carried out with trypan blue exclusion.

STUDIES OF HUMAN NATURAL KILLER CYTOTOXIC FACTOR (NKCF):

CHARACTERIZATION AND ANALYSIS OF ITS MODE OF ACTION

John R. Ortaldo, Isaac Blanca, and Ronald B. Herberman

Biological Therapeutics Branch
Biological Response Modifiers Program
National Cancer Institute
Frederick Cancer Research Facility
Frederick, Md.

SUMMARY

Soluble natural killer cytotoxic factors (NKCF) have been detected in the supernatant of normal mouse, rat, and human lymphocytes stimulated in vitro for 1 to 3 days in serum-free medium. Stimulation of large granular lymphocytes (LGL) with NK-sensitive targets or mitogens has resulted in high levels of NKCF production. Previous studies in the mouse and human systems have analyzed the cells responsible for production, specificity, and general characteristics of NKCF. In the present study, using human NKCF as a model for cytolysis by LGL, we have analyzed a variety of agents previously demonstrated to inhibit NK activity. These have included: (i) phosphorylated sugars; (ii) protease inhibitors; (iii) antibodies to rat LGL granules; (iv) Ca^{++}, and Mg^{++}; (v) lipomodulin; (vi) nucleotides; (vii) prostaglandins; and (viii) inhibitors of lysosomal enzymes. All inhibitors were tested for their effects on production of NKCF after target cell interaction, binding of NKCF to target cells, and target cell lysis (after 6-hour NKCF absorption and washing of targets). Phosphorylated sugars and antibodies to rat LGL granules were found to inhibit the lysis of targets by NKCF, whereas the other agents tested had no detectable effect (ATP, cyclic AMP, protease inhibitors, prostaglandin E_2). In regard to the production of NKCF, the data indicated that (i) the absence of calcium and magnesium, (ii) prostaglandin E_2, and (iii) ATP inhibited production, whereas phosphorylated sugars did not. Studies with these types of agents will now enable us to dissect the sites at which these agents function within the lytic process. In addition to the above studies, purification studies were performed using tritiated arginine to label NKCF to begin biochemical characterization of human NKCF. The results indicated that radiolabeled NKCF has an apparent molecular weight between 20,000 and 40,000. This material demonstrated a pattern of binding to target cells which was similar to the pattern of lysis by NKCF. In addition, the binding of this material was competitively inhibited by unlabeled NKCF preparations. Such approaches with radiolabeled NKCF should be useful for the further study of the biochemical characteristics of human NKCF and of its mechanism of action.

INTRODUCTION

During the past few years, natural killer (NK) cells have attracted considerable attention because of their potential role in antitumor defenses in humans and animals.[1] Recently, the cells responsible for NK activity in rodents and humans have been shown to be large granular lymphocytes (LGL).[2,3] However, the mechanism of their lytic activity is still poorly understood. Studies of the effects of metabolic inhibitors on NK activity support the stimulation-secretion model originally postulated[4,5] to explain the mechanism of killing by CTL.[6] In addition, Wright and Bonavida[7] have recently described a soluble factor, which is produced during the interaction of mouse spleen cells and human peripheral blood lymphocytes[7-10] and which selectively lyses NK-susceptible target cells. They termed this NK cytotoxic factor (NKCF). Although several lines of correlative evidence suggest a role for NKCF in mechanism of NK cell-mediated cytolysis, a variety of important issues still remain to be settled. In the present study, NKCF was utilized in an attempt to dissect the various steps that have been postulated to be involved in NK cell-mediated lysis. Studies were performed with a variety of agents which have been previously demonstrated to inhibit LGL-mediated cytolysis, and also we initiated biochemical characterization of human NKCF.

RESULTS

Production of NKCF by Human LGL

If NKCF is involved in the mechanism of lysis by NK cells, one would predict that the factor would be produced from isolated populations of NK cells. Therefore, LGL were tested for their ability to produce NKCF. The data in Figure 1 represent a typical experiment in which Percoll density gradient fractions containing a high percentage of LGL, upon incubation with K562, produced high levels of NKCF. In contrast, with highly purified T-cell

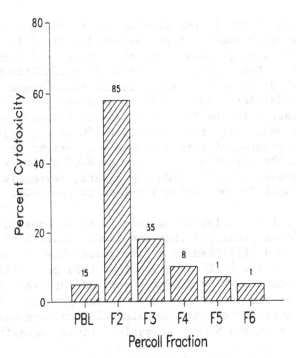

Fig. 1. Release of NKCF from Percoll fractions of human lymphocytes. Unseparated PBL or Percoll fractions of lymphocytes stimulated with K562 were tested (in a 24-hour ^{51}Cr
release assay) for their production of NKCF. Numbers
over bars represent the percent of LGL as determined by
morphological identification with Giemsa stain.

populations (or populations depleted of NK cells), release of
significant levels of NKCF activity was not seen. In addition,
the optimum release of NKCF occurred upon interaction of the LGL
with NK-sensitive targets (data not shown). Stimulation of LGL
with NK-susceptible targets, with mitogens, or membrane fragments
of such target cells resulted in a substantial release of NKCF.
In contrast, low or insignificant amounts of NKCF above those
spontaneously released by LGL were found when human NK-resistant
target cells such as RL♂1, YAC-1, and Raji were used as stimuli.
It should be noted that although stimulation of NK cells usually
was necessary for obtaining high levels of NKCF, some spontaneous

NKCF was produced by the LGL of some donors (data not shown). Table 1 summarizes some of these properties of NKCF. In addition to these general properties, some physicochemical properties have been examined. NKCF produced in serum-free conditions generally were quite stable when maintained at low temperatures (4°C or lower). In addition, they appear to be a protein in nature since they were inactivated by trypsin treatment and were quite unstable when maintained at high temperatures (56°C or higher). In addition, data presented at this Workshop (see Wright et al.) have demonstrated the glycoprotein nature of NKCF by their susceptibility to Na-periodate and reducing agents, respectively, suggesting a disulfide bond being involved in the NKCF.

If NKCF plays an important role in NK cell-mediated lysis, then it would be predicted that the factor would bind to the target cells and kill them in a time comparable to that required by intact NK cells.[11] In order to test this prediction, target cells were incubated with NKCF for various intervals at 37°C and the incubation was either continued in the presence of NKCF or the targets were washed and incubated with culture medium or in the presence of fresh NKCF. At various times thereafter, the

Table 1. Properties of NKCF

General Properties

1.	Source	LGL
2.	Effective stimuli for release	NK-sensitive targets and mitogens
3.	Lytic activity	Slow (>10 hr) and inhibited by serum proteins
4.	Specificity	Similar to that of LGL (NK cells)

Biochemical Properties

1.	Stability at	
	−20°C	weeks to months
	4°C	days to weeks
	56°C	hours
	>65°C	<10 minutes
2.	Inhibition by enzymes	Sensitive to trypsin
		Insensitive to neuraminidase

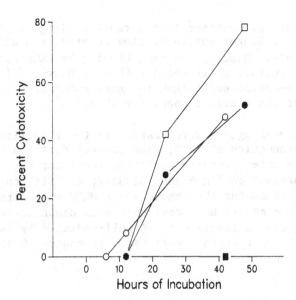

Fig. 2. Kinetics of K562 by NKCF lysis when added to assay (○),
when adsorbed into targets for 6 hr (●), or when adsorbed
for 6 hr and additional NKCF added (□), or with adsorp-
tion-depleted factor (■).

level of cytotoxicity was assessed. The data shown in Figure 2
indicate that lysis of target cells by NKCF occurred slowly,
requiring a period of incubation of approximately 48 hours (with
[111]In-labeled target cells) although twenty-four hour maximal
release has been routinely seen with ^{51}Cr targets (Fig. 3). These
kinetics of lysis were consistent for all of the supernatants
tested against [111]indium-labeled targets. In contrast, studies
on the kinetics of absorption showed that within 2 hours, and at
a maximum of between 4 and 6 hours, after incubation with NK-susceptible targets, NKCF activity was removed from supernatants.
After incubation of target cells with NKCF, the cells could be
washed and lysis proceed with kinetics similar to that observed
when the cells were maintained in the presence of NKCF (see Figure
3). In addition, supernatants previously containing NKCF were
devoid of most detectable activity after this 6-hour absorption.
However, addition of fresh NKCF increased the percentage of lysis
of target cells, indicating that maximal saturation of the target
cells by NKCF was not maintained when the cells were incubated for
several hours in the absence of factor. Overall, these results

indicated that, in contrast to the rapid killing by NK cells, NKCF requires a longer period of time to produce significant levels of lysis. However, optimal binding by NKCF can occur within short periods of incubation (2 to 4 hours of incubation), and this exposure is sufficient to cause subsequent lyis of target cells without the continued need for NKCF.

A variety of agents were tested for their ability to block either (i) production of NKCF, when present during a 24-hour period of the effector-target cell interactions; (ii) binding of NKCF, when present during 6-hour binding; or (iii) the terminal lytic phase, by adding the agents after NKCF pretreatment (Table 2). All of the agents had previously been demonstrated to inhibit post-binding events involved in NK cell-mediated lysis by human LGL. When phosphorylated sugars (such as mannose-6-phosphate),

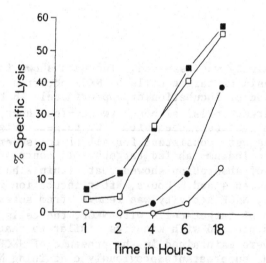

Fig. 3. Kinetics of lysis by PBL, with (■) or without (□) trypsin treatment and by NKCF, with (●) or without (o) trypsin treatment. Assay performed with ^{51}Cr-labeled K562 targets.

Table 2. Effects of Agents (Which Inhibit NK Lysis) on NKCF

Agent	Concentration Range Tested	Effect[a] on: Production	Binding	Lysis
1. Sugar-PO4				
a. Mannose-PO4	10-75 mM	−	↑	−
b. Fructose-PO4	10-75 mM	−	−	−
2. Antigranule sera	1-5 µg/ml IgG	?	↑	−↑
3. Protease inhibitors	1-100 µg/ml	−	−	−
4. CA^{++}/Mg^{++}	1-50 mM	↓	?	?
5. ATP---cAMP	1-100 mM	↓	−	−
6. PGE-2	10^{-3}-10^{-8} M	↓	−	−
7. Ammonium chloride	0-0.1 µg/ml	↓	−	−
8. Strontium chloride	0-0.1 µg/ml	↓	−	−
9. Monensin	0-0.1 µg/ml	↓	−	↓

[a]Summary of results of 5-10 experiments. "−" indicates no effect; "↓", consistent decrease in effect; "↑", consistent increase; "?", unable to determine due to technical reasons. Combinations indicate variable results, such as "−↑", that effect was no change or increase.

were tested,[12-14] they were found to inhibit binding of NKCF to target cells. However, they had no effect on NKCF production on lysis after absorption to targets. Other sugars previously shown not to inhibit NK lysis, such as fructose phosphate,[12-14] did not inhibit at any step involved with NKCF. Antisera to isolated granules from rat LGL tumors have previously been demonstrated to block the lytic effect of granules (see report by Henkart et al. in this publication). When these anti-granule antibodies were evaluated in the various steps with human NKCF, inhibition of binding was consistently seen. The effects of the antisera on production was not assessable because of the inability to remove the antibody at the end of the incubation period, as was achieved by dialysis with all the other agents tested. Interestingly, the addition of anti-rat LGL granule antibodies after absorption of NKCF resulted in variable results and often increased cell lysis. Contrary to previous reports, the protease inhibitors TLCK and TPCK (8), when tested at a variety of concentrations, were not inhibitory in the present studies.

Previous studies in a variety of cell-mediated cytotoxic systems have demonstrated the requirement for calcium and magnesium during the early events leading to lysis (6). Similarly, the presence of calcium and magnesium appear to be necessary for the production of NKCF, as demonstrated by the results of experiments performed in calcium- and magnesium-free media. However, the effects of such media on the binding and subsequent lytic phases were technically impossible to assess because of the susceptibility of the target cells to the toxic effects resulting from the absence of calcium and magnesium for extended time periods.

A wide variety of other agents which have been demonstrated to inhibit postbinding events,[1] including cyclic nucleotides, ATP, prostaglandin E_2, ammonium chloride, strontium chloride, and monensin, were tested, and all were found to inhibit the production of NKCF but not the binding of NKCF to susceptible targets. None of these agents, with the exception of monensin, affected lysis of NK-susceptible targets after they were pretreated with NKCF. It is interesting that monensin did interfere with the subsequent lysis of NK-sensitive targets by NKCF. Little is known at present regarding what occurs in the target cell after binding of the soluble cytotoxic factors. However, the internal processes of the target cells following exposure to cytotoxic molecules appear to warrant a great deal of investigation. The consistent inhibition of NKCF action by monensin suggests that receptor internalization or activation of lysosomes or some cytoskeletal changes may be involved in target cell lysis by NKCF.

Effect of Tunicamycin on Lysis by NKCF

Because phosphorylated sugars inhibit absorption of NKCF to susceptible targets, these sugars may compete with NKCF for binding to the receptors on target cells. Alternatively, NKCF might act in a lectin-like manner, reacting with phosphorylated sugars on the surface of target cells. To test this latter hypothesis, we studied the effects of NKCF on target cells pretreated with tunicamycin, which selectively inhibits the addition of asparagine-linked sugars to cell membranes.[15-18] NK-susceptible K562 target cells were pretreated for 18 hours with different doses of tunicamycin and then evaluated for tritiated glucosamine incorporation, for susceptibility to lysis by NK cells or NKCF, and for ability to absorb NKCF. The data demonstrated that treatment with tunicamycin, at levels which inhibited glycosylation but did not significantly inhibit protein synthesis, produced a significant decrease in susceptibility of K562 by lysis by NKCF and an impairment of these cells to absorb the factor (not shown). In addition, a significant decrease in the susceptibility of these cells to be lysed by intact LGL was also observed.

Combined Effects of NKCF and Proteolytic Enzyme

Whereas protease inhibitors had no detectable effect on any phase of NKCF production or activity, they have been previously reported[9] and confirmed here in parallel experiments to inhibit lysis by intact LGL. In an attempt to understand these results, we examined the effect of pretreatment of target cells with various proteolytic enzymes. Figure 3 demonstrates the typical kinetics of lysis by intact PBL or by concentrated crude NKCF, on target cells pretreated with 0.01% of highly purified trypsin. There were small but significant early increases in susceptibility to lysis by PBL when trypsin-treated targets were used. However, by 4 hours, no significant difference in lysis was seen. In contrast, with NKCF, which ordinarily induces significant lysis only after 12 hours, the trypsin-pretreated targets were lysed more rapidly and to a greater extent. Significantly greater levels of lysis were observed at both 6 and 18 hours. Less significant levels of lysis ($p > .01$ but $< .05$) at 4 hours. It should be noted that no significant toxicity was observed when low doses of trypsin were used ($<0.01\%$). However, higher doses of trypsin often resulted in toxic effects on target cells. In addition, this enzyme-enhancing effect was restricted to trypsin, whereas other enzymes tested, including chymotrypsin, lipase, neuraminidase, pronase, papain, hyaluronidase, did not result in increased lysis and often resulted in a depression or abrogation of the ability of NKCF to result in target lysis (presumably due to modification of some surface structures required for interaction with NKCF or NK cells). Based on these results, we postulate that in addition to an NKCF, a tryptic protease released by the LGL is a central and critical element in cell-mediated lysis. This hypothesis is consistent with the data that killer-cell-independent lysis is inhibited late by protease inhibitors.

Initial Biochemical Characterization of Purified NKCF

In an attempt to determine the molecular weight of NKCF and to begin purification efforts, NKCF was produced in the presence of tritiated arginine. Figure 4 demonstrates a typical profile of tritiated-arginine label in protein, based on size separation, as well as relative cytotoxic activity, measured by dilution of

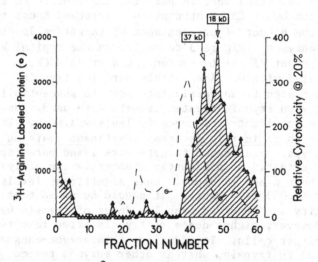

Fig. 4. Purification of ^{3}H-arginine NKCF from LGL was performed using HPLC molecular sizing. Protein profile (o) and NKCF activity (Δ) are shown. Typical experiment of 5 similar experiments. The LU 20% is the lytic unit equivalent, with the NKCF being diluted, and the lytic efficacy was calculated at 20% lysis.

cytotoxic activity, measured by dilution of purified fractions of NKCF. As consistently observed in several experiments, NKCF activity was observed in the molecular weight range between 18,000 and 40,000, with peaks of activity usually seen at approximately 20,000 and 40,000 daltons. These results suggest the possibility of polymerization of a 20,000 m.w. subunit. In addition, NKCF activity was consistently found in the void volume (e.g., far left of Figure 4), indicating some high molecular weight (>300,000 daltons) aggregates of NKCF. These fractions were prepared using high-performance liquid chromatography at neutral pH on a molecular sizing column. This purification methodology provides an approach for further purification of NKCF and use of radiolabeled factors for subsequent binding studies and/or further analysis of the mode of action of NKCF. Preliminary studies with partially purified NKCF indicate that partially purified factors induce an accelerated level of lysis, detected as early as 6 hours (data not shown). These results indicate that one reason for the slow rate of lysis by NKCF may be the purity of the factor. Therefore, more highly purified factors may minimize the differences that exist between the kinetics of lysis by intact NK cells versus NKCF.

DISCUSSION

Since the original descriptions of human and mouse NKCF,[7-11] several lines of evidence have suggested that this factor(s) might be involved in the mechanism of lysis by NK cells. Studies by Wright et al.[8] and Farran et al.[10] have indicated that NKCF is released during coculture of NK-sensitive target cells with NK cells. Although such evidence is consistent with the hypothesis that NKCF is involved in lysis by human NK cells, little or no information about the actual mechanism of lysis by human NKCF or its relationship to the mechanism of lysis by NK cells has been reported. In the present study, using inhibitors which have been demonstrated previously to inhibit NK lysis, further implications for the association of NKCF and human NK cell-mediated cytotoxicity have been examined.

First, if human NKCF plays a direct role in a mechanism of cytotoxicity by NK cells, it would be predicted that it would be produced and released by human LGL. Our experiments certainly confirm previous reports that highly purified LGL are responsible for production of NKCF as well as for NK activity.[10]

Secondly, release of NKCF should be selectively triggered by NK-susceptible targets. Our results have shown that production of NKCF was elicited mainly by NK-susceptible target cells, with

NK-insusceptible targets inducing little or no NKCF production. Thus, it is possible that the recognition receptors leading to release of NKCF and to binding to susceptible target cells may be very similar or identical.

Studies have indicated that carbohydrate moieties are involved in some post-binding events of cell-mediated lysis.[12-14] The present results are consistent with the hypothesis that inhibition of NK activity by phosphorylated sugars occurs by blocking the uptake of the lytic factor (NKCF). In addition, the pattern of inhibition of NKCF binding by various sugars was similar to that seen in studies of inhibition of lysis by intact LGL, e.g., mannose-6-phosphate inhibited whereas nonphosphorylated mannose did not. In addition, phosphorylated fructose demonstrated no significant inhibition of either NK activity or of lysis by NKCF. These parallel patterns of inhibition by sugars for NK-mediated lysis and for NKCF are consistent with the hypothesis that NKCF is involved in the mechanism of lysis by NK cells. The suscepti- bility of target cells to lysis may depend, however, on several factors, including the expression of both a specific NKCF binding site and a sugar-related site. This hypothesis is based on the fact that NKCF demonstrates considerable specificity, with lysis of NK-susceptible targets and little or no activity on NK-insus- ceptible targets. The concept that a sugar-related site is involved in NKCF binding was also supported by the observation that tunicamycin-treated target cells, whose glycosylation of surface lipoproteins or glycoproteins was blocked, demonstrate deficient binding or subsequent lysis by NKCF. These results indicate that glycosylated materials on the surface of the target are somehow required for lysis by NKCF.

Wright and Bonavida have previously demonstrated removal of the factor by NK-susceptible targets.[7-9] However, our experiments extend previous results by indicating that not only is NKCF acti- vity lost upon incubation with NK-susceptible targets, but this interaction leads to subsequent lysis. This rules out the possi- bility that loss of NKCF activity is due entirely to inactivation by the targets, since factor-independent lysis was seen. Our results also demonstrated that binding occurs gradually, with optimal binding of the preparations tested occurring by 6 hours. After this point, target cells were already programmed for subse- quent lysis, without the need for continued presence of factor, which occurred with the same kinetics as those seen in the con- tinued presence of NKCF. In contrast to the rapid killing seen by NK cells, which is detected in short-term chromium-release assays, high levels of NKCF lysis required 48 hours with [111]indium-labeled targets or 24 hours with 51 chromium-labeled targets. These re- sults are consistent with previous results obtained in both the

mouse and human[7-11]. One likely explanation for this slow cytotoxicity is that the rate of lysis of targets is largely controlled
by the concentration of available factor.

The events which occur after initial binding of NKCF to targets still remain obscure. However, the experiments performed
here may provide new insights to some of the interactions with
NKCF and targets. Inhibition of NKCF by phosphorylated sugars
is consistent with the concept that NKCF may recognize sugars on
the surface of target cells or, alternatively, bind involving
some receptor distinct from the carbohydrate moiety in the form
of a glycoprotein or a glycolipid. Although it remains to be
documented, our results with tunicamycin are consistent with the
binding of NKCF is to glycosylated residues on the target cells.
However, the relationship between the mechanisms of lysis of
targets by NKCF and by NK cells requires further investigation
before it can be concluded that NKCF is definitely involved in
the lysis by NK cells.

The possibility of producing NKCF under serum-free conditions
and regularly obtaining large amounts of activity should facilitate
its purification and biochemical characterization. The results
presented in the present studies provide information regarding the
molecular size (20-40,000 m.w., with apparently a 20,000 m.w. subunit) and potentially useful methodologies for further purification
and examination of binding, using radiolabeled NKCF. All of these
collectively should provide information for further dissection of
the mechanism of lysis by NK cells and NKCF.

REFERENCES

1. R. B. Herberman (Ed.), "NK Cells and Other Natural Effector
    Cells," Academic Press, New York (1982).
2. T. Timonen, J. R. Ortaldo, and R. B. Herberman, Characteristics
    of human large granular lymphocytes and relationship to natural-
    killer and K cells, J. Exp. Med. 153:569 (1981).
3. C. W. Reynolds, T. Timonen, and R. B. Herberman, Natural killer
    (NK) cell activity in the rat. I. Isolation and characteriza-
    tion of the effector cells, J. Immunol. 127:282 (1981).
4. J. C. Roder and T. Haliotis, A comparative analysis of the NK
    cytolytic mechanism and regulatory genes, in: "Natural Cell-
    Mediated Immunity Against Tumors," R. B. Herberman, ed.,
    Academic Press, New York (1980).
5. P. C. Quan, T. Ishizaka, and B. R. Bloom, Studies on the
    mechanism of NK cell lysis, J. Immunol. 128:1786 (1982).
6. C. S. Henney, On the mechanism of T-cell mediated cytolysis,
    Transplant. Rev. 17:37 (1973).

7. S. C. Wright and B. Bonavida, Selective lysis of NK-sensitive target cells by a soluble mediator released from murine spleen cells and human peripheral blood lymphocytes, J. Immunol. 126:1516 (1981).

8. S. C. Wright and B. Bonavida, Studies on the mechanism of natural killer (NK) cell-mediated cytotoxicity (CMC). I. Release of cytotoxic factors specific for NK-sensitive target cells (NKCF) during coculture of NK effector cells with NK target cells, J. Immunol. 129:433 (1982).

9. S. C. Wright, M. L. Weitzen, R. Kahle, G. A. Granger, and B. Bonavida, Studies on the mechanism of natural killer cytotoxicity. II. Coculture of human PBL with NK sensitive or resistant cell lines stimulates release of natural killer cytotoxic factor (NKCF) selectively cytotoxic to NK-sensitive target cells, J. Immunol. 130:2479 (1983).

10. E. Farram and S. R. Targan, Identification of human natural killer soluble cytotoxic factor(s) NKCF derived from NK-enriched lymphocyte populations: specificity of generation and killing, J. Immunol. 130:1252 (1983).

11. S. Wright and B. Bonavida, YAC1 variant clones selected for resistance to NKCF are also resistant to natural killer cell-mediated cytotoxicity. Proc. Natl. Acad. Sci. USA 80(6):1688 (1983).

12. J. T. Forbes and T. N. Oeltmann, Carbohydrate receptors in natural cell-mediated cytotoxicity, in: "NK Cells and Other Natural Effector Cells," R. B. Herberman, ed., Academic Press, New York (1982).

13. J. R. Ortaldo, T. T. Timonen, and R. B. Herberman, Inhibition of activity of human NK and K cells by simple sugars: Discrimination between binding and post-binding events, Clin. Immunol. Immunopathol. 31(3):439 (1984).

14. O. Stutman, P. Dien, R. E. Wisum, and E. C. Lattime, Natural cytotoxic cells against solid tumors in mice: blocking of cytotoxicity by D-mannose, Proc. Natl. Acad. Sci. USA 77:2895 (1980).

15. J. S. Tkacz and J. O. Lampen, Tunicamycin inhibition of polyisoprenyl-N-acetylglucosamyl pyrophosphate formation in calf liver microsomes, Biochem. Biophys. Res. Commun. 65:248 (1975).

16. P. K. Keller, D. Y. Boon, and F. C. Crum, N-acetyl glucosamine-2-phosphate transferase from hen oviduct: Solubilization, characterization, and inhibition by tunicamycin, Biochemistry 18:3946 (1979).

17. G. W. Hart, The role of asparagine-linked oligosaccharides in cellular recognition by thymic lymphocytes. Effects of tunicamycin on the mixed lymphocyte reaction, J. Biol. Chem. 257:151 (1982).

18. J. A. Werkmeister, J. C. Roder, C. Curry, and H. F. Pross, The effect of unphosphorylated and phosphorylated sugar moieties on human and mouse natural killer cell activity: is there selective inhibition at the level of target recognition and lytic acceptor site?, <u>Cell. Immunol.</u> 80:172 (1983).

DISCUSSION

Clark: In your experiment measuring the rate binding of radiolabeled NKCF to target cells, was the NKCF concentration the same as in the lytic assay?

Ortaldo: No, the radiolabeled material was HPLC purified. A similar preparation has given good target cell lysis at 8 hours.

Clark: So at the concentrations you were using to do the binding studies, the rate of target cell binding would be expected to be slower than in the lytic assay, since you are at a much lower factor concentration.

Ortaldo: Perhaps, yes.

Henney: I'm wondering if it is reasonable for a molecule with a molecular weight of 20,000 to have the features you described, i.e., a receptor-membrane complex but with the properties of a lysin as well. Could you comment on this?

Ortaldo: This is our working hypothesis, and I agree with you that the molecular weight seems small. But we must account for the well defined specificity of the factor, which does not seem to be a simple cytolytic molecule. It does not kill sheep red cells or other non-NK targets or disrupt liposomes.

Henney: Is there any evidence that your radioactive label is incorporated in the active NKCF molecule?

Ortaldo: No, we don't have direct evidence. There are a limited number of protein bands in this preparation and it does have lytic activity. We are currently trying to isolate the individual proteins.

Hudig: In your experiments on the effects of protease inhibitors on NKCF production, at what point did you remove the inhibitors?

Ortaldo: We left them in during the 18-24 hour incubation with the cells.

Hudig: TPCK and TLCK probably have a half life of about 30 minutes under theseconditions. It seems possbile that this could be related to the different results between you and Wright with regard to inhibition by these reagents. How much reagent have you used?

Ortaldo: We have used up to 100ug/ml. Beyond that we start seeing toxicity. Using our serum-free conditions we do not see any effects of these reagents on NKCF production, binding by absorption assays, or on the lytic activity.

Hudig: Then the only place you would involve proteases is at the target cell level, since target cell pretreatment makes the cells more vunerable to NKCF.

Ortaldo: Yes. Plus the small but significant enhancement of cell-mediated lysis of K562 by TPCK and TLCK pretreatment.

Clark: What is the effect of pretreating the target cells with papain?

Ortaldo: It has either no effect or diminishes the susceptibility to lysis.

Nathan: Have you examined the effect of plasminogen activator, a protease known to be produced by LGL?

Ortaldo: No, but we plan to.

M. Henkart: I would like to summarize briefly the distinctions which we see between the granule cytolysin and NKCF. First, of course, there is the large difference in the kinetics of lysis. The calcium dependence of cytolysin activity is striking, but as Susan Wright mentioned, cannot be readily tested for NKCF because of the prolonged assay. The granule cytolysin also shows a calcium inactivation, i.e., its activity is unstable in the presence of extracellular physiological levels of calcium, decaying within minutes. This is again hard to compare to NKCF, but Craig Reynolds has tried to detect an NKCF-like activity in granules which have been incubated with calcium so the cytolysin is decayed.

Reynolds: No NKCF activity was detected when these calcium-treated granules were tested in the long-term NKCF assay. As with the cytolysin, one could imagine an inhibitor might block the detection of such activity.

Ortaldo: The strongest linkage between the two activities is that the rabbit anti-granule antibodies inhibit both NKCF and the cytolysin. But we still cannot conclude the molecules are related. While there difference in kinetics is real, we and other labs are getting faster kinetics as we concentrate and purify NKCF, and the two activities seem to be getting closer. In summary, I feel that there are real similarities between the two in addition to the differences which you have mentioned.

<u>Brooks</u>: There are also differences in the molecular weights and specificities between NKCF and the cytolysin.

<u>Ortaldo</u>: There are many possible relationships between these two factors.

<u>Berke</u>: Have you looked in the EM for pore formation caused by NKCF?

<u>Ortaldo</u>: We would like to do that, but haven't had the opportunity.

AN INVESTIGATION OF THE ROLE OF SOLUBLE CYTOTOXIC FACTORS

AND REACTIVE OXYGEN INTERMEDIATES IN LYSIS BY NK CELLS

Elizabeth A. Wayner and Colin G. Brooks

Basic Immunology,
Fred Hutchinson Cancer Research Center
1124 Columbia Street
Seattle, WA 98104

INTRODUCTION

The mechanism(s) by which cytotoxic T lymphocytes (CTL) and natural killer (NK) cells lyse sensitive target cells is one of the basic questions in immunology that has remained unanswered. In the last 2-3 years, two hypotheses concerning the mechanism of cytolysis by NK cells have attracted considerable attention. According to the first hypothesis, a stable soluble cytotoxin (NKCF) is released by NK cells during their interaction with target cells, and this factor acting alone is capable of target cell lysis (Wright and Bonavida, 1982; 1983). In the second hypothesis, a crucial role for reactive oxygen intermediates (ROI) was suggested by the observation of luminol chemiluminescence (CL) during interaction between NK-enriched populations and target cells (Roder et al., 1982), and the inhibition of lysis by superoxide dismutase (SOD; Roder et al., 1982), or hydroxyl radical (OH.) scavengers (Suthanthiran et al., 1984). Whether the ROI directly inflicted damage on the target cells, as is the case in some macrophage/neutrophil cytocidal systems (Nathan et al., 1979a; b), was unclear.

Enthusiasm for both hypotheses has been considerably dampened by the failure of other laboratories to observe chemiluminescence, ROI production, or NKCF production unless the stimulating target cells are infected with mycoplasma (Koppel et al., 1984; Wayner and Brooks, 1984). A further major reservation has been the lack of unambiguous evidence that NK cells themselves are necessary and sufficient for the production of these substances. In an attempt to resolve this issue we have investigated the mechanism of lysis by cloned murine cell lines expressing NK activity. The clones we have used are in fact murine CTL which can be induced to express NK cytolytic activity, with the same specificity as splenic NK cells, by treatment with interferon (IFN) or interleukin-2 (Brooks, 1983; Brooks et al., 1983). Using a variety of experimental approaches, we failed to find any evidence for the participation of a stable soluble cytotoxin or ROI during the lysis of YAC-1 cells by such effectors.

MATERIALS AND METHODS

Mice. C57BL/6 (H-2^b), BALB/c (H-2^d), and DBA/2 (H-2^d) mice were bred at the Fred Hutchinson Cancer Research Center. CBA/J (H-2^K) and B6-C-H-2^{bm1}/ByJ (H-2^{bm1}) mice were bred at the Fred Hutchinson Cancer Research Center from stock obtained from the Jackson Laboratory (Bar Harbor, ME). Animals of both sexes were used at 8-12 wk of age.

Tumor cell lines. YAC-1 (H-2^a), a Moloney virus T cell lymphoma of A/Sn mice (Cikes et al, 1973) was used as the prototype mouse NK target. Other tumor lines used were: an NK-sensitive mouse myeloma derived from BALB/c mice, S194 (H-2^d; Horibata and Harris, 1970); an NK-sensitive clone (1C2) and an NK-resistant clone (av) of a DBA/2 derived leukemia, L5178Y (H-2^d; Fischer 1958; Durdik et al., 1980); P815 (H-2^d), an NK-resistant DBA/2 derived mastocytoma (Dunn and Potter, 1957); EL4 (H-2^b), an NK-resistant leukemia derived from C57BL mice (Gorer, 1950); and K562, a human NK-sensitive erythroleukemia (Lozio and Lozio, 1975). In vitro tumor cell lines were maintained in RPMI-1640 supplemented with 10% FBS and without any antibiotics. P815 and EL4 were maintained as ascites in syngeneic mice.

One of the mouse tumor lines, 1C2, was contaminated with mycoplasma (myc). Decontamination of 1C2 was achieved by multiple passages through syngeneic mice followed by re-establishment in culture. Mycoplasma tests were performed as described by Chen (1977).

Reagents. Methanol, ethanol, n-butanol, glycine, serine, tryptophan, thiourea, sodium benzoate, mannitol, mannose, dimethyl sulfoxide (DMSO), bovine liver catalase (20,000 U/mg) and bovine blood SOD (3100 U/mg) were obtained from Sigma, St. Louis, MO. Urea was obtained from Schwarz/Mann, Inc., Spring Valley, N.Y. 4β-phorbol 12-myristate 13-acetate (PMA) was obtained from Sigma and maintained as a stock solution at 1 mg/ml in absolute ethanol at -70 °C. Luminol (5-amino-2,3-dihydro-1,4-phthalazinedione) was obtained from Eastman Kodak, Rochester, N.Y. Luminol- saturated bovine serum albumin (BSA) was prepared by adding 0.5 g of luminol to 50 ml of 4% BSA (w/v) in water. This material was stirred in the dark at 4 °C for 18 h. It was centrifuged at 10,000 x g for 30 min, passed through 0.22 μm filters and stored in the dark at 4 °C.

Cytotoxic T lymphocyte (CTL) line. F5A4 is an antigen-dependent, many times cloned CTL line derived from a B6-C-H-2^{bm1}/ByJ anti-C57BL/6 mixed lymphocyte reaction. The preparation and propagation of such CTL clones has been described elsewhere (Brooks 1983; Brooks et al., 1983). Briefly, CTL were maintained in Click's medium supplemented with 10% fetal bovine serum (FBS, Sterile Systems, Logan, UT) and rat T cell growth factor

222

(TCGF). The latter was obtained by stimulating spleen cells with 10 µg/ml Concanavalin A (Con A; Pharmacia, Piscataway, NJ) as described (Brooks et al, 1983). After stimulation by antigen and expansion in 10% TCGF, F5A4 cells were allowed to rest for 7-10 days in 2% TCGF.

Induction of NK activity in cloned CTL. Resting F5A4 cells were induced to express NK activity by incubating 5×10^5 cells for 18-24 h in 1 ml Click's/10% FBS containing 2% TCGF and 10^4 U/ml recombinant human IFN α A/D (kindly provided by Dr. P. Trown, Hoffman-LaRoche, Nutley, NJ). The cells were then washed, dead cells were removed by centrifugation at 400g for 15 min on a cushion of Ficoll-Hypaque (density 1.077; Sigma), and the viable cells were washed again.

Cell-mediated cytotoxicity assays. NK and CTL activity was measured in RPMI-1640/10% FBS in V-bottomed microtest plates using 5×10^3 YAC-1 or EL4 target cells/well and a 4 h chromium-release assay, as described elsewhere (Wayner and Brooks, 1984). For studies of human NK activity, blood mononuclear cells (MNC) were separated on Ficoll-Hypaque, and assayed on K562 targets. For studies of mouse NK activity, spleen cell suspensions were prepared from normal CBA/J or from C57BL/6 mice injected intraperitoneally (ip) 18 h earlier with 200 µg polyinosinic: polycytidylic acid (poly I:C; Sigma), and assayed on YAC-1 targets.

For studies of macrophage-mediated cytotoxicity, the procedure of Nathan et al. (1979a, b) was followed. Briefly, C57BL/6 mice were injected ip with 0.1 ml Bacillus Calmette-Guerin vaccine (BCG; lot A-15, Trudeau Institute, Saranac City, Canada). Peritoneal exudate cells (PEC) were obtained 7-28 days later by lavage of the peritoneal cavity with HBSS/1% FBS. They were washed two times, resuspended in RPMI/5% FBS, and incubated at 2×10^5 (E:T=40:1) or 1×10^5 (E:T=20:1) cells/well in flat bottomed microtest plates for 1 h at 37 ^{o}C. The non-adherent cells were removed and the cytotoxic activity of the adherent cells, in the presence of 10 ng/ml PMA, was measured in a 4 h chromium-release assay using EL4 targets. Significant lysis of tumor cells in 4h by BCG-elicited PEC occurred only in the presence of PMA.

Cytotoxicity assay in the presence of OH. scavengers

Isotonic solutions of scavengers were prepared and appropriate dilutions made in isotonic NaCl. Fifty µl aliquots of these dilutions were added in duplicate to microplate wells, together with 100 µl of effector cells and 50 µl of target cells in RPMI-1640/10% FBS. Control wells received 50 µl isotonic NaCl. Each well was mixed three times prior to incubation.

Effect of OH. scavengers on ^{3}H-leucine incorporation

Human blood MNC were incubated at 5×10^6/ml in RPMI/5% FBS supplemented with 5×10^{-5} M 2-mercaptoethanol and 5 µg/ml Con A for 48-72hr. F5A4 cells were induced into the proliferative phase by incubation for 3d with irradiated C57BL/6 stimulator cells in Click's/10% FBS containing 10% TCGF.

223

Aliquots of 2×10^5 human Con A blasts or 10^5 alloantigen-activated F5A4 cells were incubated in leucine-free RPMI-1640 supplemented with 10% dialyzed FBS in flat-bottomed microtest plates with serial dilutions of iso-tonic OH. scavengers in isotonic NaCl for 4 h. Cultures were then labelled with 1 μCi of ^{3}H-leucine (New England Nuclear, Boston, MA) and incubated for a further 2 h. One hundred μl of 1% Triton X-100 containing 20% FBS were added to each well. After 1 min at room temperature 100 μl of 20% trichloroacetic acid was added to each well. The plates were placed at $4\,^{\circ}$C for 30 min and the precipitates then collected on glass filters using a MASH harvester.

Production of cytotoxic factor

This procedure was based on that described by Wright and Bonavida (1982, 1983) for NKCF production by spleen cells. 5×10^5 resting or IFN-treated F5A4 cells were admixed with 2.5×10^5 tumor cell stimulators in 2 ml RPMI-1640 in 16mm diameter culture wells (Costar 3524, Cambridge, MA). The medium was supplemented with 1% glutamine, 1% sodium pyruvate and 1% non-essential amino acids and was used either serum-free or with 5% FBS. After incubation at $37\,^{\circ}$C for 30 h, cell-free supernatants were pre-pared by centrifuging at 200 x g for 10 min and passing through 0.45 μm fil-ters.

Assay for cytotoxic factor

This procedure was also based on that described by Wright and Bonavida (1983) for assay of NKCF. Duplicate serial dilutions of test material in RPMI-1640 supplemented with 1% glutamine, 1% sodium pyruvate and 1% non-essential amino acids were prepared starting at 100 μl/well in flat bot-tomed microtest plates. One hundred μl containing 5×10^3 Cr-labelled YAC-1 cells in RPMI-1640/5% FBS were added to each well. The assay plates were incubated at $37\,^{\circ}$C for 18 h then 100 μl aliquots were harvested and counted.

Measurement of cytotoxic factor production during 4hr cytotoxicity assay

In this experiment two identical sets of cultures in round bottomed microtest plates were prepared. In one set, duplicate serial dilutions of res-ting or IFN-treated F5A4 effectors were admixed with 5×10^3 Cr-labelled target cells in RPMI/5% FBS supplemented with 1% glutamine, 1% sodium pyruvate and 1% non-essential amino acids. In the other identical set, effec-tors were admixed with 5×10^3 unlabelled target cells. After 4h at $37\,^{\circ}$C, 100 μl aliquots of supernatant were removed from the first set of cultures and counted for Cr-release. One hundred μl aliquots of supernatant from the second set of cultures were immediately transferred to flat-bottomed micro-plate wells containing 5×10^3 fresh Cr-labelled YAC-1 cells in 100 μl serum-free medium (giving a final FBS concentration of 2.5%). These secondary cytotoxicity cultures were incubated for 18hr, then supernatants harvested and counted.

Measurement of CL

Effector cells were washed and suspended in 750 µl of RPMI/5% FBS buffered with 10 mM HEPES in 17x60mm glass vials (VWR). Twenty µl of luminol-saturated BSA solution was added to each vial. PEC effectors were pre-incubated at 37 °C in the presence of luminol to reduce background levels of CL. CL was measured in a Beckman LS8000 scintillation counter set in the single photon mode and programmed to record cpm at 0.1 sec intervals. At T=0 the appropriate stimuli were added to the vials which were then placed in a 37 °C water bath. CL was determined at 5, 10 or 15 min intervals. Machine backgrounds $(10-20 \times 10^3$ cpm) were not subtracted. CTL and tumor cells had negligible CL, but PEC displayed a substantial background response as noted above.

RESULTS AND DISCUSSION

Expression of NK activity by IFN-treated CTL

Resting cloned CTL line F5A4 displayed lytic specificity for target cells bearing $H-2^b$ alloantigens, ie. EL4 (Fig. 1). Following incubation with 10^4 U/ml IFN for 18 h these cells, in common with all other CTL we have tested, acquired a new lytic specificity identical to that of splenic NK cells. Thus, in addition to the killing of EL4, the cells were now highly cytotoxic against NK-sensitive targets such as YAC-1, S194, and IC2 but failed to lyse NK-resistant targets such as av and P815 (Fig. 1).

Production of cytotoxic factor(s) by IFN-induced CTL

The first issue we addressed concerned the possibility that IFN-treated CTL (F5A4) might mediate lysis of NK-sensitive tumor cells via the release of soluble cytotoxic factor(s). In order to investigate this, IFN-induced F5A4

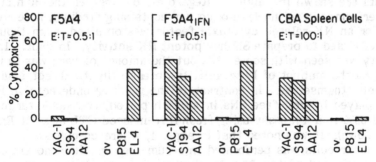

Fig. 1. Specificity of resting F5A4 cells, IFN-induced F5A4, and normal CBA/J spleen cells.

Table 1. Cytotoxic Factor Production by IFN-induced CTL.

Expt.	Effector	Target/ Stimulator	Percent cytotoxicity	
			By cells (4h assay)	By SN or lysate from same cells (18h assay)[a,b,c]
1[a]	F5A4	-	-	0
	F5A4$_{IFN}$	-	-	1
	F5A4	EL4	59	6
	F5A4$_{IFN}$	EL4	70	5
	F5A4	YAC-1	15	12
	F5A4$_{IFN}$	YAC-1	89	4
2[b]	F5A4	-	-	0
	F5A4$_{IFN}$	-	-	0
	F5A4	EL4	50	-2
	F5A4$_{IFN}$	EL4	52	-1
	F5A4	YAC-1	2	-1
	F5A4$_{IFN}$	YAC-1	66	3
3[c]	F5A4	YAC-1	6	-1
	F5A4$_{IFN}$	YAC-1	72	2

[a]Effector cells were incubated for 4h with ^{51}Cr-labelled targets at E:T ratio 2:1, or for 30h with unlabelled target cells at an effector:stimulator ratio of 2:1 in serum-free medium.

[b]Same as in expt. 1, but in medium containing 5% FBS.

[c]Effector cells incubated for 4h with ^{51}Cr-labelled targets at E:T ratio of 8:1, or frozen and thawed 2X and the cell-free lysate tested for cytotoxicity in an 18h assay.

cells expressing NK cytotoxic activity were incubated either with Cr-labelled EL4 and YAC-1 cells for 4 h or in parallel with the corresponding unlabelled tumor cells for 30 h. (It should be noted that both target cells have been rigorously established to be mycoplasma-free). Cell-free SN obtained from the latter cultures were then tested immediately after collection for ability to lyse Cr-labelled YAC-1 cells in an 18 h assay. The results of two typical experiments are shown in Table 1. Regardless of whether the 30 h stimulation was performed in serum-free or serum-containing medium, no convincing evidence for an NK-related cytotoxic factor was obtained, even though the effector cells used to prepare SN had potent NK activity. In expt. 1, slight cytotoxicity was seen with some SNs, but the amount of lysis was in inverse proportion to the amount of lytic activity observed in the direct assay with effector cells themselves. In contrast to the weak or undetectable lysis of YAC-1 displayed by cell-free SNs in an 18 h period, the same target cells were lysed 62% in a 4 h assay using fresh IFN-induced CTL at a 2:1 E:T ratio (data not shown). It was noted that in expt. 1, where co-culture of effector cells and tumor cells was performed in serum-free medium, no viable cells remained at the end of the 30 h incubation. The weak but variable toxic activity seen with the SNs derived from this experiment may therefore have been attributable to lysosomal or metabolic products released from dying cells.

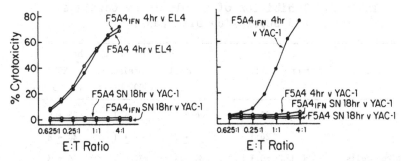

Fig. 2. Inability to detect cytotoxic activity in SN harvested from a 4 h
cytotoxicity assay and incubated immediately with fresh Cr-labelled
YAC-1 cells for 18 h.

It was also of interest to determine whether lysates from control or
IFN-induced CTL contained material cytotoxic for YAC-1 cells. One hundred μl of effector cells at 4×10^5/ml, or of cell-free lysate prepared by
freezing and thawing the cell suspension twice, were added to Cr-labelled
YAC-1 cells. Although intact effector cells could mediate >70% lysis of
YAC-1 by 4 h, no significant lytic activity could be detected in cell-free
lysates even after 18 h incubation (Table 1, expt. 3).

In a third strategy designed to elucidate whether cytotoxic factors
might mediate NK lysis, two parallel sets of cultures containing titrations of
resting and IFN-induced F5A4 cells with appropriate targets were set up in
the standard cytotoxicity assay. In the first set, Cr-labelled targets were
used to determine lytic activity directly. In the second set, unlabelled target
cells were used, and at the end of the 4 h assay, 100 μl of SN were transferred immediately to new wells containing 5×10^3 freshly labelled YAC-1
cells. These secondary cultures were then incubated for a total of 18 h
before measuring Cr release. As can be seen in Fig. 2, although high cytolytic activity was demonstrable within 4 h in the primary cultures, no activity
was detected in any of the secondary cultures.

Thus, using a variety of approaches designed to optimize the likelihood
of observing even a partially stable cytolytic factor, no evidence was obtained that such a factor was released by cloned cell lines expressing NK activity. Although the exact relationship between the NK activity expressed by
cloned CTL and that observed in vivo is unclear, the fact that the NK specificity of induced CTL is identical to that of splenic NK cells and that the NK
activity of CTL is regulated by the same lymphokines (IFN and IL-2) which
regulate splenic NK activity (Brooks, 1983), strongly supports the notion that
the NK activity of the cloned cells is physiologically relevant. Because these
cloned cell lines display extremely high NK lytic activity, and are completely
free of contaminating cell populations, our results provide compelling evidence that NK lysis is not mediated by a stable soluble cytotoxic factor.

Table 2. Inhibition of Cytolysis by Catalase and Superoxide Dismutase.

Effector	Target	E:T	% cytotoxicity at 4 hr		
			Control	Catalase (5000 U/ml)	SOD (300 U/ml)
Adherent PEC	EL4	40:1	66 ± 7[a]	1 ± 1	58 ± 5
		20:1	42 ± 7	2 ± 1	40 ± 8
Spleen cells	YAC-1	50:1	39 ± 5	32 ± 4	36 ± 3
Resting F5A4	EL4	0.5:1	25 ± 5	24 ± 4	22 ± 1
IFN-induced F5A4	YAC-1	0.5:1	35 ± 2	36 ± 5	40 ± 8
Human MNC	K562	12:1	31 ± 1	33 ± 7	41 ± 10

[a] Mean values ($\pm$SD) of 3 experiments.

Role of ROI in NK lysis

Interaction of phagocytic leukocytes with a variety of soluble or particulate stimuli triggers a cascade of enzyme-catalyzed reactions at the plasma
membrane level which rapidly culminate in a burst of oxygen consumption
and the generation of a variety of ROI. Initially, the principal ROI formed
are superoxide anions (O_2^-) and hydrogen peroxide (H_2O_2), but ROI of even
greater reactivity, including OH., singlet oxygen, and hypohalous acids, can
be generated rapidly from these primary ROI products. Considerable evidence suggests that ROI play a crucial role in the destruction of microorganisms (for review, see Badwey and Karnovsky, 1980), and tumor cells
(Nathan et al., 1979a, b) by phagocytes. We have therefore investigated in
some detail whether ROI may participate in lysis of tumor cells by NK cells.
Three NK systems were studied in parallel: lysis of K562 by human MNC,
lysis of YAC-1 by poly I:C-activated C57BL/6 spleen cells, and lysis of YAC-
1 by IFN-induced cloned CTL. BCG-activated PEC exposed in vitro to PMA,
which secrete ROI and demonstrate ROI killing (Nathan et
al., 1979a, b), were used as a positive control. Resting CTL lysis of an antigen-specific target, where participation of ROI has been excluded (Nathan et
al., 1982), was used as a negative control.

Table 2 shows that catalase, but not SOD, was a potent inhibitor of
PEC-mediated cytolysis, in agreement with previous results (Nathan et
al., 1979a, b). Catalase and SOD solutions were always prepared fresh immediately before addition to the cytotoxicity assays. At the concentration used
here, both enzymes caused approximately 50% inhibition of the luminol-dependent CL of PMA-treated PEC, and when used together completely ablated
CL (not shown). By contrast, neither enzyme inhibited any of the NK reactions. The only significant change observed was an occasional enhancement
by SOD of lysis of K562 by human MNC. This may be due to an abrogation of
the suppression of human NK function caused by monocyte-generated ROI
(Seaman et al., 1983). We were therefore unable to substantiate the claim of

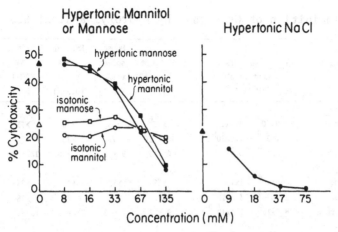

Fig. 3. Effect of hypertonicity on lysis of K562 cells by human MNC
(E:T ratio = 25:1)

Roder et al. (1982) that SOD at approximately 300U/ml could cause 75% inhibition of K562 lysis by human MNC. The results suggest that neither peroxide not superoxide plays a role in human or mouse NK-mediated lysis. The possibility that failure to inhibit might be caused by limited access of these macromolecular scavengers to the sites of interaction between NK cells and target cells cannot be excluded.

Further experiments were performed to examine whether OH. may be involved in NK-mediated lysis. Scavengers of low molecular weight, differing in their rate constants for reaction with OH., were tested for NK inhibitory activity. Preliminary experiments, in which the reagents were dissolved directly in culture medium, indicated that all scavengers were inhibitory, but it soon became clear that these effects were largely caused by alterations in the ionic strength of the medium. Fig. 3 demonstrates that when the OH. scavenger mannitol, or the sugar mannose, was dissolved directly in medium, significant inhibition was observed at concentrations as low as 33mM. By contrast, when isotonic solutions were prepared and diluted with isotonic NaCl, no significant inhibition was observed even at 135mM. Similarly, NK cytolysis could be inhibited by as little as 9mM NaCl added directly to culture medium. The exquisite sensitivity of NK cell function to ionic strength is of some interest because such small changes in tonicity would not be expected to affect cell viability (for example, tissue culture cells grow normally under such conditions). However, in terms of employing pharmacological reagents to probe the mechanisms of NK-mediated lysis, it is clearly imperative to maintain isotonic conditions.

When such precautions were taken, we obtained the results documented in Table 3. Amongst the alcohol and amino acid scavengers there was a clear inverse correlation between the concentration of scavenger required to cause 30% inhibition of cytolysis and the rate constant for reaction with OH.

Table 3. Inhibition of Cytolysis by Hydroxyl Radical Scavengers.

Scavenger	Rate constants at neutral pH $(M^{-1}s^{-1})$[a]	Human MNC v K562 (12:1)	Mouse spleen v YAC-1 (50:1)	Resting F5A4 v EL4 (0.5:1)	IFN-ind. F5A4 v YAC-1 (0.5:1)
Alcohols					
Methanol	$3.9 \times 10^8 - 8.4 \times 10^8$	>75[b]	>75	>75	>75
Ethanol	$7.2 \times 10^8 - 1.8 \times 10^9$	40 ± 20	72	>75	72
n-Butanol	$2.2 \times 10^9 - 3.4 \times 10^9$	6 ± 1	9 ± 2	14 ± 6	12 ± 8
Amino acids					
Glycine	$6 \times 10^6 - 1 \times 10^7$	>75	>75	>75	>75
Serine	$1.9 \times 10^8 - 3.2 \times 10^8$	>75	>75	>75	>75
Tryptophan	$8.5 \times 10^9 - 1.4 \times 10^{10}$	9 ± 2	7 ± 3	12 ± 2	10 ± .2
Others					
Urea	$< 7 \times 10^5$	>75	>75	>75	>75
Mannitol	$> 1 \times 10^9$	>75	>75	>75	>75
Benzoate	$3.5 \times 10^9 - 5.4 \times 10^9$	7 ± 1	11 ± 8	8 ± 2	11 ± 5
Thiourea	4.7×10^9	17 ± 3	75	28 ± 15	>75
DMSO	7×10^9	>75	>75	>75	>75

[a]Rate constants for the reaction of scavengers (except mannitol) with hydroxyl radicals in aqueous solution were taken from Anbar and Neta (1967) and Dorfman and Adams (1973). The rate constant for mannitol was from Cederbaum et al. (1977).

[b]Figures show the concentration of scavenger (mM) required for 30% inhibition of cytotoxicity. Percent lysis in control cultures lacking scavengers was always in the range 20-40%. Results are mean ± SD from 4 experiments.

Human NK activity v. K562, mouse splenic NK activity v. YAC-1, and mouse clone NK activity v. YAC-1 were all equally susceptible to inhibition. Somewhat surprisingly, specific CTL lysis of EL4 was also readily inhibited by butanol and tryptophan. These results suggested that OH. may participate in NK-mediated cytolysis, as recently suggested elsewhere (Suthanthiran, et al., 1984), and also in CTL-mediated lysis. However, when a number of other scavengers were studied, the correlation between ability to inhibit lysis and to react with OH. broke down. Thus, although benzoate and thiourea are equally reactive with OH., benzoate was a much better inhibitor of cytolysis, especially in the mouse NK systems. Furthermore, DMSO, one of the most avid OH. scavengers, had little or no inhibitory activity. Because the inhibition of NK activity failed to consistently reflect scavenger reactivity with OH., and because many of the better scavengers have broad chemical reactivity, we evaluated whether these compounds might in fact be toxic. The data in Table 4 reveal that the four scavengers which inhibited NK-mediated cytotoxicity also inhibited, at similar doses, leucine uptake by human MNC-derived Con A blasts and F5A4 cells. Thus, the ability of these compounds to inhibit NK-(and also CTL-) mediated cytolysis is unlikely to be attributable to their reaction with OH. More likely, these compounds are directly toxic to the effector cells, a conclusion that accords with that of Nathan et al. (1982), who observed morphological deterioration and loss of target cell binding capacity in CTL treated with benzoate or thiourea.

Table 4. Inhibition of Protein Synthesis
by Hydroxyl Radical Scavengers.

Scavenger	MNC blasts	F5A4
Methanol	>75[a]	>75
Ethanol	>75	>75
n-Butanol	12	50
Glycine	>75	>75
Serine	70	60
Tryptophan	1	1
Urea	70	64
Thiourea	9	27
Benzoate	12	10
DMSO	>75	>75

[a]Figures show the concentration of scavenger required for 30% inhibition of leucine uptake. Data shown are representative of 3 separate experiments.

In a further attempt to determine whether ROI might participate in NK-mediated killing, we studied the ability of cloned cells expressing NK activity to produce CL. Luminol-dependent CL is an extremely sensitive method for detecting production of ROI, including peroxide, superoxide, OH. and singlet oxygen (DeLuca, 1978) BCG-activated PEC produced a strongCL response when treated with either soluble (PMA) or particulate (mycoplasma-infected tumor cells) stimulant (Fig. 4). The sensitivity of the system was such that significant CL was produced by PMA stimulation of 500 PEC. (In

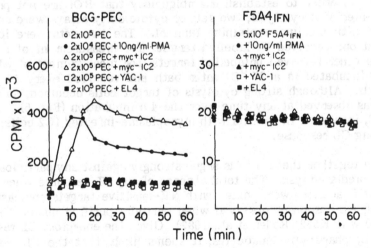

Fig. 4. Luminol-dependent chemiluminescence produced by BCG-PEC and IFN-induced F5A4 cells.

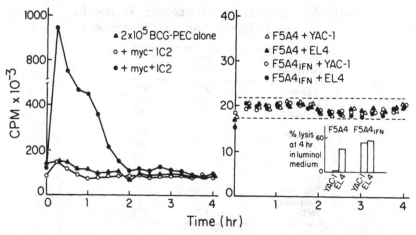

Fig. 5. Luminol-dependent chemiluminescence produced by BCG-PEC, resting
F5A4 cells, or IFN-induced F5A4 cells, when incubated with various
stimuli over a 4 h period. The straight lines in the right hand panel
indicate the range of chemiluminescence activity in control vials
containing effector cells alone. Inset shows the cytotoxic activity
of resting and IFN-treated F5A4 cells incubated in parallel vials
under identical conditions but with Cr-labelled target cells.

agreement with results recently reported by Koppel et al. (1984), we were
unable to induce any CL with a variety of mycoplasma-free tumor cells). By
contrast, IFN-induced F5A4 cells produced no detectable CL when mixed
with either specific target cells (EL4), NK targets (YAC-1), mycoplasma-
infected IC2 cells, or PMA (Fig. 4). PMA certainly interacts with F5A4 cells
because it is an extremely potent inducer of NK activity in these cells (unpublished). In order to establish unambiguously that ROI are not produced
during NK-mediated cytolysis, two sets of cytotoxicity assays were set up in
glass vials with medium containing luminol. The two sets were identical
except that one received Cr-labelled targets (for measurement of lytic activity), the other received unlabelled targets (for measurement of CL). All
vials were incubated in a 37 $^{\circ}$C water bath and removed every 15 min to
measure CL. Although strong cytolysis of target cells occurred, no significant CL was observed at any time over the 4 h incubation (Fig. 5). By contrast, PEC, incubated in parallel with mycoplasma-infected IC2 cells, generated a strong CL response.

Taken together these results argue strongly against any participation of
ROI in NK-mediated lysis. The total absence of any CL response when cloned
lines with NK activity were mixed with NK-sensitive targets contrasts with
the striking CL responses observed when partially purified human NK cells
were mixed with K562 (Roder et al., 1982). Given the enormous CL responses
generated by phagocytic leukocytes, it seems likely that the CL responses
observed by Roder et al. (1982) were caused by contaminating macrophages.
Similar conclusions have recently been reached by others (Kay et al., 1983).

SUMMARY

Using a variety of experimental approaches we have been unable to find any evidence that a monoclonal CTL line, induced to express high levels of NK activity by treatment with IFN, mediates target cell lysis by secretion of a cytotoxic factor. Thus, supernatant prepared in a variety of ways by incubating cloned killer cells with mycoplasma-free YAC-1 cells, or by freeze-thawing the killer cells themselves, were essentially devoid of lytic activity even when tested in 18hr assays. These findings substantiate at the clonal level our previous observations, that mouse splenic NK cells do not secrete detectable cytotoxic factors in the absence of mycoplasma (Wayner and Brooks, 1984). In addition, it appears that NK killing does not involve the participation of reactive oxygen intermediates. Neither catalase nor SOD were inhibitory. Inhibition observed with some OH. scavengers failed to correlate with their rate constants for reaction with OH., and was apparently due to the general toxicity of these compounds. A cloned cell line expressing potent NK activity failed to produce any luminol-reactive chemiluminescent species during incubation with target cells or with PMA.

ACKNOWLEDGEMENTS

This work was supported by PHS grant AI 15384. EAW is the recipient of a Special Fellowship of the Leukemia Society of America. We are grateful to Max Holscher for skillfull technical assistance.

REFERENCES

Anbar, M. and Neta, P. 1967. A compilation of specific rate constants for the reactions of hydrated electrons, hydrogen atoms, and hydroxyl radicals with inorganic and organic compounds in aqueous solution. Int. J. Appl. Rad. Isotopes, 18: 493.

Badwey, C. G. and Karnovsky, M. L. 1980. Active oxygen species and the functions of phagocytic leukocytes. Ann. Rev. Biochem., 49:695

Brooks, C. G. 1983. Reversible induction of natural killer cell activity in cloned murine cytotoxic T lymphocytes. Nature, 305:155

Brooks, C. G., Urdal, D. L. and Henney, C. S. 1983. Lymphokine-driven "differentiation" of cytotoxic T-cell clones into cells with NK-like specificity: correlation with display of membrane macromolecules Immunol. Rev., 72:43.

Cederbaum, A. I., Dicker, E., Rubin, E. and Cohen, G. 1977. The effect of dimethyl sulfoxide and other hydroxyl radical scavengers on the oxidation of ethanol by rat liver microsomes. Biochem. Biophys. Res. Commun., 78:1254.

Chen, T. R. 1977. In situ detection of mycoplasma contamination in cell cultures by fluorescent Hoechst 33258 stain. Exp. Cell. Res., 104:255.

Cikes, M., Friberg, S. and Klein, G. 1973. Progressive loss of H-2 antigens with concomitant increase of cell surface antigen(s) determined by Moloney leukemic virus in cultured murine lymphomas. J. Natl. Cancer

Inst., 50:347.

DeLuca, M. A. (ed.) 1978. Bioluminescence and chemiluminescence. Methods in Enzymology. Vol. LVII. Academic Press, New York.

Dorfman, L. M. and Adams, G. E. 1973. Reactivity of the hydroxyl radical in aqueous solutions. NSRDS, National Bureau of Standards, 46, (Washington, D.C.).

Dunn, T. B. and Potter, M. J. 1957. A transplantable mast cell neoplasm in the mouse. J. Natl. Cancer Inst., 18:587.

Durdik, J. M., Beck, B. N., Clark, E. A. and Henney, C. S. 1980. Characterization of a lymphoma variant selectively resistant to natural killer cells. J. Immunol., 125:683.

Fisher, G. A. 1958. Studies on the culture of leukemia cells in vitro. Ann. NY. Acad. Sci., 76:673.

Gorer, P. A. 1950. Studies in antibody response of mice to tumor inoculation. Br. J. Cancer, 4:372.

Horibata, K. and Harris, A. W. 1970. Mouse myelomas and lymphomas in culture. Exp. Cell. Res., 60:61.

Kay, H. D., Smith, D. L., Sullivan, G. Mandell, G. L., and Donowitz, G. R. 1983. Evidence for a non-oxidative mechanism of human natural killer (NK) cell cytotoxicity by using mononuclear effector cells from healthy donors and from patients with chronic granulomatous disease. J. Immunol., 131:1784.

Koppel, P., Peterhans, E., Bertoni, G., Keist, R., Groscurth, P., Wyler, R., and Keller, R. 1984. Induction of chemiluminesce during interaction of tumoricidal effector cell populations and tumor cells is dependent on the presence of mycoplasma. J. Immunol. 132:2021.

Lozio, C. B. and Lozio, B. B. 1975. Human chronic myelogenous leukemia cell line with positive Philadelphia chromosome. Blood, 45:321.

Nathan, C. F., Bruckner, L. H., Silverstein, S. C. and Cohn, Z. A. 1979a. Extracellular cytolysis by activated macrophages and granulocytes. I. Pharmacologic triggering of effector cells and the release of hydrogen peroxide. J. Exp. Med., 149:84.

Nathan, C. F., Silverstein, S. C., Bruckner, L. H. and Cohn, Z. A. 1979b. Extracellular cytolysis by macrophages and granulocytes. II. Hydrogen peroxide as a mediator of cytotoxicity. J. Exp. Med., 149:100.

Nathan, C. F., Mercer-Smith, J. A., Desantis, N. M. and Palladino, M. A. 1982. Role of oxygen in T cell mediated cytolysis. J. Immunol., 129:2164.

Roder, J. C., Helfand, S. L., Werkmeister, J., McGarry, R., Beaumont, T. J., and Duwe, A. 1982. Oxygen intermediates are triggered early in the cytolytic pathway of human NK cells. Nature, 298:569.

Seaman, W. E., Gindhart, T. D., Blackman, M. A., Dalal, B., Talal, N., and Werb, Z. 1982. Suppression of natural killing in vitro by monocytes and polymorphonuclear leukocytes. J. Clin. Invest., 69:876.

Suthanthiran, M., Solomon, S. D., Williams, P. S., Rubin, A. L., Novogrodsky, A., and Stenzel, K.H. 1984. Hydroxyl radical scavengers inhibit human natural killer cell activity. Nature, 367:276.

Wright, S. C. and Bonavida, B. 1982. Studies on the mechanism of natural killer (NK) cell-mediated cytotoxicity (CMC) I. Release of cytotoxic factors specific for NK-sensitive target cells (NKCF) during co-culture of NK effector cells with NK target cells. J. Immunol., 129:433.

Wright, S. C. and Bonavida, B. 1983. Studies on the mechanism of natural killer cytotoxicity III. Activation of NK cells by interferon augments the lytic activity of released natural killer cytotoxic factors (NKCF). J. Immunol., 130:2960.

Wayner, E. A. and Brooks, C. G. 1984. Induction of NKCF-like activity in mixed lymphocyte-tumor cell culture: direct involvement of mycoplasma infection of tumor cells. J. Immunol., 132:2135.

DISCUSSION

J. Ding-E Young: Have you tried to break your cells in a different way, other than freeze-thawing?

C. Brooks: No, that's the only way we've tried.

J. Ding-E Young: It seems to us that freeze-thawing NK cells twice wouldn't be enough to release the lytic factors from the granules.

C. Brooks: Well, using spleen cell systems, that kind of procedure has been reported to generate NKCF-like materials, so that was our rationale for using it. I agree entirely that the cold isn't sufficient to break open the granules completely, but we were more interested in the general question of whether stable cytolytic substances are released by these kinds of procedures, and they can't be, obviously.

J. Ding-E Young: You also mention some work in the literature showing that hypertonic mannitol inhibits lysis by NK cells. Do you think that would be consistent with a secretory phenomenon, since Harvey Pollard and others have shown under exactly the same conditions that you inhibit secretion by a number of different cells?

C. Brooks: Actually, I don't think I did suggest that it was in the literature. It may be, but our knowledge of this phenomenon was really spurred by some experiments that Dave Urdal did in Chris Henney's Lab a number of years ago. It is certainly intruiging that such small changes in ionic strength will inhibit NK activity. These changes would not be expected to affect the overall viability of the cells. In fact, sometimes tissue culture cells actually grow better under these altered conditions. It may be a clue as to the nature of the NK lysis itself.

G. Berke: I'd like to make a commend regarding that Suthanthiran paper in Nature. As you may recall, the authors have stated in that paper that they have checked for conjugate formation, and they found that those inhibitors did not inhibit because they were inhibiting conjugation. But in fact, they've not produced the data indicating that there was no inhibition of conjugation. Perhaps you Colin, or others in the audience, have experienced what would be the effects of benzoate, or alcohol, either methanol or ethanol, on conjugate formation by natural killer cells. Because it seems to me that this is an awfully high concentration which could retard killing activity, maybe at the expense of inhibiting conjugate formation. And in that regard, it occurs to me that a great deal of conjugate formation in natural killer cells is usually not reported in terms of hard figures.

236

People say "we looked, and it was not inhibitory", but the data usually are not documented.

I think perhaps in addition to that we need to consider how one should handle data on conjugate formation with natural killer cells, because the numbers to me seem awfully small. Great care needs to be exercised in these calculations.

B. Bonavida: It has been our experience that certain cell lines secrete inhibitory activity for NKCF. I'm wondering with your NK lines have you attempted to remove those inhibitors by dialysis or some other means? Susan Wright will present some data tomorrow on this whole issue.

C. Brooks: Well I think you're aware that when we exchanged cell lines with you and Susan that you in fact reproduced our results precisely, that the cells which were contaminated with mycoplasma, or that had been deliberately infected, would produce NKCF, whereas cell lines which had been cleaned up or had been derived from a source where they weren't infected were unable to produce NKCF. Therefore I really don't think that the issue of an inhibitor is a problem.

S. Wright: After studying a large number of cell lines, I find that many different kinds of mycoplasma-free lines can stimulate the production of NKCF. The basis for the contention that mycoplasma-infected lines stimulate the production of factors is not clear to me. According to data you've published, regarding the supernatants that are produced using mycoplasma-infected stimulators, you concluded that the cytotoxic activity was due mainly to the presence of mycoplasma organisms, since they could be removed by filtration or centrifugation. The biochemical data that I will present tomorrow show clearly that NKCF activity is due to a soluble protein or glycoprotein. So I think its not clear whether any NKCF at all is produced when you use mycoplasma infected cells.

C. Brooks: Well, in fact, we could only remove about half the activity by filtration, and the remaining activity was clearly not mycoplasma. We suggested that in view of the very potent mitogenicity of some of the strains of mycoplasma that infect these cells, one could easily get induction of various kinds of T cell products, for instance, that might be toxic in long term assays.

J. Ortaldo: I think there are a number of problems with what you're saying, one of which is alluded to on your slide. In the human system, and I think its the same in the mouse system, serum is a very potent inhibitor of NKCF. In your experiment, you have 5% serum in your assays, at least as I read your slide. I'll present data tomorrow, and Steph Targan has already published similar data, showing that serum in an assay can inhibit virtually all the NKCF activity. I don't know why, but it certainly does.

My second point concerns your argument about the kinetics of NKCF. We and Susan have similar data regarding purification. We can show lysis in 6 hours with highly purified NKCF. So I think that your arguments about it not being involved boil down to a matter of concentration.

I would not, however, argue against the contention that mycoplasma-infected targets may be a better stimulus, because many people have shown that mycoplasma-infected targets are better targets. But that doesn't say that in the absence of mycoplasma, you don't see lysis of that target or factor production.

Moreover, I don't think you can disregard the fact that PHA and Con A, with highly purified natural killer cells, both from the mouse and the human, produce this factor. So although some of your arguments are certainly valid, I don't think its an all-or-none situation, but a more quantitative issue.

C. Brooks: We've done many experiments using exactly the protocols that have been published using serum-free medium. And I should point out that the first 3 papers that were published on the NKCF phenomenon used serum in the medium, in fact, they were Marbrook culture systems.

In regard to the issue of mitogens inducing NKCF, I really haven't seen any data, except that's not been published, that shows that those factors derive from NK cells. This argument is absolutely critical, because there's no doubt that mitogens will induce cytotoxic factors from T cells. This is the lymphotoxin that Granger described years ago. So one really has to be extraordinarily careful when one is using mitogens. Especially in the long terms cultures that are used for assay of NKCF, mitogens themselves, in trace amounts, can be toxic to the tumor cells.

J. Hiserodt: In all the papers I've read on cytotoxic factor protein, the production is very dependent on responder/stimulator cell ratio, for a reason that we don't really know. But, I'm wondering if you've tried production with your clone at different ratios.

C. Brooks: We have done experiments over a wide range of cell ratios both with clones and spleen cells. I take your point, but we just simply haven't seen that.

ANALYSIS OF SEQUENTIAL SUBSTAGES OF THE NATURAL KILLER CELL LETHAL HIT

Richard L. Deem and Stephan R. Targan

Geriatric Research Education and Clinical Center Wadsworth
Veterans Administration Medical Center, Los Angeles, CA
90024 and Departments of Medicine and Microbiology and
Immunology, University of California, Los Angeles, CA 90024

INTRODUCTION

Previous studies have shown that NK cytotoxicity can be resolved
into several stages: NK-target cell binding, triggering, programming,
and killer cell independent lysis (KCIL)(1, 2). NK cells produce
soluble cytolytic factors (NKCF), which can lyse NK-sensitive targets
and have been used as another measure of the NK lethal hit (3, 4).
Since KCIL and NKCF-mediated cytolysis are independent of the NK cell,
and are inhibited by PGE_2 (5), low temperatue (1), and trypsin (6), it
was postulated that the target cell membrane probably played a crucial
role during the NK lethal hit. Several hypotheses were proposed to
explain these results. [1] Membrane fluidity/movement may play a role
in channel formation by the NK lytic complex. [2] Membrane movement
or endocytosis, requiring intact metabolic and energy transfer pathways, may be required for completion of the lethal hit. [3] Enzymatic
activity, either from target cell enzymes or a function of the NK
lytic complex itself, may be a necessary substage of the NK lethal
hit. These hypotheses were tested in this study with specific membrane crosslinking/fluidizing agents, inhibitors of energy metabolism,
and inhibitors of protease activity.

RESULTS AND DISCUSSION

Kinetic Model for the NK Lethal Hit

Glutaraldehyde, a bifunctional protein crosslinking reagent, was
chosen to examine the role of membrane movement/fluidity during the NK
lethal hit. The calcium pulse assay (1) demonstrated that 1 mM

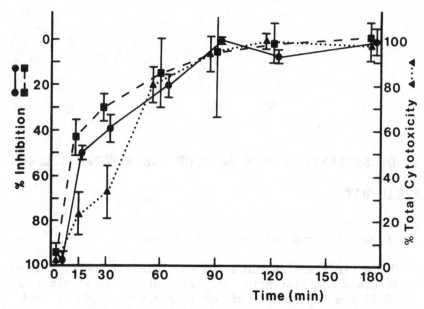

Figure 1. Kinetics of inhibition of cytolysis by 1 mM glutaraldehyde.
PBL and K562 targets were mixed at 30:1 E:T ratio and were incubated
in EGTA/Mg^{++} for 30 min at 37°C. CaCl$_2$ was then added followed at
various times by addition of (●) 10 mM EDTA or (■) 1 mM glutaraldehyde, and incubated for a total time of 3 hr. (▲) % of maximum
cytotoxicity, where maximum cytotoxicity was 45%. Bars represent SD.

glutaraldehyde inhibited cytolysis of K562 target cells at the same
level as EDTA, indicating that it blocked the programming stage of NK
cytolysis (Fig. 1). When 100 uM glutaraldehyde was added into an NKCF
assay (6), cytolysis of L929 target cells was inhibited (7). Pretreatment of L929 target cells but not pretreatment of NKCF with 100
uM glutaraldehyde inhibited NKCF-mediated cytolysis (7), indicating
that glutaraldehyde was affecting the target cell directly. The cold
target competition assay (6) was performed to determine if glutaraldehyde was altering the NKCF receptor. Glutaraldehyde pretreated K562
and L929 cold target cells were not able to compete as well as untreated cold target cells to inhibit lysis of labeled L929 targets
(Fig. 2). To comfirm these results, cold target absorption of NKCF
was performed at 4°C, to eliminate the possibility that glutaraldehyde
was inhibiting endocytic uptake of NKCF. Again, glutaraldehyde pretreated K562 target cells were not able to absorb NKCF activity as
well as untreated target cells (Fig. 3). Thus, the earliest substage
of the NK lethal hit, lytic complex/NKCF binding, was inhibited by
glutaraldehyde. This inhibition was due to its direct crosslinking
effect upon the NKCF receptor.

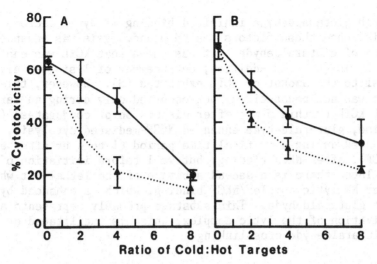

Figure 2. Cold target competition of L929 target cells with A, L929 cold target cells and B, K562 cold target cells. (▲), untreated cold target cells; (●), cold target cells pretreated 2 hr with 100 uM glutaraldehyde. Bars represent SD.

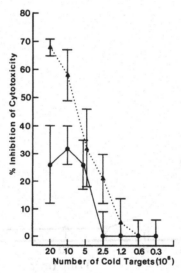

Figure 3. Inhibition of cytotoxicity by cold target absorption of NKCF with untreated and glutaraldehyde pretreated K562 target cells. Cold K562 targets were untreated or incubated in 100 uM glutaraldehyde for 2 hr at 37°C. Cold targets were washed 3 times and increasing numbers (in 450 ul) were added to 300 ul NKCF and incubated 5 hr at 4°C. The centrifuged supernatants were diluted and added to labeled L929 target cells for 18 hr. (▲), control K562 cold targets; (●), glutaraldehyde pretreated K562 cold targets. Control cytotoxicity was 20 ± 2%. Bars represent SD.

Although glutaraldehyde inhibited binding of lytic factors to target cells, once these factors became bound, lysis was enhanced by the addition of glutaraldehyde. It was shown that KCIL was enhanced by 13 ± 3% lysis (8). In addition, enhancement of lysis was directly proportional to the amount of KCIL exhibited (8). However, this enhancement was not nonspecific, but occurred only during an early substage of KCIL (within 5 min after dispersion of conjugates) (Fig. 4). Likewise, glutaraldehyde enhanced NKCF-mediated cytolysis, but only when added during a critical time period (1 to 4 hr after addition of NKCF), after NKCF binding, but well before initiation of lysis (Fig. 5). Thus, there is a second substage of the lethal hit which occurs after NK lytic complex/NKCF binding, which is enhanced by the addition of glutaraldehyde. This substage probably represents assembly or activation of the lytic complex, which is facilitated or stabilized by glutaraldehyde crosslinking.

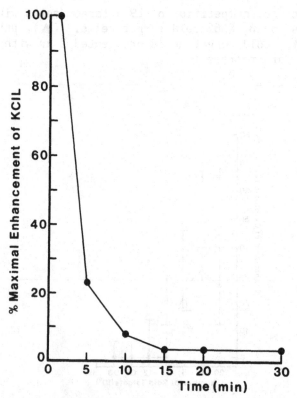

Figure 4. Kinetics of enhancement of KCIL by glutaraldehyde after dispersion of conjugates. PBL and K562 targets were mixed at 40:1 E:T ratio and incubated in EGTA/Mg^{++} for 30 min at 37°C, followed by addition of CaCl$_2$ for 20 min. Glutaraldehyde (1 mM) was added at various times after dispersion of conjugates and percent cytotoxicity was determined after a total incubation time of 90 min. Maximal enhancement of KCIL was 13%.

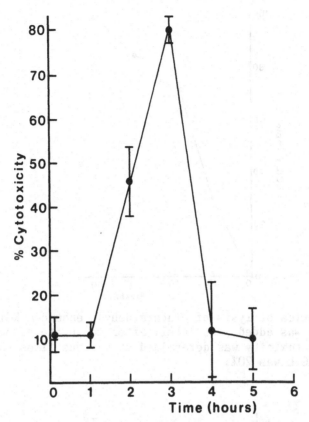

Figure 5. Critical time for enhancement of NKCF-mediated cytolysis by glutaraldehyde. NKCF (180 ul) was added to L929 target cells followed by addition of 20 ul of 200 uM glutaraldehyde (final concentration 20 uM) at hourly intervals. Control lysis (no glutaraldehyde added) was 8 ± 3%. Bars represent standard deviation.

It has been hypothesized that NKCF lacks a focusing molecule of the assembled NK lytic complex, and that this deficiency accounts for the slow rate of lysis of NKCF compared to direct NK cytolysis (6). It is possible that glutaraldehyde may act to replace the function of the focusing molecule by crosslinking membrane-bound NKCF into a more effective lytic complex. Alternatively, glutaraldehyde may stabilize membrane-bound NKCF to increase the number of effective lesions produced. It has been shown that glutaraldehyde can stabilize lymphotoxin (9), and although it does not stabilize free NKCF (7), it may stabilize NKCF once it becomes bound to the target cell membrane.

Following the glutaraldehyde enhanceable stage is a stage during which little or no lysis occurs, and yet glutaraldehyde is unable to enhance lysis. In KCIL, this stage occurs 5 to 15 min after dispersion of target-effector conjugates (Fig. 4 & 6). In an L929 assay, this effector stage occurs 5 to 10 hr after addition of NKCF (Fig. 5).

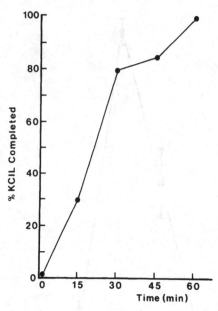

Figure 6. Kinetics of lysis of glutaraldehyde enhanced KCIL. Glutaraldehyde (1 mM) was added immediately after conjugate dispersion and the percent cytotoxicity was determined at various times thereafter. Total percent KCIL was 20%.

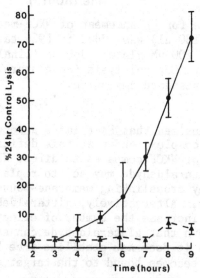

Figure 7. Kinetics of NKCF-mediated cytolysis with and without glutaraldehyde. NKCF (180 ul) was bound to L929 target cells for 2 hr at 37°C, followed by addition of either (▲) 20 ul media or (●) 20 ul 100 uM glutaraldehyde (final concentration 10 uM). Wells were harvested at hourly intervals. 24 hr conrol lysis was 43 ± 3%. Bars represent SD.

The terminal stage of the NK lethal hit, the lysis stage, is also unaffected by glutaraldehyde. In KCIL, the majority of lysis occurs between 15 and 30 min after conjugate dispersion and is completed by 45 min (Fig. 6). Thus, the kinetics of lysis of glutaraldehyde-enhanced KCIL are nearly identical to the kinetics of KCIL without the addition of glutaraldehyde (1). NKCF-mediated lysis is much slower, with nearly all lysis occurring 11 to 14 hr after addition of NKCF (data not shown). However, glutaraldehyde can significantly accelerate the rate of NKCF-mediated lysis (Fig. 7), indicating that its effects may represent more than simple stabilization of membrane-bound NKCF.

In summary, the NK lethal hit can be divided into 4 substages based upon modulation by glutaraldehyde (Table 1). The first substage, the lytic factor binding stage, is inhibited by glutaraldehyde. Although programming for lysis was inhibited by addition of glutaraldehyde, it has not be determined if this was due to inhibition of triggering, inhibition of lytic factor release or alteration of the lytic factor binding receptor. It is clear that glutaraldehyde blocks NKCF-mediated lysis early by crosslinking the NKCF receptor to prevent NKCF binding. The second substage, assembly/activation, occurs immediately after lytic factor binding (the beginning of KCIL or 2 hr after addition of NKCF) and is enhanced by glutaraldehyde. This enhancement of lysis is specific and is directly related to the crosslinking time of various concentrations of glutaraldehyde (8). Following this stage is the effector substage, during which little or no lysis occurs, but is not affected by glutaraldehyde. The terminal stage of the NK lethal hit, lysis, is also unaffected by glutaraldehyde.

Table 1. Functional Substages of the NK Lethal Hit

Substage	NKCF-mediated Cytolysis		Killer Cell Independent Lysis	
	Time (hr)	Glut. Effect	Time (min)	Glut. Effect
1. Binding	0 - 2	inhibits	n/a	inhibits?
2. Assembly/ Activation	2 - 5	enhances	0 - 5	enhances
3. Effector	5 - 10	none	5 - 15	none
4. Lysis	10 - 15	none	15 - 45	none

Analysis of Chemical Crosslinking-Mediated Enhancement of the NK Lethal Hit

In order to analyze the mechanism by which glutaraldehyde enhanced lysis of the assembly/activation substage of the NK lethal hit, several specific chemical crosslinking reagents were chosen for study. Low concentrations of glutaraldehyde enhanced KCIL and NKCF-mediated cytolysis but had no effect upon NKCF binding (although higher concentrations of glutaraldehyde inhibited NKCF binding) (Table 2). Malonaldehyde, a bifunctional crosslinking aldehyde, also enhanced NKCF-mediated cytolysis, but had no effect upon KCIL (Table 2). Malonaldehyde is a smaller molecule than glutaraldehyde and crosslinks over shorter distances. In addition, it crosslinks more slowly and less effectively than glutaraldehyde (10). This probably accounts for malonaldehyde's lack of enhancement of KCIL, since the critical time period for enhancement of KCIL is only 5 min. Monofunctional aldehydes also crosslink slowly and incompletely (10). Thus, formaldehyde and acetaldehyde had little or no effect upon KCIL or NKCF-mediated cytolysis (Table 2). Crotonaldehyde, a monofunctional unsaturated molecule, is more reactive than other monofunctional aldehydes (11), but had no effect upon KCIL, although it did inhibit NKCF-mediated lysis (Table 2). The noncrosslinking aldehydes, butryaldehyde and valeraldehyde, had no effect upon KCIL or NKCF-mediated cytolysis (Table 2). Thus, it appears that crosslinking and not just the presence of an aldehyde functional group is required for enhancement of lysis during the NK lethal hit. It is also likely that the speed of crosslinking is important and that a certain minimum crosslinking distance may be required for enhancement of the lethal hit (The bifunctional reagents crosslink more effectively and over a longer distance than monofunctional reagents and enhance lysis more effectively.).

Although glutaraldehyde crosslinks primary amino groups, particularly lysine, it can also crosslink other functional groups, such as tyrosyl, histidyl, and sulfhydryl groups (12). Because of this lack of specificity by aldehyde crosslinking reagents, more specific reagents were tested. The bis-imidates are very specific protein crosslinking reagents which react only with primary amino groups (13). All the bis-imidates tested, dimethyl suberimidate, dimethyl pimelimidate, and dimethyl adipimidate, enhanced KCIL slightly but inconsistantly. This is probably due to the reaction rate of the imidates with proteins. Although the imidates react within a few minutes, the intermediate products which are formed, have a half life of 5 to 30 min (13). Thus, it is likely that most cross-links are not formed during the first critical 5 minutes of KCIL. However, all the bis-imidates tested enhanced NKCF-mediated cytolysis nearly as well as glutaraldehyde.

Osmium tetroxide enhanced KCIL, although variably, and inhibited NKCF-mediated cytolysis, probably by affecting the NKCF receptor

Table 2. Effect of Crosslinkers Upon NKCF-Mediated Cytolysis and KCIL

Concentration	Reagent	Primary Crosslinking Specificity	% Change From Control		
			NKCF +[a] Pretreated L929	NKCF +[a] Reagent	Reagent[b] in KCIL
10 uM	Glutaraldehyde	a-amino, lysine	0 ± 6	190 ± 10	209 ± 20
4 mM	Malonaldehyde	a-amino	-1 ± 7	177 ± 9	-32 ± 14
170 uM	Formaldehyde	a-amino	0 ± 6	19 ± 9	7 ± 22
2.3 mM	Acetaldehyde	a-amino	-10 ± 4	35 ± 8	-18 ± 26
140 uM	Crotonaldehyde	a-amino	-65 ± 3	-42 ± 7	12 ± 19
1.4 mM	Butryaldehyde	none	-6 ± 7	13 ± 3	-23 ± 18
1.2 mM	Valeraldehyde	none	-5 ± 3	-10 ± 6	8 ± 32
1.8 mM	Dimethyl Suberimidate	a-amino	3 ± 10	190 ± 18	44 ± 20
1.9 mM	Dimethyl Pimelimidate	a-amino	135 ± 21	161 ± 6	25 ± 50
2.0 mM	Dimethyl Adipimidate	a-amino	3 ± 7	139 ± 10	26 ± 29
40 uM	Osmium tetroxide	unsaturated lipids	-55 ± 11	-71 ± 6	125 ± 52
10 ug/ml	Concanavalin A	D-glucose, D-mannose	77 ± 7	168 ± 9	4 ± 34
10 ug/ml	Wheat Germ Agglutinin	N-acetyl-D-glucosamine	61 ± 12	135 ± 12	ND
100 ug/ml	Peanut Agglutinin	D-galactose	ND	-1 ± 6	ND
100 ug/ml	Soy Bean Agglutinin	D-galactose, N-acetyl-D-galactosamine	ND	-2 ± 3	ND

[a] Mean ± S.E.M. for 3 experiments. Control cytotoxicity was 31 ± 3%.
[b] Mean ± S.E.M. for 3 to 35 experiments. Control KCIL was 10.5 ± 1.4%.

(Table 2). Although osmium tetroxide primarily crosslinks unsaturated lipids, it can crosslink or cleave (by oxidation) proteins (14), and is especially reactive toward the amino acids tryptophan, cysteine, and histidine (15). Therefore, whether or not lipid crosslinking is involved during enhancement of the lethal hit remains to be determined.

Lectins can crosslink biological membranes by binding to glycoproteins. Concanavalin A (con A) (specificity: D-mannose, D-glucose) did not enhance KCIL (Table 2), but this would be expected, since its crosslinking activity requires Ca^{++} and Mn^{++} (16), which are removed during the EDTA dispersion technique. However, NKCF-mediated cytolysis was enhanced significantly (Table 2). Likewise, wheat germ agglutinin (WGA) (specificity: N-acetyl-D-glucosamine) enhanced NKCF-mediated lysis, whereas lectins with specificty for D-galactose, peanut agglutinin (PNA) and soybean agglutinin (SBA) had no effect (Table 2). It should be noted that pretreatment of L929 target cells with con A or WGA also enhanced NKCF-mediated lysis (Table 2). This enhancement was not due to enhanced NKCF binding by these lectin crosslinked targets, since lectin pretreated cold target cells were not more effective than control cold targets in a cold target competition assay (data not shown). Thus, it appears that crosslinking of the target cell membrane with specificity for glucose residues may be important during enhancement of the lethal hit.

These data suggest that enhancement of NKCF-mediated lysis probably results from crosslinking of proteins or glycoproteins on the target cell membrane. Since pretreatment with some crosslinking reagents resulted in enhancement of cytolysis, it is possible that generalized crosslinking of the membrane may in some way facilitate the action of NKCF.

Effect of Pharmacologic Agents Upon Substages of the NK Lethal Hit

As noted previously, the lytic factor binding stage is inhibited by crosslinking agents, which can modify the NKCF receptor. These reagents include glutaraldehyde, osmium tetroxide, and crotonaldehyde.

Reagents that break disulfide bonds, such as 2-mercaptoethanol (2-ME) and dithiothietol (DTT), inhibited NKCF-mediated lysis nearly completely and KCIL partially (Table 3). In addition, 2-ME inhibits beyond calcium-dependent events in a calcium pulse assay, suggesting that 2-ME inhibits at a very early stage of KCIL (5). Kinetic addition of 2-ME into an L929 assay showed that inhibition of lysis decreased almost immediately after addition of NKCF, indicating that these reagents affect an early process of NKCF-mediated lysis (Fig. 8). This early inhibition is even more evident during glutaraldehyde enhanced NKCF-mediated lysis, where inhibition decreased from nearly 100% to less than 10% in 5 hr (Fig. 9). Thus, it appears that 2-ME

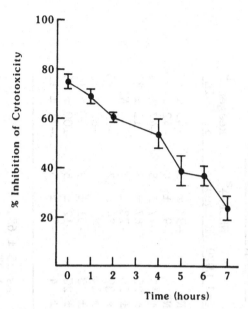

Figure 8. Kinetics of inhibition of NKCF-mediated cytolysis by 5 mM 2-ME. NKCF was added to labeled L929 target cells followed at various times by addition of 2-ME. All wells were harvested at 18 hr. Bars represent SD.

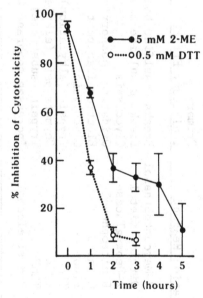

Figure 9. Kinetics of inhibition of glutaraldehyde-enhanced NKCF-mediated cytolysis by 5 mM 2-ME and 0.5 mM DTT. NKCF was bound to L929 target cells for 2 hr followed by removal of NKCF and addition of 10 mM glutaraldehyde. 2-ME and DTT were added at hourly intervals and all wells were harvested at 18 hr. Bars represent SD.

Table 3. Effect of Pharmacologic Mediators Upon NKCF-Mediated Cytolysis and KCIL

Concentration Reagent	Primary Inhibitory Effect	% Change From Control		
		NKCF +[a] Pretreated L929	NKCF +[a] Reagent	Reagent[b] in KCIL
5.0 mM 2-Mercaptoethanol	Breaks disulfide bonds	ND	-97 ± 3	-45 ± 12
0.5 mM Dithiothrietol	Breaks disulfide bonds	ND	-95 ± 4	-42 ± 14
50 mM 2-Deoxyglucose	Glycolysis	-33 ± 15	-77 ± 5	-47 ± 12
10 mM Dinitrophenol	Oxidative Phosporylation	6 ± 20	-67 ± 7	12 ± 23
1.0 mM Cyanide	Electron Transport	-40 ± 16	-73 ± 7	ND
50 mM Fluoride	Glycolysis	19 ± 39	-34 ± 12	-23 ± 15
0.5 mM TLCK	Trypsin (alkylation)	-32 ± 14	-88 ± 9	-80 ± 23
0.5 mM TPCK	Chymotrypsin (alkylation)	-25 ± 8	-51 ± 9	-90 ± 15
0.5 mM TLME	Trypsin (substrate)	-31 ± 20	-12 ± 5	-100 ± 49
12 mM Benzyl alcohol	Increases membrane fluidity	0 ± 4	-99 ± 5	-71 ± 12

[a]Mean ± S.E.M. for 3 to 10 experiments. Control cytotoxicity was 35 ± 6%.
[b]Mean ± S.E.M. for 3 to 8 experiments. Control KCIL was 11.2 ± 1.7%.

and DTT inhibit during an early phase of the assembly/activation substage. Since KCIL is so rapid, it seems likely that these reagents do
not totally inhibit KCIL because this stage occurs within minutes
after conjugate dispersion.

To test whether intact energy metabolic processes are required in
the target cell during the NK lethal hit, several inhibitors of glycolysis, oxidative phosphorylation and electron transport were chosen
for study. These inhibitors had little or no effect upon KCIL,
probably beacause depletion of intracellular ATP levels requires
several hours (17), whereas KCIL is completed within 45 min. All the
reagents tested inhibited NKCF-mediated cytolysis 30 to 80%. The
effects of pretreatment of L929 target cells with dinitrophenol (DNP)
and fluoride were totally reversible, whereas the effects of 2-deoxy-
glucose and cyanide were only partially reversible. Analysis of the
kinetics of inhibition of these metabolic inhibitors has shown that
they inhibit maximally through 4 hr (data not shown). Thus, they
probably inhibit until late in the assembly/activation substage of the
lethal hit, although this is uncertain because of the delay of action
of these agents. Thus, it seems likely that some energy requiring
process is involved during completion of the lethal hit. This process
may require membrane movement or endocytosis of the lytic complex.

It has been shown that inhibitors of serine protease activity can
inhibit CTL cytotoxicity (18) and ADCC (19), but the stage at which
these inhibitors act has not been adequately defined. All inhibitors
of serine protease activity tested in this study, TLCK, TPCK, and TLME
inhibited KCIL nearly completely. TLCK and TPCK (irreversible alkylating agents) inhibited NKCF-mediated lysis, whereas the competitive
trypsin inhibitor, TLME, had little effect. Pretreatment of L929
target cells with these inhibitors partially inhibited NKCF-mediated
cytotoxicity, indicating that a target cell originating protease may
be involved in the lethal hit. In addition, it has been found that
pretreatment of NKCF with these inhibitors and dialysis had no effect
upon its ability to lyse L929 target cells. Kinetic analysis of
inhibition of NKCF-mediated lysis has shown that TLCK inhibits maximally through 6 hr and continues to inhibit until the beginning of
lysis (data not shown). These data suggest that protease activity is
require late in the NK lethal hit, probably during the effector
substage.

Since crosslinking of the target cell membrane resulted in
enhancement of the lethal hit, it was postulated that the opposite
effect, increasing membrane fluidty, might inhibit the NK lethal hit.
The neutral anesthetic, benzyl alcohol was chosen because of its
specific fluidizing effect upon the lipid bilayer of biological
membranes (20). This reagent inhibited direct NK cytotoxicity completely, although pretreatment of target or effector cells had no
effect (data not shown). Likewise, both KCIL and NKCF-mediated lysis
were inhibited, and pretreatment of L929 target cells had no effect

upon NKCF-mediated lysis (Table 3). Analysis of the kinetics of
inhibition of benzyl alcohol showed that it completely inhibited
NKCF-mediated cytolysis through 8 hr (data not shown). In addition, a
benzyl alcohol pulse experiment has shown that addition (for up to 5
hours) and removal of benzyl alcohol to L929 targets prebound 2 hr
with NKCF had no effect upon subsequent lysis. Thus, benzyl alcohol
effects only the late substages of the NK lethal hit (effector and
lysis substages). Since NK lysis may involve formation of transmembrane channels (21), it is possible that benzyl alcohol's fluidizing
effect may disrupt these channels to prevent lysis. Alternatively,
benzyl alcohol may inhibit some required enzymatic activity by
changing conformations of integral membrane proteins, as has been
shown to occur for the enzyme adenylate cyclase (22). In addition,
benzyl alcohol has been shown to inhibit fusion of endocytic vesicles
(23), which may be required for completion of the lethal hit.

CONCLUSIONS

The terminal stage of the NK cytolysis has been studied kinetically using KCIL and NKCF-mediated cytolysis. There appear to be at
least 4 substages of the lethal hit based upon modulation by pharmacologic agents (Fig. 10). The binding substage is inhibited only
early by certain crosslinking reagents. Immediately after binding is
the assembly/activation substage, which is inhibited early by agents
that break disulfide bonds. In addition, chemical crosslinking agents

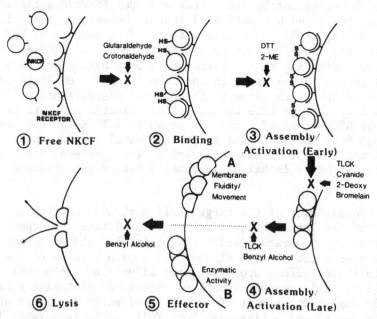

Figure 10. Model for substages of the NK lethal hit.

enhance lysis at this substage, suggesting that complex formation or polymerization of subunits may be required for completion of the lethal hit. Inhibitors of energy metabolism inhibit late in this substage, suggesting a role for membrane movement/endocytosis. The effector substage is inhibited by inhibitors of serine protease activity, suggesting a role for enzymatic activity during the later substages of the lethal hit. The effector and lysis substages are inhibited by benzyl alcohol, which may inhibit by fluidizing the membrane to disrupt NK lytic factor-induced transmembrane channels.

ACKNOWLEDGEMENTS

We wish to thank Dr. Michael D. Brogan for his contribution on the effect of protease inhibitors upon the NK lethal hit and Adrene Niederlehner for her contribution on the effect of inhibitors of energy metabolism upon the NK lethal hit.

REFERENCES

1. Hiserodt, J.C., L.J. Britvan, and S.R. Targan. 1982. Characterization of the cytolytic reaction mechanism of the human natural killer (NK) lymphocyte: resolution into binding, programming, and killer cell-independent steps. J. Immunol. 129: 1782.
2. Targan, S.R. and W. Newman. 1983. Definition of a "Trigger" stage in the NK cytolytic reaction sequence by a monoclonal antibody to the glycoprotein T-200. J. Immunol. 131: 1149.
3. Wright, S.C. and B. Bonavida. 1982. Studies on the mechanism of natural killer (NK) cell-mediated cytotoxicity (CMC). I. Release of cytotoxic factors specific for NK-sensitive target cells (NKCF) during co-culture of NK effector cells with NK target cells. J. Immunol. 129: 433.
4. Farrum, E. and S.R. Targan. 1983. Identification of human natural killer soluble factors (NKCF) derived from NK-enriched lymphocyte populations: specificity of generation and killing. J. Immunol. 130: 1252.
5. Hiserodt, J.C., L. Britvan, and S.R. Targan. 1982. Differential effects of various pharmocologic agents on the cytolytic reaction mechanism of the human natural killer lymphocyte: further resolution of programming for lysis and KCIL into discrete stages. J. Immunol. 129: 2266.
6. Hiserodt, J.C., L. Britvan, and S.R. Targan. 1983. Studies on the mechanism of the human natural killer cell lethal hit: analysis of the mechanism of protease inhibition of the lethal hit. J. Immunol. 131: 2705.
7. Deem, R.L. and S.R. Targan. 1984. Sequential substages of natural killer cell-derived cytolytic factor (NKCF)-mediated cytolysis as defined by glutaraldehyde modulation of the target cell. J. Immunol. 133: in press.

8. Deem, R.L. and S.R. Targan. 1984. Evidence of a dynamic role of the target cell membrane during the early stages of the natural killer cell lethal hit. J. Immunol. **133**: in press.

9. Devlin, J.J., R.S. Yamamoto, and G.A. Granger. 1981. Stabilization and functional studies of high-molecular weight murine lymphotoxins. Cell. Immunol. **61**: 22.

10. Bowes, J.H. and C.W. Cater. 1965. The reaction of glutaraldehyde with proteins and other biological materials. J. Roy. Micro. Soc. **85**: 193

11. Flitney, F.W. 1965. The time course of fixation of albumin by formaldehyde, glutaraldehyde, acrolein and other higher aldehydes. J. Roy. Micro. Soc. **85**:353.

12. Richards, F.M. and J.R. Knowles. 1968. Glutaraldehyde as a protein cross-linking reagent. J. Mol. Biol. **37**: 231.

13. Peters, K. and F.M. Knowles. 1977. Chemical cross-linking: reagents and problems in studies of membrane structure. Ann. Rev. Biochem. **46**: 523.

14. Hopwood, D. 1969. Fixation of proteins by osmium tetroxide, potassium dichromate and potassium permanganate. Histochimie **18**: 250

15. Bahr, G.F. 1954. Osmium tetroxide and ruthenium tetroxide and their reactions with biologically important substances. Exptl. Cell Res. **7**: 457.

16. Goldstein, I.J. and C.E. Hayes. 1976. The lectins: carbohydrate-binding proteins of plants and animals. Arch. Biochem. Biophys. **173**: 127.

17. Silverstein, S.C., R.M. Steinman, and Z.A. Cohn. 1977. Endocytosis. Ann. Rev. Biochem. **46**: 669.

18. Chang, T.W. and H.E. Eisen. 1980. Effects of N-tosyl-L-lysyl-chloromethylketone on the activity of cytotoxic T lymphocytes. J. Immunol. **124**: 1028.

19. Trinchieri, G. and M. DeMarchi. 1976. Antibody dependent cell-mediated cytotoxicity in humans. III. Effect of protease inhibitors and substrates. J. Immunol. **116**: 885.

20. T. Shibata, Y. Sugiura, and S. Iwayanagi. 1982. Effects of benzyl alcohol on phosphatidylcholine lamellar phase with different water contents. Chem. Phys. Lipids **31**: 105.

21. Podack, E.R. and G. Dennert. 1983. Assembly of two types of tubules with putative cytolytic function by cloned natural killer cells. Nature **302**: 442.

22. Needham, L., A.D. Whetton, and M.D. Houslay. 1982. The local anaesthetic and bilayer fluidizing agent, benzyl alcohol decreases the thermostability of the integral membrane protein adenylate cyclase. FEBS Lett. **140**: 85.

23. Tolleshaug, H. and T. Berg. 1982. Evidence for the selective inhibition of fusion between endocytic vesicles and lysosomes by benzyl alcohol. Biochem. Pharmac. **31**: 593.

DISCUSSION

Adams: Do you think that the NKCF binding site is internalized and goes through the endosome-lysosome cycle? This would be supported by your data and Ortaldo's data that the binding is very low at 4° and that you get significant uptake only at 37°. Have you looked at lysosome-active agents to see if they block uptake?

Targan: We have looked with monensin and this does indeed block. We are now looking to see if we can bypass this after it has been taken up. But it also possible that it is uptake.

Adams: It is possible that the agent acts on the membrane but is broken down in the lysosomes.

Herberman: Any comments on the uptake question from those studying channel formation?

Young: There is precedent with certain toxins for a requirement for internalization and acidification.

Bhakdi: One has to dinstinguish between the channels which form after acidification with diptheria toxin and the channels formed by complement and probably lymphocyte granules. There is a different mechanism here, and we have only data on elimination of the complement channels from Mayer's lab which could be due to an endosomal process. But all this awaits further experimentation.

Young: There probably differences in channel structure in the two situations.

Podack: With regard to temperature dependence, I would like to mention that C9 polymerization is strongly temperature dependent. Below 20° it is not measurable. So the assembly of cytolysins themselves can be temperature dependent.

Berke: The temperature effects and the inhibitors such as cyanide bear on the question of whether NKCF induces a selective ionic permeability increase or a large pore which is non-specific. If the latter were the case, such temperature or cyanide effects would not be predicted. If low temperatures were blocking the assembly of pore structures, this should be observable in the electron microscope.

Podack: Others have shown that once the poly C9 channel is formed, you can drop the temperature and you will not close the channel.

Berke: Yet efflux of cellular constitutents of nucleated cells drops, as I will show tomorrow.

Brooks: I am confused by John Ortaldo's statement that NKCF is very sensitive to serum, while your NKCF is generated and asayed in 10% serum. So what is the relationship of your NKCF to his?

Targan: In my lab we have made NKCF with and without serum, and it seems to be dependent on the batch. I suspect that the human NKCF's studied by the three labs are similar.

Brooks: Is anything that kills K562 an NKCF?

Targan: NKCF has its own specificity which is similar to NK cells. As the biochemical work progresses it should be possible to make a more meaningful comparison.

Reynolds: You have hypothesized that glutaraldehyde crosslinks target cell surface molecules. Is it possible that glutaraldehyde inhibits target cell repair processes so they cannot repair the damage?

Targan: We thought this was a possibility before we studied the kinetics, but because of the timing we observe we regard this as unlikely.

Sitkovsky: Is there a correlation between membrane crosslinking by SDS gels and the effect you describe?

Targan: All we have done is to look at the ability of the cells to patch and cap, and here we do see a correlation.

THE LIPOXYGENASE PATHWAY IN THE HUMAN NK CELL SYSTEM

Mikael Jondal, Charlotte Kullman, Jan-Åke Lindgren*and
Paolo Rossi
Department of Immunology
*Department of Physiological Chemistry
Karolinska Institutet, 104 01 Stockholm, Sweden

INTRODUCTION

Induction of cell-mediated cytotoxicity requires trans-membrane
signalling as in other lymphocyte activation systems. Earlier
studies have pointed to the importance of arachidonic acid (AA)
metabolites in regulating different cytotxicity systems (1-4a+4b).
In the human NK cell system Seaman recently showed that antagonists
of lipoxygenation such as nordihydroquaiaretic acid (NDGA) and
3-amino-1-m-(trifluoromethyl)-phenyl-2-pyrazoline (BW 755C) rapidly
supress killing (5) and Suthanthiran et al that other anti-oxidants
which scavenge hydroxyl radicals are suppressive (6). Hattori
et al have demonstrated that purified lipomodulin, which selectivly
inhibit phospholipase A_2 activity, also inhibit NK cell killing
(7). Using virally infected adenoma cells as target cells, Rola-
Pleszynski demonstrated induction of NK cell activity with leukotriene B_4 (LTB_4) (8).

In the T cell system the importance of the lipoxygenase pathways
have been suggested by several different observations. Interlukin 1
dependent, mitogen induced thymocyte proliferation depends on intact lipoxygenase activity (9) as does T lymphocyte migration (10)
and induction of T cell suppressor activity (11). Goetzl have reported
that T lymphocytes produce products of the 5-lipoxygenase pathway
such as 5-HETE and LTB_4 (12) using freshly isolated and purified
human T lymphocytes. However, the purity of the used cell populations
(between 77-86% as estimated by surface markers) may not be sufficient to conclusively determine the location of this metabolic
pathway. The unequivocal demonstration of lipoxygenase products in
normal lymphoid cells, i.e. cloned and growth factor propagated,
is still missing.

AA can be metabolized either into prostaglandins and thromboxanes through the cyclooxygenase pathway or into different lipoxygenase products including H (P)ETE) acids and leukotriens $LTA_4-B_4-C_4-D_4-E_4$ (13). Cyclooxygenase products such as prostaglandins are in general considered immunosuppressive through the induction of cyclic AMP via external cell surface receptors (14, 15). There is no convincing data that cyclooxygenase activity is necessary for NK cell activity. However, as mentioned above, lipoxygenation of AA appears to be involved in the activation of both NK cells and other lymphocyte functions. During trans-membrane signalling the release of AA is linked to an increase in membrane phospholipid turn-over, Ca^{2+} mobilization and increased levels of cyclic GMP (cGMP) (16). AA can be released from the membrane either from inositol phospholipid through phospholipase C and diacylglycerol lipase activation or from phosphatidylcholine and phosphatidyethanolamine through phospholipase A_2 cleavage (16). Alternatively AA may be taken up from external sources, T lymphocytes release AA during activation which may be used by monocytes for the production of eicosanoids (17).

Lipoxygenation of AA occur at sites adjacent to the double bonds present in the molecule, in human leucocytes at C-5, C-12 and C-15 leading to formation of unstable HPETE and more stable HETE acids (13). The unstable epoxide LTA_4 is consequently metabolized either into the $LTC_4-D_4-E_4$ pathway or into LTB_4 and related products. LTB_4 has potent chemotactic properties (18, 19), increase leukocyte adherence (20) and degranulate neutrophilic cells at low concentrations (19, 21).

In the present work we have approached the following questions.
1) Are the lipoxygenase inhibitors used active at specific concentrations and can NK cell activity thus be reconstituted into the system with purified lipoxygenase products ?
2) Which lipoxygenase products are needed for the triggering event ?
3) What metabolic step is controlled by those metabolites ?,
4) Is NK-like killing mediated by herpesvirus Ateles transformed T cell lines (22a), inhibited by NDGA to the same extent as normal NK cells ? If so, this would indicate that lipoxygenation occurs in NK effector cells and not in contaminating non-lymphoid monocytic/ granulocytic cells.

MATERIAL AND METHODS

Isolation and fractionation of NK cells.

NK cells were isolated from fresh peripheral blood using Ficoll-Isopaque density gradients. Adherent cells were removed from density gradient isolated cells using nylon wool columns as earlier described (14). In such non-adherent cell preparations the majority of cells expressed T cell markers and between 5-15 % NK cell markers. In some ezperiments purified NK cells were used, obtained either through Percoll gradient fractionation or through the "panning method". Panned cells usually contained the highest number of NK cells as investigated by surface markers or target binding capacity (14).

Cytotoxicity assay

^{51}Cr release assays were used in standard 96 well microplates with 10^4 labelled target cells with a final volume of 150 ul in each well (14). Tests were done in duplicated in RPMI 1640 medium supplemented with 10 fetal calf serum and antibiotics for a time period of 3 h with human NK cells and for 6 h with HVA transformed killer T cell lines. 50 ul supernatant was harvested from each well and amount released radioisotope calculated according to the standard formula (14). Target cell lines used were the standard targets K-562 derived from erythroleukemia (22 b) and Molt-4 derived acute lymphocytic leukemia (23).

Lipoxygenase inhibitors and cyclic nucleotides

Nordihydroguaiarectic acid (NDGA) was purchased from Sigma 5, 8, 11, 14-eicosatetraynoic acid (ETYA) from Hoffman-LaRoche indometacin from Dumex as a sodium salt ("Confortid") and 3-amino-1-m-(trifluoromethyl) phenyl-2-pyrazoline (BW 755C) was obtained from Wellcome Research Laboratories. N^2, O^2'-dibutyrylguanosine-3':5'-cyclic monophosphoric acid (dB-cGMP) and N^6, O^2- dibutyryladenosine 3':5'-cyclic monophosphate (dB-cAMP) were obtained from Sigma (nr D 3510 and D 0627 resepctively).

Preparation of HETE acids, LTB_4 and related metabolites

Lipoxygenase metabolites were isolated from human leukocyte suspentions after incubation with ionophore A 23187 and arachidonic acid (14 b). Briefly, the incubations were terminated by addition of 3 volumes ethanol. After filtration and evaporation of the ethanol, the remaining water phase was extracted with diethyl ether at pH 3. Thereafter the extract was purified on a silica acid column, eluted with diethyl ether / hexane (10/90 and 40/60; v/v) and methanol/ethyl acetate (5/95 v/v). The two last fractions containing monohydroxy and dihydroxy/trihydroxy acids respectively, were subjected to reverse phase - high performance liquid (RP-HPLC) chromatography. The dihydroxy and trihydroxy acids were methylated and further purified on straight phase (SP)-HPLC followed by hydrolysis with LiOH. 20-COOH-LTB_4 was further purified in two steps using RP-HPLC (21). The compounds were quantitated by UV spectroscopy.

RESULTS

Suppression of NK cell killing by inhibition of AA lipoxygenation

Four different lipoxygenase inhibitors were used in standard cytotoxicity tests in several repeated experiments. Figure 1 report
representative experiment in which NK cells were enriched for by
using the panning technique with OKT3 treated cells. In this way
OKT3 positive cells will remain bound to the solid matrix and the
OKT3-population can be harvested in an unmodulated form. OKT3-
cells obtained this way, contain most of the NK cell activity and
the target binding cells (TBC). All four different inhibitors
suppressed NK cell lysis with NDGA active at approximately 4 times
higher concentration to obtain similar 50 % inhibition levels.
BW 755C required even a slightly higher concentration as compared
to ETYA and indometacin. In repeat experiment the ID_{50} level varied
between 5 to 50 uM with NDGA depending on the activation level of
the effector cell population and on the age (oxidation level)
of the inhibitor. In the target binding assay, cellular interactions were investigated at the start of the ^{51}Cr release assay
using the solidified agarose test method (24). At inhibitor concentrations above 125 uM there was a decrease in the target binding
capacity of the NK cell population but below that concentration
undisturbed effector target cell conjugation occured.

Reconstitution of NK cell activity to NDGA suppressed cells, with
LTB_4 and other lipoxygenase products

Part of NK cytotoxicity suppressed by NDGA could be reconstituted to the system with purified LTB_4 (Fogire 2). The reconstitution curve was optimal at 1 - 100 pM approaching control
levels at both higher and lower concentration. Reconstitution was
more complete at lower NDGA concentrations. LTB_4 is derived from
the epoxide LTA_4 by enzymatic hydrolysis (13). LTA_4 can also be
non-enzymatically converted to isomeric forms such as 12-epi-
6-trans-LTB_4 and 6-trans-LTB_4 and 20-COOH-LTB_4 (26, 27). In LTB_4
activated systems the isomeric forms are usually considered inactive and the omega oxidized forms to have variable effects in
different responses (26,27). In the present system it has found
that 12 epi, 6-trans-LTB_4 and 6-trans-LTB_4 were as efficient as
LTB_4, to restore the lytic ability in NDGA inhibited cells
(Table 1). The omega oxidized LTB_4 analogues 20-OH-LTB_4 and 20-
COOH-LTB_4 were considerably less potent in restoring NK cell
activity. 5-HETE, 12-HETE and 15-HETE:s were also tested in
several repeat experiments for restoring NK killing to NDGA
inhibited cells (Table 2). All three HETE:s could reconstitute
lysis at similar optimal concentration of 10^{-11} to 10^{-12} M
with highest reconstitution with 5-HETE (28.0% of control) and
lowest with 15-HETE (17.6 % of control).

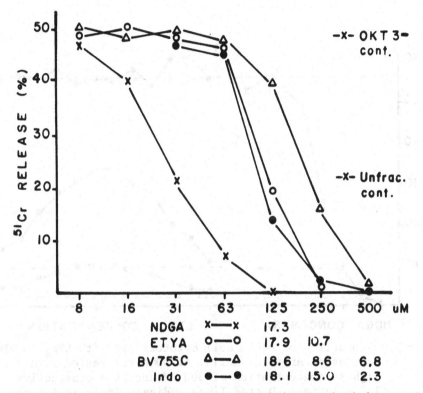

NDGA	x—x	17.3		
ETYA	o—o	17.9	10.7	
BV755C	△—△	18.6	8.6	6.8
Indo	●—●	18.1	15.0	2.3

Figure 1. Suppression of NK cell cytotoxicity by inhibitors of AA lipoxygenation. ^{51}Cr release and target cell binding capacity was tested with an OKT3-negative effector cell population. TBC values (as % of whole cell population) are given for the three highest concentrations, control TBC 18.1 %.

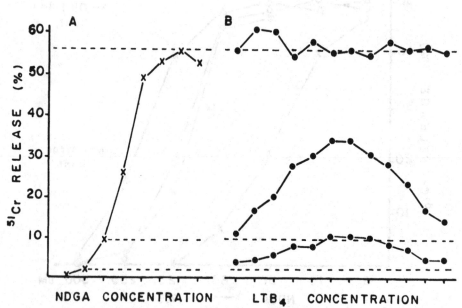

Figure 2. Reconstitution of NK cell cytotoxicity with LTB$_4$ to NDGA
suppressed effector cells. A. NDGA was tested with
highest concentration of 300 uM and at 8 consecutive
1:2 dilutions. Dotted lines indicate lysis at 150 and
75 uM and upper control. B. LTB$_4$ was added with an
initial concentration of 10^{-6} and with 8 consecutive
1:10 concentrations.

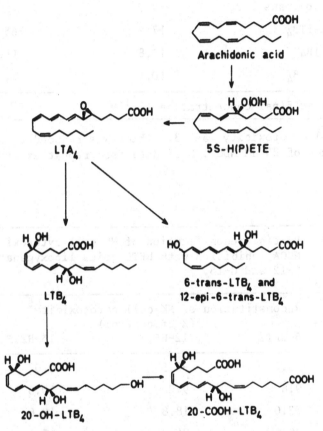

Figure 3. Formation of LTB$_4$ and related metabolites from AA. 6-trans-LTB$_4$ and 12-epi, 6-trans-LTB$_4$ are formed non-enzymatically and 20-OH-LTB$_4$ and 20-COOH-LTB$_4$ enzymatically

Table 1. Partial reconstitution of NK cell cytotoxicity after NDGA inhibition with LTB_4 and analogues 12-epi, 6-trans-LTB_4, 6-trans-LTB_4, 20-OH-LTB_a and 20-COOH-LTB_4

Metabolite[§]	NK cytotoxicity[&] ($\%^{51}Cr$ release)	Reconstitution (% of cont)
LTB_4	33.2	64.6
12-epi, 6-trans-LTB_4	18.9	72.3
6-trans-LTB_4	17.9	65.3
20-OH-LTB_4	10.8	11.5
20-COOH-LTB_4	10.6	14.1

[§]Tested at final concentration 10^{-11}M.

[&]Control cytotoxicity was 23.9 which was reduced to 8.9 in the presence of 25 uM NDGA. Mean data from repeat experiments are given.

Table 2. Partial reconstitution of NK cell cytotoxicity after NDGA inhibition with HETE acids lipoxygenated at C-5, C-12 and C-15.

HETE Conc (M)	Reconstitution of NK cell cytotoxicity[§] (% of control)		
	5-HETE	12-HETE	15-HETE
10^{-7}	-5.0	-2.5	0.0
10^{-8}	9.6	9.2	10.5
10^{-9}	23.0	18.8	12.6
10^{-10}	26.4	24.3	15.5
10^{-11}	27.2	23.8	17.6
10^{-12}	28.0	26.8	16.3
10^{-13}	22.6	25.9	15.9
10^{-14}	14.6	16.7	7.9

[§]Control cytotoxicity was 32.2 which was reduced to in the presence of 25 uM NDGA. Mean data from repeat experiments are given.

Reconstitution of NK cell activity to NDGA inhibited cells with cyclic nucleotides

dB-cGMP and dB-cAMP were tested for their capacity to restore NK lysis to NDGA suppressed cells. One representative experiment is given in Figure 4 demonstrating that both nucleotides were competent to restore lysis to high levels. Control experiments with butyrate were negative (data not shown).

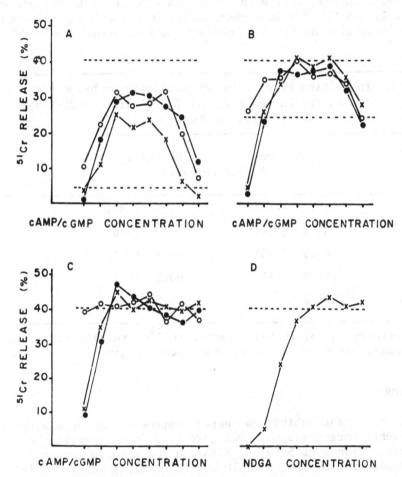

Figure 4. Reconstitution of NK cell cytotoxicity to NDGA suppressed effector cells with cyclic nucleotides. NDGA was used starting from 150 uM with 8 consecutive 1:2 dilutions (D). Cyclic nucleotides were used starting from 10^{-4} with 8 consecutive 1:10 dilutions. Filled circles indicate dB-cAMP, open circles dB-cGMP and crosses a combination of dB-cAMP and dB-cGMP. Upper dotted line indicate control lysis (C) and lower lines, killing at 75 (A) and at 37.5 uM NDGA (B) respectively.

Inhibition of NK-like cytotoxicity by herpesvirus Ateles transformed marmoset T cell lines.

Herpesvirus Ateles transform marmoset T cells into continuously growing lines that express a killer function similar to marmoset NK cells (22 a). Using standard targets from the human NK system, HVA transformed cells predominantly kill leukemic T cell lines such as Molt-4 whereas other targets such as K-562 are virtually resistant (22a). The HVA transformed cell line 77-DR-2 was used against Molt-4 target cells in parallell with fresh human NK cells in the presence of NDGA. It was found that 77-DR-2 cells were equally sensitive to NDGA inhibition as fresh NK cells from peripheral blood (Table 3).

Table 3. Inhibition of cellular cytotoxicity by herpesvirus Ateles tranformed marmoset T cell line 77-DR-2 against Molt-4 target cells by NDGA.

NDGA conc (M)	77-DR-2 cells[§] ($\%$ ^{51}Cr release)		NK cells	
75	10.2	(−86)	7.3	(−87)
37.5	35.8	(−50)	34.5	(−46)
18.8	60.9	(−15)	50.6	(−21)
9.4	70.9	(+1)	60.5	(−5)
control	71.3		64.0	

[§]Cytotoxicity was estimated by standard ^{51}Cr release method in a 6 h assay. One representative experiment is given.

DISCUSSION

All lipoxygenase inhibitors tested suppressed NK lysis although at different concentrations. NDGA gave 50 % inhibition in the concentration range of 5-50 uM, ETYA and indometacin required higher concentrations and BW 755C was found least active. This ranking order is similar to what Salari et al found for inhibition of 5-lipoxygenase activation (28) and thus supports the view that the NK inhibition seen depend on lipoxygenase inhibition and not on unrelated toxic side-effects. NDGA is 5-lipoxygenase selective with human leucocytes and platelets whereas ETYA and BW 755C is equally active against cyclocooxygenase and lipoxygenase enzymes (28). Indometacin is highly cyclooxygenase specific at lower concentrations (below 10^{-6}M) but also active against lipoxygenase enzymes at higher concentrations. Inhibition with NDGA up to 125 uM did not cause toxic effects on the target cells cultured alone without NK cells present (data not shown), thus the ID_{50} concentration for NDGA was far from toxicity level. However, with the other inhibitors, NK cell suppresion was seen rather close to toxic concentrations, suggesting that caution is needed in interpreting these results. With NDGA it was also found that inhibition was irreversible after short-term treatment and extensive washing of effector cells (data not shown). As NDGA was the preferable inhibitor in the present system it was further used in this study.

NDGA is an anti-oxidant with the capacity to scavenge free oxygen radicals (29). If compatible with the irreversible nature of this inhibitor, this could partly explain its mode if action as lipoxygenation leads to the formation of radicals (30,31). It is clear however, that NDGA does not at all suppress the capacity of isolated NK cells to conjugate to target cells (Figure 1) in line with earlier findings (5). Thus the lipoxygenase dependent event in NK cell lysis is not related to initial binding but rather to triggering of the lytic machinery.

As mentioned above lipoxygenation can occur at different positions in AA and further metabolic processing depend on the enzyme content of the host cell. In fact, the complexity of this system, both as far as formed metabolites and their mode of action is concerned, is much greater than presently defined. New metabolites and functions are being defined (32). As LTB_4 has earlier been shown to influence several leucocyte functions, including degranulation of lytic enzymes, we found it logical to initially investigate if NDGA inhibition of NK lysis depended on a selective LTB_4 inhibition. As it was found that NK lysis could be reconstituted to NDGA inhibited cells with not only LTB_4 but also with the isomeric forms 12-epi, 6-trans-LTB_4 and 6-trans-LTB_4, that are usually considered to be biologically inactive, we further tested the influence of different HETE:s in the system and found that especially 5-HETE nad 12-HETE also could reconstitute. These findings indicate that there is no LTB_4 specificity in the NK system as has earlier been described in polymorphonuclear cells with specific LTB_4 receptors (33).

This lack of LTB_4 specificity and the positive results with HETE acids suggested a more primitive mechanism at work, possibly related to cyclic nucleotides as extensively investigated and discussed by Hadden and Coffey and others (34). For the early response to mitogens Hadden and Coffey have suggested that H(P)ETE acids function via direct activation of gyanyl cyclase (35) as has also been directly shown by Graff et al with guinea pig spleen derived enzymes (36). Indeed, we found strong reconstitution of NK cell killing in NDGA inhibited cells using both dB-cGMP and dB-cAMP (Figure 4). The positive effect of dB-cAMP was surprising considering the postulated opposed influence of this cyclic nucleotid to cGMP.

However, high concentrations of dB-cAMP were consistently NK cell suppressive as earlier reported. This suppression depend on defect target cell conjugation in the human NK system (14). Also, the finer inter-relationship between cGMP and cAMP is not well understood and cAMP have a role in positive signalling as defined in the stimulus-secretion model. Thus, although the present dB-AMP data should be regarded with caution it is fully possible that the low concentrations found optimal for NK reconstitution are physiologically inductive, alternatively the dB-cAMP reconstitution may be an in vitro artifact that does not occur normally.

In summary, the present work demonstrate that the 5-lipoxy-selective inhibitor NDGA inhibits NK lysis at non-toxic concentrations by interfering with lytic triggering at the post-conjugation stage. This inhibition may depend on the capacity of NDGA to prevent the formation of lipoxygenation products such as H(P)ETE acids and further leukotrienes (such as LTB_4) and related structures. As dB-cGMP reconstitute NDGA inhibited Nk cell cytotoxicity, as well as the various lipoxygenase metabolites, it is possible that the function of these metabolites is related to the formation of inductive cyclic nucleotides. Further work measuring cGMP levels in isolated NK cells stimulated with defined metabolites is needed to clarify this question although it has been shown that membrane-bound guanyl cyclase is activated in human peripheral blood lymphocytes by AA and 5-HETE (35). Also, the demonstration of the lipoxygenase pathway in cloned lymphoid cells with standard biochemical methods is lacking as well as a characterization of formed lymphoid metabolites.

REFERENCES

1 T Hoffman, F Hirata, P Bougnoux, B A Fraser, R H Goldfarb, R B Herberman and J Axelrod. Phospholipid methylation and phospholipase A_2 activation in cytotoxicity by human antural killer cells. Proc Natl Acad Sci USA 78: 3839, 1981
2 P C Quan, T Ishizaka and B R Bloom . Studies on the mechanism of NK cell lysis. J Immunol 128:1786, 1982
3 Berke G. Recent advances and questions in lymphocytotoxicity. In: Regulatory Mechanisms in Lymphocyte Activation. Ed E. Lucas. Academic Press, NY p 812, 1977.
4a Y Kobayashi, J-I Sawada and T Osawa. Activation of membrane phoshpolipase by guinea pgi lymphotoxin (GLT). J Immunol 122:1791, 1979.
4b U Ramstedt, C N Serhan, U Lundberg,H Wigzell and B Samuelsson. Inhibition of human natural killer cell activity by 14,15-dihydroxy-4, 8, 10, 12-eicosatetraenoic acid (14, 15-D_1HETE) PNS in press.
5 W E Seaman. Human natural killer cell activity is reversibley inhibited by antagonists of lipoxygenation. J Immunol 131: 2953, 1983

6   Suthanthiran, S D Solomon, P S Williams, A L Rubin,
       A Novogrodsky and K H Stenzel. Hydroxyl radical scavengers
       inhibit human natural killer cell activity. Nature 307:276,
       1984

7   Hattori, F Hirata, T Hoffman, A Hizuta and R B Herberman.
       Inhibition of human natural killer (NK) activity and antibody-
       dependent cellular cytotoxicity (ADCC) by lipomodulin, a
       phospholipase inhibitory protein. J Immunol 131:662, 1983

8   Rola-Pleszczynski, L Gagnon and P Sirois. Leukotriene B_4
       augments human natural cytotoxic cell activity. Biochem
       Biophys Res Com. 113: 531, 1983

9   Dinarello, S O Marnoy and L J Rosenwasser. Role of arachidonate
       metabolism in the immunoregulatory function of human leukocytic
       pyrogen/lymphocyte-activating factor/interleukin 1. J Immunol,
       130 :890, 1983

10   Payan and E J Goetzl. The dependence of human T lymphocyte mig-
       ration on the 5-lipoxygenation of endogenous arachidonic acid.
       J Clin Immunol, 1:266, 1981.

11   Rola-Pleszczynski, P Borgeat and P Sirois. Leukotriene B_4 induces
       human suppressor lymphocytes. Biochem Biophys Res Comm, 108:1531,
       1982.

12   Goetzl. Selective feed-back inhibition of the 5-lipoxygenation
       of arachidonic acid in human T lymphocytes. Biochem Biophys Res
       Comm, 101, 344, 1981.

13   Samuelsson. Leukotrienes: Mediators of immediate hypersensitivity
       reactions and inflammation. Science, 220:568, 1983.

14a   Ullberg, Jondal M, Lanefelt F and Fredholm B. Inhibition of human
       NK cell cytotoxicity by induction of cyclic AMP depends on impaired
       target cell recognition. Scan J Immunol, 17:365, 1983.

14b   Lindgren, Hansson G and Samuelsson B. Formation of novel hydroxy-
       lated eicosatetraenoic acids in preparations of human polymorpho-
       nuclear leukocytes. FEBS lett, 128, 329, 1981.

15   Shenker and I Grey. Cyclic nucleotide metabolism during lymphocyte
       transformation. 43: 11, 1979.

16   Nishizuka. The role of protein kinase C in cell surface signal
       transduction and tumor promotion. Nature, 308, 693, 1984.

17   Goldyne and Stobo J D. Human monocytes synthesize eicosanoids
       from T lymphocyte derived arachidonic acid. Prostaglandins, 24:
       623, 1982.

18   Ford-Hutchinson, M A Bray, M V Doing, M E Shiply and J H Smith
       Nature, 286:264, 1980.

19   Goetzl, and W C Picket. The human PMN leukocyte chemotactic ac-
       tivity of complex hydroxy-eicosatetraenoic acids (HETEs). J
       Immunol, 125:1789, 1980.

20   Palmblad, C Malmsten, A M Uden, O Rådmark, L engstedt and B Sam-
       uelsson. Leukotriene B_4 is a potent and stereospecific stimulator
       of neutrophil chemotaxis and adherence. Blood, 58:658, 1981.

21   Feinmark, J Å Lindgren, H Claesson, C Malmsten and B Samuelsson.
       Stimulation of human leukocyte degranulation by leokotriene B_4
       and its oxidized metabolites. FEBS lett, 136: 141, 1981.

22a Johnson D R and Jondal M. Herpesvirus-transformed cytotoxic T cell lines. Nature, 291:81, 1981.

22b Lozzio C B and Lozzio B B. Cytotoxicity of a factor isolated from human spleen. J Natl Cancer Inst. 50:535, 1973.

23 Minowada J, Ohnuma T and Moore G E. Rosette-forming human lymphoid cell lines. J Natl Cancer Inst, 49:891, 1972.

24 Grimm E A, Thoma J A and Bonavida B B. Mechanism of cell-mediated cytotoxicity at single cell level. J Immunol, 123, 2870, 1979.

25 Lindgren J Å, Hansson G and Samuelsson B. Formation of novel hydroxylated eicosatetraenoic acids in preparations of human polymorphonuclear leukocytes. FEBS lett, 128:329, 1981.

26 Feinmark S J, Lindgren J Å, Claesson H, Malsten C and Samuelsson B. Stimulation of human leukocyte degranulation by leukotriene B_4 and its omega-oxidized metabolites. FEBS lett, 136:141, 1981.

27 Hansson G, Lindgren J Å, Dahlen S-E, Hedqvist P and Samuelsson B. Identification and biological activity of novel omega-oxidized metabolites of leukotrienes B_4 from human leukocytes. FEBS lett, 130, 107, 1981.

28 Salari H, Braquet P and Borgeat P. Comparative effects of indometacin, acetylenic acids, 15-HETE, nordihydroguaiaretic acid and BW755C on the metabolism of arachidonic acid in human leukocytes and platelets. Prostaglandins Leukotrienes and Medicine, 13:53, 1984.

29 Bokoch G M and Reed P W. Evidence for inhibition of leukotriene A_4 synthesis by 5,8,11,14-eicosatetraenoic acid in guinea pig polymorphonuclear leukocytes. J Biol Chem, 256:4156, 1981.

30 Hamberg M. Studies on the formation and degradation of unsaturated fatty acid hydroperoxides. Prostaglandins Leukotrienes and Medicine, 13:27, 1984.

31 Lands W E. Biological consequences of fatty acid oxegenase reaction mechanism. Prostaglandins Leukotrienes and Medicine, 13, 35, 1984.

32 Serhan C N, Hamberg M, and Samuelsson B. Trihydroxytetraenes: A novel series of compounds formed from arachidonic acid in human leukocytes, 118:943, 1984.

33 Goldman D W and Goetzl E J. Eur J Immunol, 129:1600, 1983.

34 Hadden J W and Coffey R G. Cyclic nucleotides in mitogen-induced lymphocyte proliferation. Immunol Today, 3, 299, 1982.

35 Coffey R G and Hadden J W. Arachidonate and metabolites in mitogen activation of lymphocyte guanylate cyclase. Advances in Immun pharmacol, Pergamon Press, 1981.

36 Graff G, Stephenson J H, Glass D B, Haddox M K and Nelson D Goldberg. Activation of soluble splenic cell guanylate cyclase by prostaglandin endoperoxids and fatty acid hydroperoxides. J Biol Chem, 253:7662, 1978.

A SERINE PROTEINASE AS A "TRIGGER" FOR HUMAN NATURAL

KILLER LYMPHOCYTE-MEDIATED CYTOLYSIS

Dorothy Hudig, Lory Minning[*] and Doug Redelman

Department of Microbiology
School of Medicine
University of Nevada, Reno
Reno, Nevada   89557-0046

INTRODUCTION

The nature of the lesion created by cytotoxic lymphoyctes is not yet known. However, current evidence is consistent with insertion of a hydrophobic pore or channel into the membrane of the target cell. The sieving properties (1,2) and morphological appearance (3,4,5) of the membranes of dead target cells are similar but not identical to the properties of erythrocyte membranes after complement attack. Efforts to determine whether or not the lymphocyte-mediated lesions could be composed of complement or complement-like proteins have been negative (6,7) or substantially inconclusive (8). We approached the problem in a different manner, reasoning that if there were similarities between complement- and lymphocyte-mediated lesions, then a serine dependent proteinase cascade could regulate the lymphocyte system in a manner similar to the regulation characterized by complement proteinases D and Bb or Clr, Cls, and C2a.

We have accumulated considerable evidence that serine proteinase activity is required for both human NK (9,10) and mouse T (11,12) lymphocyte-mediated cytotoxicity. This proteinase activity has an aromatic amino acid specificity of cleavage (10,12). A summary of the NK findings and of data indicating that this proteinase is unlikely to play a role in either lymphocyte-target binding or killer cell-independed cytolyis follows.

---

*UC San Diego Cancer Center, T-011, La Jolla, CA. 92093

METHODS

All experiments were performed with the peripheral blood mononuclear cells of normal human donors as effector lymphocytes and with ^{51}Cr-labeled K562 cells as targets (10,13), except where otherwise indicated. Concentrations of inhibitors that resulted in a two-fold decrease of killer cell activity as determined by lytic units were termed ID_{50}s (10,14). The sources for all inhibitors and other reagents can be found in reference 10.

Conjugates were formed at room temperature at 1:1 or 2:1 lymphocyte to target ratios by 40g centrifugation (10) and kept on ice until ready to count by light microscopy.

The cloned human cell line 6G12.1 was established by limiting dilution from a cell line that was originally stimulated with phytohemagglutinin. This cell line was T cell growth factor dependent; recloned once at limiting dilution; maintained in continuous culture without appreciable loss of NK-like activity for over a year; cytotoxic to K562, Molt 4, U937 but not Jurkat cells; and OK T3$^+$, OK T4$^-$, OK T8$^+$, and HNK-1$^-$.

RESULTS

Inhibition of NK with Class-Specific and Substrate-Restrictive Inhibitors of Proteinases

NK is inhibited by the serine class-specific proteinase inhibitors phenylmethylsulfonylfluoride (PMSF) and diisopropylfuorophosphate (DFP). It is also inhibited by the plasma antiproteinase alpha-1-antichymotrypsin, which reacts only with serine dependent proteinases that have aromatic amino acid specificity of cleavage. Although all three reagents react with the active site serine of the proteinases in question, it is necessary to weight the value of these data in the light of additional considerations. PMSF can also act as a less specific alkylating agent (15), and commercial preparations of DFP contain thiol-reactive contaminants (16). We have found that non-penetrating reagents which react with cell surface thiol groups can block cell-mediated cytotoxicity (11,17). In contrast, the reagent alpha-1-antichymotrypsin has no other known reactivity other than with chymotrypsin-like enzymes. Thus the data with alpha-1-antichymotrypsin has the greatest value, and the data with the other two reagents provide supportive but not conclusive evidence for a requirement for a serine dependent proteinase in NK.

In addition, we have used alternate substrates for proteinases which can compete the activity of proteinases of several different classes, but yield valuable information concerning substrate specificity. The ester and amide synthetic substrates containing aromatic amino acids compete NK when present in the NK assays, whereas similar derivatives containing basic or aliphatic amino acids do not compete NK (10). Furthermore, the esters compete NK better than the amides, and the L-enantiomers compete better than the D-enantiomers (10), at concentrations similar to those that would compete activity of chymotrypsin-like enzymes.

The substrate specificity of the activity required for NK is also confirmed by the relative efficacy of selected fungal inhibitors of proteinases.

These data are summarized in the following two tables:

Table I. Representative Inhibitors of Serine Dependent Proteinases which Inhibit Human NK

Reagent	ID_{50} (mM)	Origin of inhibitor	Comments
Irreversible proteinase inhibitors:			
Phenylmethyl-sulfonyl fluor-ide (PMSF)	0.5	synthetic	Reacts with serine in proteinase active site
Diisopropyl-florophosphate	2.0	synthetic	Reacts with serine in proteinase active site
A-1-Antichymo-trypsin	0.01	plasma	Couples covalently and stochiometrically to proteinase active site serine
Reversible proteinase inhibitors:			
Chymostatin	25 ug/ml	fungal	Looses reactivity in aqueous solutions
AcTyrOEt	0.4	synthetic	Acts as competitive, alternate substrate

Table II. Inhibitors of Serine Dependent Proteinases which Do
Not Inhibit Human NK

Irreversible proteinase inhibitors: None

Reversible proteinase inhibitors:

Basic Pancreatic Trypsin Inhibitor, Kunitz (BPTI)	pancreas	Preferentially inhibits enzymes with basic a.a. specificity
Leupeptin, Antipain	fungal	Both serine and sulfhydryl proteinases, basic a.a. specificity
AcLysOMe	synthetic	Proteinases with basic a.a. specificity
AcGlyOMe	synthetic	Proteinases with aliphatic a.a.

With these probes we have acquired additional information concerning the NK-associated proteinase. Although the plasma antiproteinase alpha-1-antichymotrypsin reacts covalently and irreversibly with appropriate proteinases, pretreatment of cytotoxic lymphocytes with this or other plasma antiproteinases did not result in subsequent inhibition of cytolysis. The inhibitor had to be present during killing. Thus, prior to killing, the cytotoxicity-associated proteinase is either not activated, or not available to these macromolecular plasma antiproteinases which are all larger than 50,000 Daltons. Furthermore, the similarities between the ID_{50}s for NK and the K_ms and K_is of the reagents for chymotrypsin imply that the natural substrate for the NK activity cannot be in great excess of the K_m of this natural substrate for the NK enzyme or competition of NK would not be observed. This implication is more consistent with a proteinase of refined specificity rather than one of promiscuous appetite that could digest all the proteins of the target cell surface.

Proteinase Activity Is Not Needed for Lymphocyte-Target Cell Binding

A regent that blocks cell-mediated cytotoxicity as measured by ultimate ^{51}Cr release can block killing at target cell binding, at the phase termed the lethal hit, or at the events that are restricted to the target cell after the killer lymphocyte dissociates itself. We have used cloned NK-like cells for this experiment to obviate the problems caused by the low frequency of killer cells among the population of fresh human mononuclear cells that bind to K562 cells. With the clone 6G12.1, we observed that the frequency of initial target-binding cells was not reduced in the presence of concentrations of the alternate substrate tyrosine ethyl ester (TyrOEt) that greatly diminished killer cell activity (figure 1). Thus, under conditions in which proteolytic acitivity would have been blocked, initial binding of effector and targets was not blocked. Even at the end of the assay at 37° C, the cloned cells remained firmly attached to the K562 targets in the presence of TyrOEt (figure 2A and 2B). Although there remains the possibility that the avidity of binding was imperceptibly decreased, the simplest explanation is that TyrOEt inhibits lymphocyte events that follow binding.

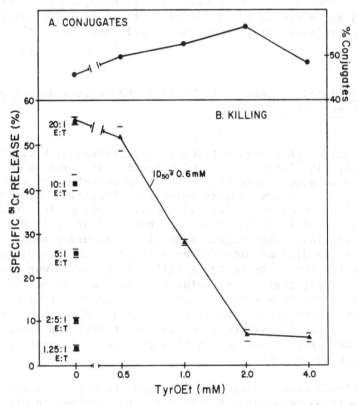

Figure 1. The alternate substrate TyrOEt blocks killing but not binding of cloned 6G12.1 NK-like cells. The control killing is at several E:T ratios is indicated by the filled squares. This 15 hour assay was to K562 cells.

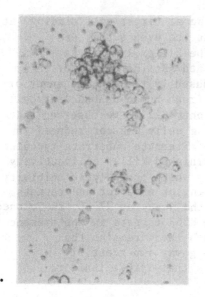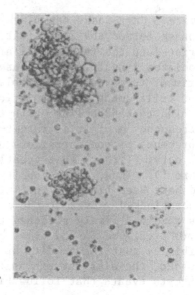

A.   B.

Figure 2.   Clone 6G12.1 cells with K562 targets, in the absence (A, E:T=3.5:1) and presence (B, E:T=14:1), of 1.5 mM TyrOEt at the end of the ^{51}Cr release assay. The large cells are K562 cells.

The NK-Associated Proteinase Is Unlikely to Mediate Direct Damage to the Target Cells.

Extremely high concentrations of proteinases with extremely broad specificity (pronase), or with specificity restricted to selected amino acids wherever available in proteins but not restricted to exclusive protein substrates (trypsin, chymotrypsin and papain) do not effect ^{51}Cr release from K562 cells. Even at concentrations of 1 mg/ml and after 4 hours, K562 cells did not release ^{51}Cr (10). The enzymes were effective under these experimental conditions because the ability of these radiolabeled, enzyme treated target cells to be killed by NK cells was competely abrogated. Thus, there is no evidence that the presence of such a nonspecific proteinase would result in release of label. Furthermore, since pronase treatment would be expected to remove all available protein external to the target cell membrane, it is unlikely that simple destruction of any target cell surface protein would result in cell death.

Additional experiments have been made to determine whether the proteinase is active on the target after the lymphocyte dissociates from the target, during the killer cell-independent stage of

276

cytolysis. In these experiments, killing was arrested after 30 minutes of cytolyis at 37° C. At this time either medium or the alternate proteinase substrate AcTyrOEt was added. Three hours later the experiments were harvested. It was expected that if AcTyrOEt affected the killer cell-independent stages, ^{51}Cr release would be lower in the presence of AcTyrOEt than in the presence of only medium. A combination of sodium azide and 2-deoxyglucose (10 mM and 25 mM, respectively) was used to arrest killing rather than EDTA, since chelation of Ca^{++} would be expected to reduce the proteolytic activity of many serine dependent proteinases as well as block the continued killing of lymphocytes. This combination of metabolic inhibitors totally blocks NK when added at room temperature after conjugate formation and prior to the onset of cytotoxicity (0 hr of assay). These metabolic inhibitors would not be expected to affect serine proteinase activity. The results are consistent with no role for this proteinase activity in the killer cell independent stages of cytolysis (Table 3).

Table III. Addition of the Alternate Proteinase Substrate AcTyrOEt after Arrest of Lymphocyte-Dependent Functions of NK Cytolysis Did Not Reduce Subsequent ^{51}Cr Release.

Reagent Added	Time of Addition of AcTyrOEt[a]	Lytic Units per 10^6 PBL
Medium	0 hr.	2.0
2.0 mM AcTyrOEt	0 hr.	0.25
Medium	0.5 hr.	2.0
2.0 mM AcTyrOEt	0.5 hr.	2.0

[a]In all cases, azide and 2-deoxyglucose were added after 30 minutes of incubation.

DISCUSSION

The immediate implications of the data from each approach were discussed within the preceding text. Activity of a serine dependent proteinase with an aromatic amino acid specificity appears to be esssential for NK cytotoxicity. However, this proteinase and its natural substrate remain to be identified and

isolated. Furthermore, there is indication that this proteinase is
is activated or exposed only during the post-binding events of NK
lymphocyte-mediated cytolysis. The evidence for selective
activation and the unknown nature of the natural substrate will
make this NK-associated proteinase difficult to isolate and/or
identify from among proteinases that may be isolated from killer
lymphocytes.

Evaluation of these experiments in the context of other
biological systems in which proteinases play crucial roles provides
a basis for speculation. A serine dependent proteinase of
identical class and substrate specificity to the NK activity is
required for mast cell degranulation (18, 19). Chymase, a serine
dependent proteinase with aromatic amino acid specificity of
cleavage, has been isolated from mast cell granules (20), and can
also "trigger" degranulation of mast cells when the enzyme is added
exogenously to the cells (21). At this time, we consider it a
strong possibility that the proteolytic activity implicated in NK
has a similar function, i.e., to initiate release of the final NK
lytic substance from granules. It is also possible that this
proteinase activity may initiate formation of the lytic substance
from a prolytic substance.

ACKNOWLEDGMENTS

This work was supported in part by NIH CA28196 and CA38942
(D.H) and NIH CA/AI24450 and CA38396 (D.R.).

REFERENCES

1. Henney, C.S. 1973. Studies on the mechanisms of
    lymphocyte-mediated cytotoxicity. II. The use of various
    cell markers to study cytolytic events. J. Immunol. 110: 73.

2. Simone, C., and P. Henkart. 1980. Permeability changes in-
    duced in erythrocyte ghosts by antibody-dependent cytotoxic
    effector cells: Evidence for pores. J. Immunol. 124: 954.

3. Dourmashkin, R.R., P. Deteix, C.B. Simone, and P. Henkart.
    1980. Electron microscopic demonstration of lesions in target
    cell membranes associated with antibody-dependent cellular
    cytotoxicity. Clin. Exp. Immunol. 42: 554.

4. Henkart, M., and P.A. Henkart. 1982. "Lymphocyte-mediated
    cytolysis as a secretory phenomenon". In, Mechanisms of
    Cell-Mediated Cytotoxicity, edited by W.R. Clark and P.
    Golstein. Plenum Press, N.Y. P 227.

278

5. Podack, E., and G. Dennert. 1983. Cell-mediated cytolysis: Assembly of two types of tubules with putative cytolytic function by cloned natural killer cells. Nature 302: 442.

6. Henney, C.S., and M.M. Mayer. 1971. Specific cytolytic activity of lymphocytes: Effect of antibodies to C2, C3, and C5. Cell. Immunol. 2: 702.

7. van Boxel, J.A., W.E. Paul, J. Green, and M.M. Frank. 1974. Antibody-dependent lymphoid cell-mediated cytotoxicity: Role of complement. J. Immunol. 112: 398.

8. Sundsmo, J., and H.J. Muller-Eberhard. 1979. Neoantigens of the complement membrane attack complex on cytotoxic human peripheral blood lymphocytes. J. Immunol. 122: 2371.

9. Hudig, D., T. Haverty, C. Fulcher, D. Redelman, and J. Mendelsohn. 1981. Inhibition of human natural cytotoxicity by macromolecular antiproteinases. J. Immunol. 126: 1569.

10. Hudig, D., D.D. Redelman, and L. Minning. Requisite proteinase activity for human lymphocyte-mediated natural cytotoxicity (NK): Serine dependence and aromatic amino acid specificity of cleavage. J. Immunol., 1984.

11. Redelman, D., and D. Hudig. 1980. The mechanisms of cell-mediated cytotoxicity. I. Killing by murine cytotoxic T lymphocytes requires cell surface thiols and activated protease. J. Immunol. 124: 870.

12. Redelman, D., and D. Hudig. 1983. The mechanism of cell-mediated cytotoxicity. III. Protease-specific inhibitors preferentially block later events in CTL-mediated lisis than do inhibitors of methylation or thiol-specific reagents. Cell. Immunol. 81: 9.

13. Rice, C., D. Hudig, R.S. Newton, and J. Mendelsohn. 1981. Effect of unsaturated fatty acids on human lymphocytes. Disparate influences of oleic and lilnolenic acids on natural cytotoxicity. Clin. Immunol. Immunopath. 20: 389.

14. Hudig, D., D. Redelman, and L. Minning. 1982. "Evidence for proteases with specificity of cleavage at aromatic amino acids in human natural cell-mediated cytotoxicity". In, NK Cells and Other Natural Effector Cells, edited by R.B. Herberman. Academic Press, N.Y. P. 923.

15. Whitaker, J.R., and J. Perez-Villasenor. 1967. Chemical modification of papain. I. Reaction with chloromethyl ketones of phenylalanine and lysine and with phenylmethyl-sulfonyl fluoride. Arch. Biochem. Biophys. 124: 70.

16. Gould, N.R., and I.E. Liener. 1965. Reaction of ficin with diisopropylphosphofluoridate. Evidence for a comtaminating inhibitor. Biochemistry 4: 90.

17. Hudig, D., D. Redelman, and L. Minning. 1982. "Cell surface thiols in human natural cell-mediated cytotoxicity. In, NK Cells and Other Natural Effector Cells, edited by R.B. Herberman, Academic Press, N.Y. P. 1021.

18. Ishizaka, T. 1982. Biochemical analysis of triggering signals induced by bridging of IgE receptors. Fed. Proc. 14: 17.

19. Austen, K.F., and W.E. Brocklehurst. 1961. Anaphylaxis in chopped guinea pig lung. I. Effect of peptidase substrates and inhibitors. J. Exp. Med. 113: 521.

20. Benditt, E.P., and M. Arase. 1959. An enzyme in mast cells with properties like chymotrypsin. J. Exp. Med. 110: 451.

21. Schick, B., K.F. Austin, and L.B. Schwartz. 1994. Activation of rat serosal mast cells by chymase, an endogenous secretory granule protease. J. Immunol. 132: 2571.

THE MECHANISM OF LEUKOREGULIN ENHANCEMENT OF TARGET CELL SUSCEPTIBILITY TO NK CELL MEDIATED CYTOTOXICITY IN HUMANS

Janet H. Ransom[1], Charles H. Evans[2],
Richard P. McCabe[1], and M. G. Hanna, Jr.[1]

[1]Litton Institute of Applied Biotechnology, 1330 Piccard
Drive, Rockville, Maryland 20850
[2]Div. of Cancer Etiology, National Cancer Inst., Bldg. 37
Rm. 2A17, Bethesda, Maryland 20205

Leukoregulin is an anticancer immunologic hormone or lymphokine whose actions include the inhibition of tumor cell growth and lysis of tumor cells either directly or indirectly by stimulating target cell sensitivity to lysis mediated by natural killer (NK) cells (1,2,3). Only a few cell types are directly lysed by leukoregulin and lysis requires very large leukoregulin concentrations. Leuko-regulin enhancement of target sensitivity to NK cell cytolysis, how-ever, occurs in the presence of small concentrations of leukoregulin for carcinoma, sarcoma, and leukemia tumor cells (4). Therefore, the primary in vivo means of tumor destruction may be through the combined action of leukoregulin and NK cells.

Until recently, lymphotoxin was attributed with the anticancer activities now identified as due to leukoregulin (2,4). Classically defined lymphotoxin directly induces the cytolytic destruction of murine L cells (5). We recently have found that human and hamster lymphotoxin preparations contain at least one additional lymphokine biochemically separable from lymphotoxin which causes the growth inhibition and enhanced tumor cell susceptibility to NK-mediated cytotoxicity (4,6) of human or hamster tumor cells, respectively. This new lymphokine was termed leukoregulin. Moreover, purified human lymphotoxin did not display any antihuman tumor cell cytotoxic activities.

The mechanism of leukoregulin enhancement of susceptibility of target cell cytolysis was examined during the several discrete steps of NK cell-mediated cytolysis, which include recognition and binding to target cells, alterations induced in target cells ("programming for lysis"), and target cell-NK cell dissociation whereupon the destruction of the target commences.

Kinetics of Leukoregulin Mediated Enhancement of Target Cell Susceptibility to NK Cytotoxicity

Incubation of K562 human erythroleukemia cells with human leukoregulin (obtained by stimulating human peripheral blood mono-nuclear leukocytes with phytohemagglutinin) for 5 minutes is suffi-cient to augment target cell sensitivity to NK-mediated cytotoxicity (3). Maximum sensitization occurs by 2 hours and this change in cellular physiology is transitory with re-establishment of the basal state by 72 hours. Interferon-induced resistance of target cells to NK cytotoxicity is not detectable until after 30 min. of exposure to interferon. Moreover, leukoregulin in the presence of interferon remains able to sensitize target cells to NK cytotoxicity. Thus, leukoregulin rapidly induces an increased sensitivity to NK cytotox-icity in NK responsive target cells exposed to the lymphokine. Leukoregulin, however, does not induce NK susceptibility in cells not normally responsive to NK cytotoxicity.

Leukoregulin Enhancement of Target Cell-NK Cell Conjugate Formation

K562 cells were incubated in media or media containing leuko-regulin for 1 hour at 37°C and then washed. NK-enriched human lym-phocytes (Ficol-Hypaque isolated, nylon wool nonadherent peripheral blood lymphocytes) were mixed with K562 cells at a 1:1 ratio, centri-fuged and the number of K562-NK cell conjugates enumerated as de-scribed by Grimm and Bonavida (7). Leukoregulin treatment of K562 cells enhanced conjugate formation by 45%. Possible explanations for the enhanced conjugate formation include, 1) leukoregulin may have increased K562 cell surface NK cell receptor expression by enhancing de novo receptor synthesis and 2) leukoregulin may have altered the cell surface conformation such that the receptor struc-ture was more accessible to NK cells. Leukoregulin does influence cell surface receptor expression because leukoregulin treatment of K562 cells causes a marked decrease in transferrin receptor expres-sion measured by quantitating the binding of monoclonal antibody to the transferrin receptor. This observation in itself is an interest-ing paradox to be resolved because the transferrin receptor is a putative receptor for NK cells (8,9), yet leukoregulin which enhances target cell sensitivity to NK mediated cytotoxicity causes a decrease in transferrin receptor expression.

Leukoregulin Alteration in Target Cell Plasma Membrane Permeability

Changes in K562 cell membrane permeability caused by leukoregu-lin were measured by flow cytometric analysis (4). When leukoregulin is added to K562 cells, the narrow angle forward light scatter of the cells decreases, propidium iodide fluorochromasia increases, and fluorescein diacetate (FDA) fluorochromasia decreases (Figure 1). The change in narrow angle forward light scatter reflects a change in cell shape and/or size with a decrease in cell volume confirmed by cell volume analysis on a Coulter Counter. The increase in propidium iodide fluorochromasia reflects an increase in membrane permeability as propidium iodide enters the cell and intercalates with nucleic acid. The decrease in FDA fluorochromasia also reflects increased membrane permeability as the fluorescent intracellular fluorescein diffuses out of the cell. These flow cytometric quantifiable leukoregulin induced changes are detectable 5 min. after the treatment of K562 cells and are maximal by 2 hours. Alpha, beta and gamma interferon and lymphotoxin do not induce any of these changes in cell surface conformation or plasma membrane permeability during this time period.

The relationship between leukoregulin directed changes in target cell surface conformation and plasma membrane permeability and mechanism of NK cytotoxicity was further examined by mixing target cells and effector lymphocytes and determining whether the leukoregulin directed changes are an intrinsic part of the cytolytic process (3). When narrow angle forward light scatter and FDA fluorescent signals are analyzed simultaneously by dual parameter flow cytometric analysis, the patterns of K562 and NK cells are clearly different. Analysis two hours into the NK cytotoxicity reaction demonstrates that cell surface conformation and plasma membrane permeability changes of K562 cells increase directly with the concentration of natural killer cells and are identical to those alterations induced by leukoregulin alone (Figure 2). K562 cells displaying leukoregulin specific cell surface alterations during a NK reaction, moreover, have been isolated by flow cytometric cell sorting and shown to reestablish their basal state. Thus, the plasma membrane permeability changes at this point in the NK cytotoxicity reaction are reversible. This "instantaneous" measurement of target cell surface changes provides strong evidence for the participation of leukoregulin as an integral component of NK-mediated cytotoxicity.

The Relationship Between Leukoregulin and NK Cytotoxic Factors (NKFC)

Leukoregulin is present in the culture media of NK cells stimulated with phytohemagglutinin. NKCF similarly can be induced by mitogen stimulation of lymphocytes or can be detected in the culture media of NK cells mixed with target cells. The difference between NKCF and leukoregulin is that NKCF has specificity for NK responsive targets (9), while leukoregulin affects a variety of tumor cell targets and is 10-fold more cytotoxic for several colon adenocarcinoma cell lines than for K562 cells. Yet the colon adenocarcinomas are relatively insensitive to NK cells. Therefore, leukoregulin is distinct from and plays a different role in the NK cytotoxic reaction than does NKCF.

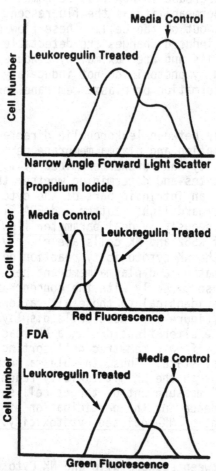

Fig. 1.   Flow cytometric analysis of leukoregulin induced cell surface conformation and plasma membrane permeability changes
in K562 cells. K562 cells were incubated 1 hour at 37°C
with 10 units of purified leukoregulin. The cells were
washed and suspended in either 0.2 µg propidium iodide/ml
RPMI 1640 or 6.25 µg FDA/ml RPMI 1640. After 5 min. the
cells were analyzed on a flow cytometer using 488 nm
wavelength for excitation.

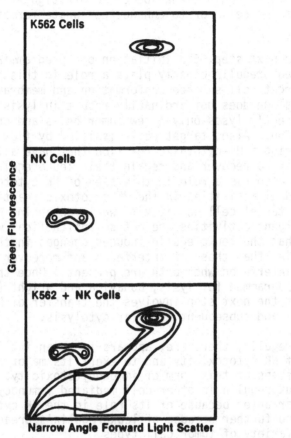

Fig. 2. Dual parameter contour plots of the flow cytometric analysis of K562 cells during an NK cytotoxic reaction. K562 cells were incubated with human nylon wool nonadherent peripheral blood lymphocytes at a ratio of 25 lymphocytes per K562 cell for 2 hours. The cells were centrifuged, resuspended in FDA and analyzed as in Figure 1. The box surrounds the region in which K562 cells exposed to leukoregulin appear.

Theoretical Role of Leukoregulin in NK Cell Mediated Cytotoxicity

It has been postulated that NK cell mediated cytotoxicity is a multistep process which can be separated into discrete events (10). Initially the NK cell recognizes and binds to an appropriate target. Leukoregulin, either exogenously present or endogenously secreted by the NK cell, enhances NK cell-target cell conjugate formation. The resultant effect could either be to form a tighter association between the conjugating cells or to enhance conjugate formation by nearby cells.

In the next step, the initiation or "programming" for lysis occurs. Leukoregulin clearly plays a role in this process by altering the target cell surface conformation and membrane permeability. This step alone does not ordinarily result in lysis because leukoregulin directly lyses only a few tumor cells and only at high concentration. Also, target cells isolated by flow cytometric sorting during a NK-cytotoxic reaction that have altered membrane permeability do recover and regain their leukoregulin responsiveness. Interferon also has a role in this step of NK cytotoxicity. Interferon has dual activities in the NK cytotoxic reaction, that of decreasing target cell sensitivity while enhancing NK cell reactivity. These divergent activities are not so antithetical when one considers the fact that the leukoregulin-induced changes in the target cell occur earlier than those of interferon and moreover supersede the effect of interferon when both are present. Once the target cell has been programmed for lysis, Bonavida and Wright (10) have suggested that the next step involves the transfer of NKCF to the target cell and subsequent cellular cytolysis.

Leukoregulin, therefore, appears to be an intrinsic molecular mediator of NK cytotoxicity and to exert its major actions during the early steps of this form of immunocytotoxicity. Studying the role of leukoregulin in other cell mediated immunocytotoxic reactions is warranted because of its role in the NK cytotoxicity reaction and further because of leukoregulin's breadth of reactivity against a variety of tumor cell types.

REFERENCES

1. Ransom, J.H., L.S. Cleveland, R.P. McCabe, and M.G. Hanna, Jr. Human gastrointestinal carcinoma cells are highly susceptible to the growth inhibitory effects of the immunologic hormone leukoregulin. Proc. Amer. Assoc. Cancer Res. 25:236 (1984).
2. Cleveland, L.S., J.H. Ransom, and C.H. Evans. Leukoregulin: A new anticancer lymphokine distinct from lymphotoxin and interferon. Fed. Proc. 43:1931 (1984).

3. Evans, C.H., J.H. Ransom, and J.A. Heinbaugh. Leukoregulin: A molecular mediator of natural killer cell cytotoxicity. Proc. Amer. Assoc. Cancer Res. 25:268 (1984).
4. Ransom, J.H., J.A. Heinbaugh, and C.H. Evans. Leukoregulin: identification of an anticancer immunologic hormone distinct from lymphotoxin and interferon (submitted for publication, 1984).
5. Granger, G.A., and W.P. Kolb. Lymphocyte in vitro cytotoxicity: mechanisms of immune and non-immune small lymphocyte mediated target L cell destruction. J. Immunol. 101:111 (1968).
6. Ransom, J.H., and C.H. Evans. Molecular characterization of Syrian hamster lymphotoxin's anticarcinogenic and growth inhibitory activities. Cancer Res. 43:5222 (1983).
7. Grimm, E., and B. Bonavida. Mechanism of cell-mediated cytotoxicity at the single cell level. I. Estimation of cytotoxic T lymphocyte frequency and relative lytic efficiency. J. Immunol. 123:2861 (1979).
8. Baines, M.G., F.L. LaFleur, and B.E. Holbein. Involvement of the transferrin and transferrin receptors in human natural killer effector:target interaction. Immunol. Letters 7:51 (1983).
9. Wright, S.C., M.L. Weitzen, R. Kahle, G.A. Granger, and B. Bonavida. Studies on the mechanism of natural killer cytotoxicity. II. Coculture of human PBL with NK-sensitive or resistant cell lines stimulates release of natural killer cytotoxic factors (NKCF) selectively cytotoxic to NK-sensitive target cells. J. Immunol. 130:2479 (1983).
10. Bonavida, B., and S.C. Wright. Soluble cytotoxic factors and the mechanism of NK cell mediated cytotoxicity. Adv. Exp. Med. Biol. 146:379 (1982).

SECTION 4. THE ROLE OF MEMBRANE COMPONENTS IN CTL FUNCTION

INTRODUCTION

In past several years, a number of different cell surface
molecules have been found to be functionally important for cytotoxic T lymphocytes. As described in Mechanisms in Cell-Mediated
Cytotoxicity, the groups of Martz and Springer, and of Golstein
and Pierres, produced monoclonal antibodies against the antigen
now generally called LFA-1. Subsequent observations have confirmed the importance of this molecule in lymphocyte
interactions, and the first two chapters in this section are
devoted to these studies. The cell surface antigens Lyt 2/T8 and
L3T4/T4 have also been the investigated intensively with respect
to their role in T cell functions involving recognition of MHC
class 1 and 2 antigens. MacDonald and collaborators discussed
their early experience with CTL and anti-Lyt 2 in Mechanisms in
Cell-Mediated Cytotoxicity, and in this section provide a summary
of their recent findings, along with related chapters by Ware and
Reade, and by Palladino, et al. A third and distinct group of
CTL surface molecules important in cytotoxic function is the human T3 antigen, which is present as part of a complex with the
antigen receptor. Tsoukas and collaborators summarize their
findings on this system in this section.

In addition to observing the functional effects of antibodies against cell surface proteins, more biochemical
approaches are being applied to the study of lymphocyte membranes
with the hopes of defining those components important for cytotoxic function. The basic biochemical studies of Mescher and
Apgar on lymphoid cell membranes reveal the existence of a novel
membrane skeletal structural network which may well have direct
functional importance. By comparing the surface membrane
proteins of cloned CTL and helper cells, Gately and collaborators
have been able to show that CTL may contain unique components
which may be related to the cytotoxic function.

The final two chapters in this section deal with the nature
of the surface molecules involved in target cell recognition by
CTL. Bonavida, et al. examine those cases where the normal CTL
antigen receptor is bypassed by lectins or other means, while
Sitkovsky and collaborators utilize a novel biochemical approach
to identify "contact proteins" at the CTL-target interface.

LYMPHOCYTE FUNCTION-ASSOCIATED ANTIGENS:

REGULATION OF LYMPHOCYTE ADHESIONS IN VITRO AND IMMUNITY IN VIVO

Eric Martz and Stanislaw H. Gromkowski*

Department of Microbiology
University of Massachusetts
Amherst MA 01003

ABSTRACT

Antibodies to most cytolytic T lymphocyte (CTL) external membrane antigens have no effect on CTL-mediated killing in the absence of complement. However, antibodies which do inhibit killing have now been identified for 7 distinct molecular sites. Antibodies to 6 of these "lymphocyte function-associated antigens" (LFAs, also called "blocking sites") inhibit when bound to the CTL, and to the 7th, when bound to the target cell. Mouse homologs have been identified for only 4 of the 7 human LFAs. 5 (probably 6) of the blocking sites inhibit by interfering with adhesion formation between the CTL and the target cell; the exception is T3. None of the presently identified blocking sites are believed to be lethal hit structures (CTL "toxin").

Reduction of target cell H-2 alloantigen density by pretreatment with papain reduces CTL-target functional "affinity", and increases susceptibility to inhibition 100-fold for anti-Lyt-2,3 and 10-fold for anti-LFA-1. This is consistent with the hypothesis that Lyt-2,3 aids in recognition of class 1 MHC antigens, perhaps by strengthening intercellular adhesion.

On the other hand, LFA-1 appears to function differently. Trypsin pretreatment of target cells has little effect on MHC antigens or CTL-target affinity, yet still increases by 10-fold susceptibility to inhibition by anti-LFA-1. This is seen in both

---

*Present address: Ludwig Institute for Cancer Research, Chemin des Boveresses, CH-1066 Epalinges s/Lausanne, Switzerland.

human and mouse CTL systems. These results suggest the existence
of a non-MHC target structure which participates in the adhesion-
strengthening function of LFA-1, and which is trypsin (and papain)
sensitive: the "trypsin-sensitive counter blocker" (TSCB). LFA-3
may be the human TSCB.

The roles of these LFAs in intercellular adhesion extend to
more general cell adhesions. Anti-LFA-1 and anti-LFA-3 weaken the
spontaneous adhesions which form between cells of the human B cell
line JY. These homotypic adhesions are not initiated by
immunologic recognition.

Anti-LFA-1 is more potent at prolonging allograft survival in
vivo than are anti-Lyt-2,3, anti-T200, anti-Thy-1, or anti-I-A.
Thus, the potent anti-adhesion properties of LFA-1 seen in vitro
may lead to useful immunotherapy in the clinic.

INTRODUCTION

Monoclonal antibodies (MAb) which inhibit (or augment)
cytolytic T lymphocyte (CTL)-mediated killing have been described
as defining "lymphocyte function-associated antigens" or LFAs
(Davignon et. al., 1981). Antibodies to most CTL and target
antigens neither inhibit nor augment killing (Shinohara and Sachs,
1979; Davignon et al., 1981; Martz et al., 1982); hence, LFAs or
blocking sites represent a minority of the glycoproteins expressed
on CTL and target cells. Using a related and somewhat more
specific terminology, antigens on the surfaces of cytolytic T
lymphocytes (CTL) and target cells can be categorized into
"blocking sites" or "non-blocking sites". When antibody specific
for a single molecule significantly inhibits (typically by 40-90%)
CTL-mediated killing in the absence of complement, then that
molecule may be designated a "blocking site". This is most
convincing when the antibody is monoclonal, and immunoprecipitates
a single membrane glycoprotein.

At the time of the First International Workshop on Mechanisms
of Cell-Mediated Cytotoxicity (September, 1981), immunologists were
at the beginning of a wave of discoveries of blocking sites. The
idea of identifying functional CTL molecules by screening for
monoclonal antibodies was still new, but was in full swing. At
that time, only one blocking site was well recognized, mouse Lyt-
2,3 (Shinohara and Sachs, 1979; Nakayama et al., 1979). The wave of
discoveries ended (temporarily, we hope) in 1982, with a total of
six distinct CTL blocking sites and one target cell blocking site
having been described, summarized in Figure 1. We have recently
reviewed this topic (Martz et al., 1983), and that paper may be
consulted for citation of the original works describing the sites
listed in Figure 1. The mouse homolog of human T4, designated

L3T4, was not described until 1983 (Dialynas et al.). Human LFA-2 was described in 1982 (Sanchez-Madrid et al.), and later recognized to be the sheep red cell receptor, also designated T11 or Leu-5 (however, OKT11A MAb does not block killing; Krensky et al., 1983). In fact, Fast et al. (1981) had earlier shown partial inhibition of CTL-mediated killing with monoclonal anti-R_{srbc} antibody 9.6.

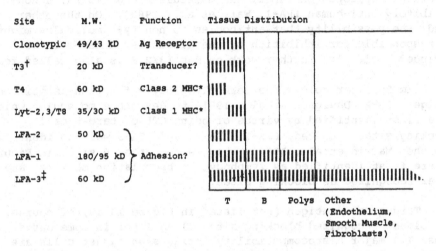

Site	M.W.	Function	Tissue Distribution
Clonotypic	49/43 kD	Ag Receptor	
T3[†]	20 kD	Transducer?	
T4	60 kD	Class 2 MHC*	
Lyt-2,3/T8	35/30 kD	Class 1 MHC*	
LFA-2	50 kD		
LFA-1	180/95 kD	Adhesion?	
LFA-3[‡]	60 kD		

                                        T   B   Polys Other
                                                       (Endothelium,
                                                        Smooth Muscle,
                                                        Fibroblasts)

* Assist in recognition of MHC antigens on target cell.

[†] αT3 MAb is mitogenic, and does not block conjugate formation.
   T3 comodulates with the clonotypic antigen receptor.

[‡] Target cell blocking site (all others are CTL blocking sites).

Fig. 1. Blocking Sites for CTL-Mediated Killing

[According to the new "cluster of differentiation" nomenclature (Bernard et al., 1984) T3 is CD3, T4 is CD4, T8 is CD8, and LFA-2 is CD2.]

Recently, it has been shown that some antibodies to the human T3 antigen can augment CTL-mediated killing (see H. Spits and coworkers elsewhere in this Volume). T1 may also be an LFA, since anti-T1 has recently been reported to induce T helper cells to release factors which induce B cell proliferation (Thomas et al., 1984).

It remains unclear whether or not T200 (also known as Ly-5 or the common leucocyte antigen) is a CTL blocking site (which would bring the total to 7). One early report (Nakayama et al., 1979) and one recent study (Harp et al., 1984) show inhibition of CTL-mediated killing by conventional alloantisera to Ly-5. Also, Gunther Dennert (Salk Institute, La Jolla CA, unpublished data, personal communication) has observed inhibition of CTL-mediated killing by the rat anti-mouse T200 MAb I3/2.3 described by Omary et al. (1980). However, Minato et al. (1980) and Brooks et al. (1982) saw no inhibition by conventional anti-Ly-5 alloantiserum. Also, two other rat monoclonal antibodies to mouse T200 failed to inhibit killing (Davignon et al., 1981). Of course, some monoclonals to LFAs do not inhibit killing, and thus are said to define non-functional epitopes on functional molecules (e.g. TS2/4, a non-inhibitory anti-human LFA-1, Ware et al., 1983). On the other hand, the possibility that antibodies to non Ly-5 molecules might be responsible for inhibition by the alloantisera needs to be excluded. Clearly, further work on MAb I3/2.3 is also called for.

Tim Springer coined the term "lymphocyte function-associated antigen" (LFA, Davignon et al., 1981) to designate molecules which were first identified by virtue of being CTL or target cell blocking sites. Indeed, LFA-1, LFA-2, and LFA-3 were so identified (Sanchez-Madrid et al., 1982), whereas the other 4 sites in Figure 1 were first identified as lymphocyte subpopulation markers, and later recognized as blocking sites.

Target cell antigen (not listed in Figure 1) is, of course, the oldest recognized blocking site. Class I (or in some cases class II) major histocompatibility antigens on target cells are blocking sites by virtue of being part or all of the specific antigen recognized by the CTL. Antisera specific for target cell H-2 were shown to block allospecific CTL nearly 20 years ago by Brunner et al. (1966), this in fact before CTL were shown to be T cells with anti-θ serum plus complement (Cerottini et al., 1970).

It is of particular interest that one target cell membrane glycoprotein, LFA-3, which does not appear to be part of the known antigen complex recognized by the CTL, is nevertheless a blocking site. Although LFA-3 is expressed on the CTL (and all other cells tested to date), the inhibitory effect of anti-LFA-3 antibody is mediated largely by binding to the target cell (based on experiments in which either the CTL or the target cells are precoated with MAb, then washed, Krensky et al., 1983). In this respect, anti-LFA-3 differs from all of the other blocking sites listed in Figure 1.

Mouse homologs have not yet been described for 3 of the 7 human sites listed in Figure 1: T3, LFA-2, and LFA-3. Note, however, that Gunter et al. (1984) have recently raised the possibility of homology between Thy-1 and T3. The slower progress in identifying mouse LFAs, as contrasted with human LFAs, is likely

294

explained by the fact that the former are identified with closely related allogeneic, rat or hamster monoclonal antibodies, while the latter are identified with much more phylogenetically distant mouse monoclonal antibodies. On the assumption that most of the yet-to-be-identified LFAs are structures conserved during evolution, murine immunologists are likely hindered by the fact that monoclonal antibody technology is best developed in murine species. Extension of monoclonal antibody technology to more distant species such as bovines (Srikumaran et al., 1983) would doubtless benefit the study of conserved functional antigens in murine species.

Antibodies to 5 of the blocking sites in Figure 1 inhibit the formation of strong adhesions between CTL and target cells, as judged by microscopic scoring of CTL-target conjugates (reviewed in Martz et al., 1983; see also Krensky et al., 1984). Antibodies to clonotypic putative antigen receptors have apparently not been tested, but would be expected to do the same. The well documented exception is anti-T3 antibody, which uniquely blocks killing without impairing conjugate formation (see, for example, Tsoukas elsewhere in this Volume).

Note that there exist at the present time no monoclonal antibodies which are believed to inhibit CTL-mediated killing by binding to lethal hit structures. This is in contrast to certain conventional xeno antisera which appear to be able to inhibit death of the target cell even when applied after completion of the lethal hit (Hiserodt and Bonavida, 1981; see also Hiserodt elsewhere in this Volume; for detailed discussion, see Martz et al., 1983). Henkart (elsewhere in this Volume) has been able to inhibit NK but not CTL-mediated killing with antisera to the granule constituents from effector lymphocytes.

BLOCKING VS. CTL-TARGET AFFINITY

Several years ago, our own results plus those from other laboratories (MacDonald et al., 1982) led us to hypothesize that susceptibility to inhibition by monoclonal antibody is inversely related to CTL-target affinity. Thus, we predicted that if the functional affinity between CTL and targets were experimentally reduced, less antibody would be needed to produce, say, 50% inhibition of CTL-mediated killing.

We reasoned that pretreatment of the target cells with papain, so as to remove most of the H-2 antigen, would reduce their affinity for allo-specific CTL (Gromkowski et al., 1983). In order to verify that affinity was reduced, we used the post-dispersion lysis assay (Martz, 1977). This quantitates the percentage of the target cells which form shear-resistant adhesions to CTL during a 5 min incubation (Fig. 2). [Admittedly, this is not a totally satisfactory way to estimate strength of adhesion or functional "affinity". However, the elegant binding assay developed by Balk and Mescher (1981) requires more than an hour to reach equilibrium, during which time significant replacement of H-2 would occur.] Removal with papain of over 90% of the target cell (P815) H-2 had little effect on killing in a conventional 2 hr ^{51}Cr release assay. This may have resulted from some replacement during the assay, since about 70% inhibition was seen when the assay time was reduced to 10 min (using 90:1 lymphocytes/targets). As expected, and consistent with reduced CTL-target affinity, post-dipsersion lysis following a 5 min incubation was reduced 50 to 98%.

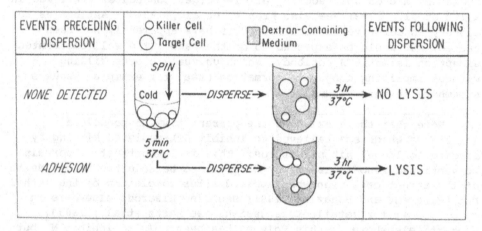

Figure 2. Post-dispersion lysis assay used to estimate relative strength of CTL-target adhesion. The percentage of target cells releasing ^{51}Cr during the 3 hr post-dispersion incubation represents the percentage which formed vortex dispersion-resistant adhesions with CTL during the 5 min pre-dispersion incubation. A reduction in the percentage of lysis was taken as an indication of reduced CTL-target affinity. Results are summarized in Table I. For details of this assay, see Gromkowski et al., 1983.

As indicated in Table I, papain pretreatment of target cells produced dramatic reductions in the concentrations of anti-Lyt-2,3 and anti-LFA-1 required for a given level of inhibition. MacDonald et al. (elsewhere in this Volume) found a similar result when the effective H-2 density was reduced with anti-H-2 antibody. These results are consistent with our working hypothesis (see Conclusions below).

Table I.

Effects of Protease Pretreatment of P815

Target Cells on Mouse CTL-Mediated Killing

Target Pretreatment:	Papain	Trypsin
2 hr Killing:	unchanged	unchanged
10 min Killing:	REDUCED	unchanged
5 min Adhesion:	REDUCED	slightly reduced
Class 1 MHC Antigen:	REMOVED	spared
Increased Suscept. to Inhibition by: αLyt-2,3:	<u>100 fold</u>	none
αLFA-1:	10 fold	10 fold

This Table summarizes data from Gromkowski
et al. 1983 and 1984a.

LFA-1 FUNCTION: INVOLVEMENT OF A TRYPSIN-SENSITIVE TARGET CELL MOLECULE

To address the possibility that H-2 was not the only relevant molecule being affected by papain, we examined the effects of trypsin (Gromkowski et al., 1984a). As expected (see Table I), H-2 was not removed by trypsin, and killing of trypsin-pretreated target cells (washed with trypsin inhibitor before the killing assay) was not diminished, even in a 10-min assay. Post-dispersion lysis was reduced about 25%, consistent with the idea that trypsin produced a smaller reduction in CTL-target affinity than did papain.

In marked contrast with the effect of papain, trypsin pretreatment of targets did not increase the susceptibility of the killing to inhibition by anti-Lyt-2,3. This was expected, and is consistent with the working hypothesis. However, to our suprise, susceptibility to inhibition by anti-LFA-1 was increased about 10-fold by trypsin pretreatment of the targets (see Table I), much as

it was by papain. This result provided a new functional
distinction between Lyt-2,3 and LFA-1. [MacDonald et al. (1982)
earlier provided a distinction by showing that some CTL clones are
susceptible to inhibition by LFA-1 but not Lyt-2,3.]

We considered what molecules might be removed by trypsin to
produce this effect. The P815 target cells used in these studies
express a low level of LFA-1, and this is trypsin-sensitive (S. H.
Gromkowski, W. Heagy, and E. Martz, unpublished data). However,
inhibition of killing requires saturation of the LFA-1 on the CTL;
binding of antibody to target cell LFA-1 alone does not inhibit
killing (Gromkowski and Martz, unpublished data; cf. Krensky et
al., 1983). Therefore, the concentration of anti-LFA-1 needed for
inhibition of CTL function could be increased as a result of target
cell LFA-1 competing for the intentionally limited supply of anti-
LFA-1 in a "sensitivity to blocking" assay. Removal of target cell
LFA-1 with trypsin could thus increase inhibition by removing this
competition. To test this possibility, we precoated P815 target
cells with anti-LFA-1 MAb, which prevented target cell LFA-1 from
competing for subsequently added limiting amounts of anti-LFA-1.
Yet we found that precoating did not increase the inhibition of
killing by the latter antibody. This result excluded the
possibility that the trypsin effect was mediated by its removal of
target cell LFA-1 (Gromkowski et al., 1984a).

The augmentation of anti-LFA-1 inhibition observed with
trypsinized targets suggests participation of a previously
unidentified non-H-2 target cell molecule. Removal or inactivation
of this putative molecule by trypsin makes blocking by anti-LFA-1
easier. Hence, when intact, the molecule must have a "counter
blocking" activity (we use "counter" rather than "anti" to avoid
confusion with "antibodies"). Consequently, an operational term
for this putative molecule is the "trypsin-sensitive counter
blocker" (TSCB, Gromkowski et al., 1984a; Martz et al., 1983).

CONCLUSIONS FOR THE MOUSE CTL SYSTEM

These results suggest the following tentative conclusions:

   1. The density of target cell class I H-2 antigens is
   crucial in determining the functional affinity between
   allospecific CTL and the targets. Other trypsin-
   sensitive target cell molecules may also be involved.

   2. Susceptibility of CTL-mediated killing to inhibition
   by anti-Lyt-2,3 is inversely related to CTL-target
   functional affinity. This does not appear to be the case
   for anti-LFA-1.

3. Lyt-2,3, but not LFA-1, is likely to be involved in the recognition of class I MHC antigens. [But see Hünig (1984) for a different conclusion.]

4. The function of LFA-1 is regulated by a non-MHC target cell molecule, the "trypsin-sensitive counter blocker" (TSCB).

Our conclusion 2 is in the same vein as one reached by Biddison et al. (1984), who saw an inverse relation between susceptibility of human CTL-mediated killing (allospecific for class II SB antigens) to inhibition by anti-T4 MAb and CTL-target affinity quantitated by the suspension equilibrium binding assay of Balk and Mescher (1981). Similarly, Marrack et al. (1983) saw an inverse relationship between inhibition by anti-L3T4 of IL2 release from T cell hybridomas and their affinity for antigen. The latter was quantitated by the reciprocal concentration of antigen (ovalbumin) needed for responsiveness.

Both Lyt-2,3 and LFA-1 seem likely to provide an "adhesion strengthening" function. LFA-1 might do this by binding to a natural ligand on the target cell (and perhaps, vice versa, target cell LFA-1 binding to a ligand on the CTL). This ligand might be the TSCB. However, a TSCB consistent with our data could exist regardless of whether or not it is a ligand for LFA-1. Thus, the question of whether or not CTL LFA-1 binds to a ligand on the target cell is independent from the question about the existence of a TSCB molecule.

What is the TSCB? We have already mentioned evidence which excludes target cell LFA-1 from this role. An attractive possibility would be LFA-3 (or its mouse homolog, yet to be identified). As mentioned above, anti-LFA-3 MAb inhibits CTL-mediated killing when only the target cell is pretreated with MAb. Pretreatment of the CTL is not inhibitory. LFA-3 is a 60 kD molecule with no evident relationship to MHC antigens. Moreover, anti-LFA-3 and anti-LFA-1 inhibit killing synergistically (Krensky et al., 1983). It was with the question of the relationship between the TSCB and LFA-3 in mind that we extended target trypsinization studies from the mouse to the human CTL system.

FUNCTIONAL DISTINCTIONS BETWEEN LFA-1, LFA-2, AND LFA-3 IN THE HUMAN CTL SYSTEM

In the human CTL system, our functional results with anti-LFA-1 and trypsin were very similar to those in the mouse (Gromkowski et al., 1984b). Trypsin pretreatment did not reduce the densities of HLA-A,B,C or HLA-DR, and reduced only slightly the density of the LFA-1 epitope recognized by the blocking MAb TS1/18. Also consistent with results in the mouse system, killing of trypsinized target cells was 10-fold more sensitive to inhibition by anti-LFA-1 (Figure 3).

Indeed, LFA-3 was about half-removed by a concentration of trypsin which produced the plateau-level 10-fold increase in sensitivity to inhibition of killing by anti-LFA-1. With 3-fold more trypsin, LFA-3 was completely removed. Thus, the trypsin-sensitivity of LFA-3 is consistent with the hypothesis that it is the TSCB. However, a definitive answer regarding this relationship awaits further work.

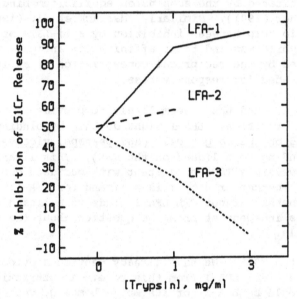

Figure 3. Effect of Target Trypsinization on Inhibition of Human CTL-Mediated Killing by Anti-LFA Antibodies. ^{51}Cr-labeled JY cells were pretreated with trypsin at the concentrations indicated in the presence of 2% fetal calf serum for 30 min, then rinsed in soy bean trypsin inhibitor. Cultured CTL were pretreated for 35 min in MAb (anti-LFA-1 = TS1/18; anti-LFA-2 = TS2/18; anti-LFA-3 = TS2/9), and target cells were added (without removing excess MAb) for 2 hr. Data are replotted from Gromkowski et al. (1984b).

Unexpectedly, we found striking functional differences for the effects of target trypsinization on inhibition by anti-LFA-1, anti-LFA-2, and anti-LFA-3 (Figure 3). Inhibition by anti-LFA-2 was not affected by target trypsinization. This helps to exclude the idea that trypsin might produce some nonspecific disturbance in, for example, cell charge or cytoskeleton which would increase blocking by any inhibitory antibody. [Neither did target trypsinization ever convert a non-blocking antibody into a blocking antibody.]

Inhibition by anti-LFA-3 was abolished by target trypsinization (Figure 3). If LFA-3 were an adhesion strengthening ligand for LFA-1, then we would predict that reduction in LFA-3 density would increase (steric) blocking by a given level of anti-LFA-3. Since we observed the opposite, another explanation is needed. (Keep in mind that the question of whether LFA-3 is a ligand for LFA-1 is independent of whether it is the TSCB.) LFA-3 might not normally be a direct participant in cell-cell adhesion. Instead, it could be a receptor for an unidentified agonist such that anti-LFA-3 triggers the delivery of an adhesion-inhibitory signal to the cell. This model would predict that reduction in LFA-3 density would be accompanied by a reduced inhibitory effect of anti-LFA-3, as we observed. It would also predict the observed lack of effect of LFA-3 removal on killing.

LFA-1 AND LFA-3 REGULATE NON-IMMUNOLOGIC HOMOTYPIC ADHESIONS OF HUMAN B LYMPHOCYTES

As shown in Figure 1, LFA-1 is widely expressed on lymphoid and myeloid cells. LFA-3 is expressed on every cell type tested to date (Krensky et al., 1983). Hence, it occurred to us that the abilities of these sites to regulate intercellular adhesions might not be limited to the heterotypic (e.g. CTL to target) adhesions triggered by immunologic antigen recognition which have been the focus of past studies.

Human B lymphocyte cell lines established in tissue culture tend to form spontaneous aggregates. The Epstein-Barr virus transformed cell line JY forms particularly large aggregates, easily reaching more than 500 microns in diameter and containing over 10^5 cells. Such aggregates form spontaneously overnight from a starting population of single cells. The adhesions are weaker than those between CTL and specific targets, since they can be broken by vortexing or vigorous swirling of the culture medium.

Anti-LFA-1 MAb greatly weakens the adhesions between JY cells (Gromkowski et al., 1984c). In the presence of the MAb, smaller looser-looking aggregates form, but they are broken into single cells by gentle swirling. Addition of anti-LFA-1 MAb to existing aggregates weakens them within a few hours so that they disintegrate upon gentle swirling (Figure 4). Anti-LFA-3 MAb also has a weakening effect, although much less dramatic. Control MAbs to HLA-A,B,C or HLA-DR did not weaken aggregates.

Unlike the antigen-specific adhesions previously shown to be

301

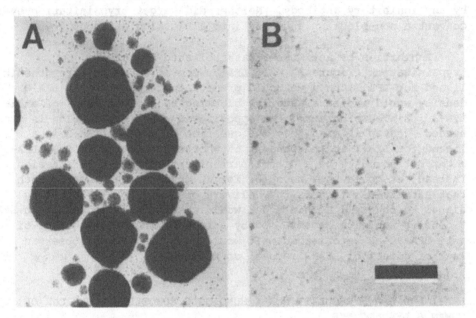

Figure 4. Anti-LFA-1 weakens spontaneous homotypic adhesions of JY human B cells. 7 x 10^4 JY cells (dispersed into single cells by vortexing) were cultured in 0.5 ml RPMI 1640 with 5% fetal calf serum in a 1.5 cm diameter polystyrene tissue culture well. After 3 days, aggregates had formed as shown in panel A. The photograph was taken after jiggling the plate so as to pile the largest aggregates into the field of view (4x objective). The scale bar in panel B signifies 500 μm. The larger aggregates in panel A are about 500 μm in diameter and contain about 50,000 cells each. Central cells do not become necrotic under these conditions. 50 μl of a culture supernantant from anti-LFA-1 hybridoma TS1/18 was added, bringing the MAb concentration to 5 μg/ml, and the cultures were swirled and returned to 37°. After 2.3 hr further incubation, the aggregates in the well containing anti-LFA-1 had largely disingegrated; a few small loose ones remained. The wells were shaken by hand for 15 sec; this caused complete disintegration of the aggregates in anti-LFA-1 (panel B), and had no effect on the aggregates in control wells.

inhibited by anti-LFA-1, these JY-JY cell-cell adhesions are presumably not triggered by an immunologic recognition of antigen, and occur between like cells (homotypic adhesion). Similar effects of anti-LFA-1 on mouse T and B cells had been noted by Pierres et al. (1981). The effect on JY adhesion is the first effect on human B cells seen for these MAbs. The regulation of cell-cell adhesions by LFA-1 and LFA-3 thus appears to extend to more general, non-immunologic adhesions of lymphoid cells.

POTENT IMMUNOSUPPRESSIVE EFFECT OF ANTI-LFA-1 IN VIVO

The foregoing data have demonstrated that anti-LFA-1 has unusual effects on cell interactions in vitro, even among inhibitory MAbs to the various other blocking sites. This led us to ask whether it might also have unusual effects in vivo. Heagy et al. (1984) compared the effects of several CTL-blocking MAbs in mice using two systems: rejection of semi-allogeneic P815 (H-2^d) tumor cells by A/J (H-2^a) mice, and the growth of syngeneic S1509a tumor cells in A/J mice. In both cases, tumor cells were injected subcutaneously, and tumor size was monitored by calipering.

Anti-LFA-1 was more potent at prolonging tumor allograft survival than were anti-Lyt-2,3, anti-T200, anti-Thy-1, anti-I-A, or anti-H-2K,D (Figure 5). Anti-LFA-1 (100 μg/day i.p. for the first 5 days) prolonged survival by 11 days (from 16 to 27 days). It increased the peak tumor area by 100%. None of the other antibodies prolonged survival for more than 5 days, or increased peak area by more than 40%. Anti-LFA-1 also accelerated the rate of growth of the syngeneic tumor more than did the other MAbs. Interestingly, the acceleration was cancelled when the anti-LFA-1 was mixed with anti-I-J MAb (the latter having previously been shown to retard S1509a tumor growth in A/J mice, Drebin et al., 1983).

Clearly, anti-LFA-1 has potential for immunosuppressive use in the clinic. The basis for its high immunosuppressive potency compared to other anti-lymphocyte MAbs may reside in a unique ability to inhibit intercellular adhesion interactions. This may inhibit both the primary immune response in vivo, as well as the ability of effector cells, once formed, to exit from the vasculature into the target tissue.

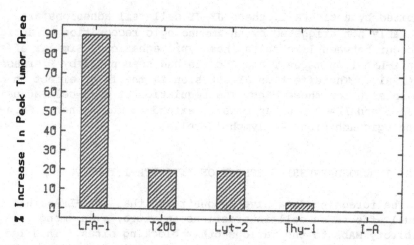

Figure 5. Effects of MAbs on allogeneic tumor growth in vivo. A/J
mice received 5 x 10[5] P815 cells subcutaneously in the back. Groups
of 6 were injected with MAb to the antigen indicated on the
abcissa: anti-LFA-1 = M17/4; anti-T200 = M1/9.3; anti-Lyt-2,3 =
M12/5; anti-Thy-1 = M5/49; anti-I-A = M5/114; controls, M1/69.HK
(does not bind to mouse cells). All MAbs were IgG2a except control
and anti-I-A were IgG2b. 100 μg Ig/day was injected i.p for the
first 5 days after tumor injection. Tumors were calipered daily.
Peak area in controls was 70 mm^2 on day 9; tumors were rejected
(less than 25 mm^2) on day 19. Peak areas for experimental mice were
achieved on days 9-15, and rejections were completed on days 19-31.
Data are replotted from Heagy et al. (1984).

REFERENCES

Balk, S., P., and Mescher, M. F., 1981, Specific reversal of
    cytolytic T cell-target cell functional binding is induced
    by free target cells. J. Immunol., 127:51.
Bernard, A., Bernstein, I., Boumsell, L., Dausset, J., Evans, R.,
    Hansen, J., Haynes, B., Kersey, J., Knapp, W., McMichael,
    A., Milstein, C., Reinherz, E., Ritts, R. E., and
    Schlossman, S. F., 1984, Differentiation human leucocyte
    antigens: a proposed nomenclature. Immunol. Today, 5:158.
Biddison, W. E., Rao, P. E., Talle, M. A., Goldstein, G., and Shaw,
    S., 1984, Possible involvement of the T4 molecule in T cell
    recognition of class II HLA antigens. Evidence from studies
    of CTL-target cell binding. J. Exp. Med., 159:783.

Brooks, C. G., Kuribayashi, K., Sale, G. E., and Henney, C. S., 1982, Characterization of five cloned murine cell lines showing high cytolytic activity against YAC-1 cells. J. Immunol., 128:2326.

Brunner, K. T., Mauel, J., and Schindler, R., 1967, Inhibitory effect of isoantibody on in vivo sensitization and on the in vitro cytotoxic action of immune lymphocytes. Nature, 213:1246.

Cerottini, J.-C., Nordin, A. A., and Brunner, K. T., 1970, Specific in vitro cytotoxicity of thymus-derived lymphocytes sensitized to alloantigens. Nature, 228:1308.

Davignon, D., Martz, E., Reynolds, T., Kürzinger, K., and Springer, T. A., 1981, Lymphocyte function-associated antigen one (LFA-1): a surface antigen distinct from Lyt-2/3 that participates in T lymphocyte-mediated killing. Proc. Nat. Acad. Sci. USA, 78:4535.

Dialynas, D. P., Quan, Z. S., Wall, K. A., Pierres, A., Quintans, J., Loken, M. R., Pierres, M., and Fitch, F. W., 1983, Characterization of the murine T cell surface molecule, designated L3T4, identified by monoclonal antibody GK1.5: similarity of L3T4 to the human Leu-3/T4 molecule. J. Immunol., 131:2445.

Drebin, J. A., Waltenbaugh, C., Schatten, S., and Greene, M. I., 1983, Inhibition of tumor growth in F_1 hybrids by in vivo administration of monoclonal anti-I-J antibodies reactive with either parental haplotype. J. Immunol., 130:505.

Fast, L. D., Hansen, J. A., and Newman, W., 1981, Evidence for T cell nature and heterogeneity within natural killer (NK) and antibody-dependent cellular cytotoxicity (ADCC) effectors: A comparison with cytolytic T lymphocytes (CTL). J. Immunol., 127:448.

Gromkowski, S. H., Heagy, W. E., Sanchez-Madrid, F., Springer, T. A., and Martz, E., 1983, Blocking of CTL-mediated killing by monoclonal antibodies to LFA-1 and Lyt-2,3 I. Increased susceptibility to blocking after papain treatment of target cells. J. Immunol., 130:2546.

Gromkowski, S. H., Heagy, W. H., and Martz, E., 1984a, Blocking of CTL-mediated killing by monoclonal antibodies to LFA-1 and Lyt-2,3 II. Evidence that trypsin pretreatment of target cells removes a non-H-2 molecule important in killing. Submitted for publication.

Gromkowski, S. H., Krensky, A., Martz, E., and Burakoff, S. J., 1984b, Functional distinctions between the LFA-1, LFA-2, and LFA-3 membrane proteins on human CTL are revealed with trypsin pretreated target cells. J. Immunol., in press.

Gromkowski, S. H., Krensky, A. M., Burakoff, S. J., and Martz, E., 1984c, LFA-1 and LFA-3 membrane molecules regulate cell-cell adhesions of human B cells. Submitted for publication.

Gunter, K. C., Malek, T. R., and Shevach, E. M., 1984, T cell-activating properties of an anti-Thy-1 monoclonal antibody. J. Exp. Med., 159:716.

Harp, J. A., Davis, B. S., and Ewald, S. J., 1984, Inhibition of T
cell responses to alloantigens and polyclonal mitogens by Ly-
5 antisera. J. Immunol., 133:10.

Heagy, W., Waltenbaugh, C., and Martz, E., 1984, Potent ability of
anti-LFA-1 monoclonal antibody to prolong allograft
survival. Transplantation, 37:520.

Hiserodt, J. C., and Bonavida, B., 1981, Studies on the induction
and expression of T cell-mediated immunity: XI. Inhibition
of the "Lethal Hit" in T cell-mediated cytotoxicity by
heterologous rat antiserum made against alloimmune cytotoxic
T lymphocytes. J. Immunol., 126:256.

Hünig, T., 1984, Monoclonal anti-Lyt-2.2 antibody blocks lectin-
dependent cellular cytotoxicity of H-2-negative target
cells. J. Exp. Med., 159:551.

Krensky, A. M., Robbins, E., Springer, T. A., and Burakoff, S. J.,
1984, LFA-1, LFA-2, and LFA-3 antigens are involved in CTL-
target conjugation. J. Immunol., 132:2180.

Krensky, A. M., Sanchez-Madrid, F., Robbins, E., Nagy, J. A.,
Springer, T. A., and Burakoff, S. J., 1983, The functional
significance, distribution, and structure of LFA-1, LFA-2,
and LFA-3: Cell surface antigens associated with CTL-target
interactions. J. Immunol., 131:611.

MacDonald, H. R., Glasebrook, A. L., and Cerottini, J.-C., 1982,
Clonal heterogeneity in the functional requirement for Lyt-
2/3 molecules on cytolytic T lymphocytes: analysis by
antibody blocking and selective trypsinization. J. Exp.
Med., 156:1711.

Marrack, P., Endres, R., Shimonkevitz, R., Zlotnik, A., Dialynas,
D., Fitch, F., and Kappler, J., 1983, The major
histocompatibility complex-restricted antigen receptor on T
cells. II. Role of the L3T4 product. J. Exp. Med.,
158:1077.

Martz, E., 1975, Early steps in specific tumor cell lysis by
sensitized mouse T-lymphocytes I. Resolution and
characterization. J. Immunol., 115:261.

Martz, E., Davignon, D., Kürzinger, K., and Springer, T. A., 1982,
The molecular basis for cytolytic T lymphocyte function:
analysis with blocking monoclonal antibodies. Adv. Exptl.
Biol. Med., 146:447.

Martz, E., Heagy, W., and Gromkowski, S. H., 1983, The mechanism of
CTL-mediated killing: Monoclonal antibody analysis of the
roles of killer and target cell membrane proteins. Immunol.
Rev., 72:73.

Minato, N., Reid, L., Cantor, H., Lengyel, P., and Bloom, B. R.,
1980, Mode of regulation of natural killer cell activity by
interferon. J. Exp. Med., 152:124.

Nakayama, E., Shiku, H., Stockert, E., Oettgen, H. F., and Old, L.
J., 1979, Cytotoxic T cells: Lyt phenotype and blocking of
killing activity by Lyt antisera. Proc. Natl. Acad. Sci.
USA, 76:1977.

Omary, M. B., Trowbridge, I. S., and Scheid, M. P., 1980, T200 cell surface glycoprotein of the mouse. Polymorphism defined by the Ly-5 system of alloantigens. J. Exp. Med., 151:1311.

Pierres, M., Goridis, C., and Golstein, P., 1981, Inhibition of murine T cell-mediated cytolysis and T cell proliferation by a rat monoclonal antibody immunoprecipitating two lymphoid cell surface polypeptides of 94,000 and 180,000 molecular weight. Eur. J. Immunol., 12:60.

Sanchez-Madrid, F., Krensky, A. M., Ware, C. F., Robbins, E., Strominger, J. L., Burakoff, S. J., and Springer, T. A., 1982, Three distinct antigens associated with human T lymphocyte-mediated cytolysis: LFA-1, LFA-2, and LFA-3. Proc. Nat. Acad. Sci. USA, 79:7489.

Shinohara, N., and Sachs, D. H., 1979, Mouse alloantibodies capable of blocking cytotoxic T-cell function I. Relationship between the antigen reactive with blocking antibodies and the Lyt-2 locus. J. Exp. Med., 150:432.

Srikumaran, S., Guidry, A. J., and Goldsby, R. A., 1983, Production and characterization of monoclonal bovine immunoglobulins G1, G2 and M from bovine x murine hybridomas. Vet. Immunol. Immunopathol., 5:323.

Thomas, Y., Glickman, E., DeMartino, J., Wang, J., Goldstein, G., and Chess, L., 1984, Biologic functions of the OKT1 cell surface antigen I. The T1 molecule is involved in helper function. J. Immunol., 133:724.

Ware, C. F., Sanchez-Madrid, F., Krensky, A. M., Burakoff, S. J., Strominger, J. L., and Springer, T. A., 1983, Human lymphocyte function associated antigen-1 (LFA-1): Identification of multiple antigenic epitopes and their relationship to CTL-mediated cytotoxicity. J. Immunol., 131:1182.

DISCUSSION

B. Bonavida: Do you have any evidence that the TSCB (trypsin sensitive counter blocker) is not papain sensitive?

E. Martz: No, in fact we believe it is.

B. Bonavida: So actually it could be a papain as well as a trypsin sensitive molecule.

E. Martz: Yes.

B. Bonavida: What was the recovery rate of this molecule?

E. Martz: Several hours.

T. Springer: Work in my laboratory leads to a very similar conclusion on the involvement of LFA-1 in cell-cell adherance. When we took JY cells and rotated them at several hundred RPM, they fell apart into single cells. However, if you then add phorbol ester the cells form adhesions which are resistant to the shear force. If you add anti-LFA-1 antibody to the system the shear resistant aggregates are completely broken up into single cells.

Our interpretation of the CTL data actually is that blocking by anti-LFA-1 may not always be unidirectional. In the original experiments that we did together [with Martz] we were working with mouse anti-rat killer cells -- there, clearly anti-LFA-1 antibody was blocking because it was binding to the effector cells. It was impossible for it to bind to the target cells which were of the same species. But we have some preliminary evidence that if LFA-1 is absent on the effector cells -- we have some LFA-1 negative patients -- anti-LFA-1 antibody added to the target cells can decrease killing in some cases. So in fact it may be a bidirectional interaction but in most cases I think that LFA-1 on the effector cell is contributing much more to the avidity than LFA-1 on the target cell.

E. Martz: I would certainly agree with those points. The effects on the JY cells strongly suggest that the antibody (inaudible) must be having some effects on the target cell. Actually, Misha Sitkovsky will present some data which will show effects on target cells.

P. Golstein: One way of testing whether the monoclonal antibody acts on killer cells or target cells is to preincubate either killers or target cells, and then wash out, and then mix and see what happens. Now with anti-LFA-1 antibodies if you preincubate the killer cells then you get block, but the block is not complete. If you preincubate the target cells and wash out then usually you do not get block. If now, having preincubated the killer cells, you also preincubate the target cells, then you complete the block. In other words, you have LFA-1 determinants on the target cells which play a role in adhesion, but in order to see this role, you have to neutralize the LFA-1 determinants on the effector cells.

E. Martz: We also have similar data, that pretreatment of both the killer and the target is more effective than pretreatment of one. We believe that this result could be accounted for by the fact that if you don't pretreat the target, it can simply serve as an antibody sink, able to remove antibody from the killer cell. Therefore the interpretation of that experiment could still be that the action is primarily on the CTL.

C. Nathan (?): Eric, I wonder if either you or Tim has had a chance to compare the LFA-1 family to the cell adhesion molecules described by Gerry Edelman's lab, specifically N-CAM and L-CAM.

E. Martz: I see no evident molecular relationship. I think Edelman's work is quite pretty. These LFA molecules appear to be expressed only on leucocytes, lymphoid or monocyte myeloid type cells.

T. Springer: I agree with that. We have looked with our anti-beta subunit antibodies which pick up not only LFA-1 but other members of this family and they clearly don't stain neuronal cells in the brain.

J. Russell: Does anti-LFA-1 have any effect on the growth properties of the cells?

E. Martz: We haven't looked in the JY system. However, in our early experiments, Tim showed that anti-LFA-1 was not able to block proliferation in the mixed lymphocyte assay once the antigenic triggering had occured. When the antibody was added at day 2 or 3, it was unable to block LPS-induced proliferation. So there's good evidence in the mouse system that anti-LFA-1 does not affect cell proliferation once its turned on.

(unidentified): Have you tried the in vivo experiments with LFA-1 negative tumors?

E. Martz: Sarcoma 1509a, for which we observed accelerated growth in syngeneic mice, is an LFA-1 negative tumor, at least as far as one can tell by FACS analysis.

G. Berke: I was cautioned at times that when we're using trypsin on cells to use acetylated trypsin, since trypsin is somewhat tricky: it may stick on cells, and in fact affect the

other cell. So I'd like to suggest that you do those experiments
by testing the effect of acetylated trypsin (you can get it from
Sigma) to exclude the possibility that that sort of deblocking is
actually a reverse trypsin effect on the part of the killer cell.

[Editor's comment added later by E. Martz: the trypsinized
target cells were washed in soy bean trypsin inhibitor before being
exposed to the effector cells.]

THE FUNCTION OF LFA-1 IN CELL-MEDIATED KILLING AND ADHESION: STUDIES ON HERITABLE LFA-1, Mac-1 DEFICIENCY AND ON LYMPHOID CELL SELF-AGGREGATION

Timothy A. Springer, Robert Rothlein, Donald C. Anderson, Steven J. Burakoff, and Alan M. Krensky

Dana-Farber Cancer Istitute, Harvard Medical School
Boston, Massachusetts 02115
Baylor College of Medicine, Houston, TX 77030
Stanford University, Stanford, CA 94395

INTRODUCTION

Lymphocyte function associated antigen-1 (LFA-1) is a cell surface glycoprotein identified in mouse and human by monoclonal antibodies which inhibit cytolytic T lymphocyte (CTL) mediated cytolysis (1-5). LFA-1 contains noncovalently associated α and β subunits of M_r = 180,000 and 95,000, respectively. Anti-LFA-1 monoclonal antibodies (MAb) inhibit cytolysis by CTL and NK cells as well as proliferative responses to mitogens, alloantigens, and soluble antigens. LFA-1 is broadly distributed on leukocytes, including lymphocytes, granulocytes, and monocytes, but is not expressed on a number of other somatic cells. Anti-LFA-1 monoclonal antibodies inhibit conjugate formation between CTL and targets (1,6,7); therefore, LFA-1 may be instrumental in cell-cell adhesion.

Recently, a number of patients with recurring, life-threatening infections were found to be deficient in LFA-1 and two other surface molecules which utilize the same β subunit, Mac-1 and p150,95 (8-11). This experiment of nature offered another means of testing the functional importance of LFA-1. We have previously suggested that LFA-1 acts as a cell adhesion molecule which can synergize with antigen-specific receptors in CTL-mediated killing, Fc receptors in antibody-dependent cellular cytotoxicity, or other receptors in natural killing to increase the avidity of cell-cell interactions (5,12,13). In addition to this, however, was raised the possibility that LFA-1 was not involved in adhesion, but that binding of anti-LFA-1 MAb provided a nonspecific "off" signal to effector cells (14).

311

The LFA-1-deficient patients provide a means of discriminating between these possibilities. Further experiments are also described in which it is shown that LFA-1 can mediate homotypic adhesion between cells. The results in both cases demonstrate the importance of LFA-1 in leukocyte cell-cell adhesion. Both findings also suggest that LFA-1 on target cells, as well as on effector cells, can contribute to adhesion reactions.

Mac-1, LFA-1, p150,95 IMMUNODEFICIENCY

We have investigated three patients with this disease (8-10). The αM and β subunits of Mac-1, the αL and β subunits of LFA-1, and at least the β subunit of p150,95 are deficient on the surface of patient leukocytes. Deficiency appears to be quantitative rather than qualitative, with two patients expressing about 0.5% and one patient about 5% of normal amounts on granulocytes and mononuclear cells. Quantitation by immunofluorescent flow cytometry of subunits on granulocytes from parents of these patients shows approximately half-normal surface expression. Together with absence of any evidence of mosaicism due to X chromosome inactivation in the mothers' leukocytes, the data demonstrate autosomal recessive inheritance. It appears that the primary deficiency in patient cells is of the common β subunit. Patient lymphocytes biosynthesize normal amounts of LFA-1 α chain intracellular precursor; however, it does not mature or become surface expressed (9). It appears that association with the β subunit is required for surface expression.

FUNCTIONAL ASSESSMENTS OF LFA-1 DEFICIENT LYMPHOCYTES

To examine allospecific lysis, peripheral blood lymphocytes (PBL) from LFA-1 deficient patients, family members, and unrelated individuals were stimulated with the EBV-transformed B cell line, JY. Mismatches occurred at a number of HLA loci. After six days, cells were harvested and tested for cytolysis of ^{51}Cr-labeled JY cells (Table I). All LFA-1 deficient individuals showed abnormally low levels of cytolysis of JY cells. Lytic unit calculations showed that patient 1 gave less than 10% of control lysis; patient 2 was less than 15% of control levels. In one preliminary experiment, patient 4 was approximately 50% of control levels of cytolysis (not shown). The proliferative response to JY by patient cells was 30% to 50% of normal (data not shown). Since all effector cells were adjusted to the same concentration before the CTL assay, the deficiency in cytolysis was not secondary to a failure to proliferate. Although primary human mixed lymphocyte cultures contain both specific CTL and non-specific NK cells, anti-HLA-A,B,C (w6/32) and OKT3 monoclonal antibody blocking experiments showed that greater than 50% of the JY cytolysis was allospecific and mediated by OKT3[+] CTL (data not shown).

Table I. Primary Cytolysis on Specific and Natural Killing Targets[a]

E:T[b]	Specific Killing			Natural Killing		
	100:1	25:1	6:1	100:1	25:1	6:1
	JY ^{51}Cr release (%)			K562 ^{51}Cr release (%)		
Patient 1	10	8	2	14	7	0
Mother 1	45	33	15	55	46	18
Father 1	52	49	33	67	51	27
Control 1	84	72	56	80	83	72
Patient 2	16	14	9	18	11	8
Mother 2	38	23	9	35	25	20
Father 2	53	36	29	77	55	59
Control 2	76	65	64	90	87	88

a. Cytolysis by primary cultures (6 days) of peripheral blood
lymphocytes is shown as percentage specific release in a 3-4 hour
assay (5). HLA types are patient 1: HLA-A2,w32; Bw35,w51; Cw4;
DR3,4; mother 1: HLA-A2,2; B27,w51; Cw1; DR3,?: father 1: HLA-A3,
w32; B7,w35; Cw4,7; DR2,4; patient 2: HLA-A1,2; B14,14; Cw7,w8;
DR1,w6; mother 2: HLA-A1,w23; B14,w57; Cw3,w7; DRw6,w9; father 2:
HLA-A2,28; B14,w62; Cw1,w8; DR1,?; JY: HLA-A2,2; B7,7; DR4,6.
b. Effector: target ratio.

To assess natural killing, PBL from LFA-1 deficient individuals,
their families, and unrelated controls were cultured alone or with
JY cells for six days. Natural killing was assessed on the K562
erythroleukemia cell line (HLA negative). All LFA-1 deficient
individuals showed low levels of NK cell-mediated cytolysis
compared to that of family members and unrelated indivuals (Table I).

PBL were also tested for proliferation after stimulation with
the lectin phytohemagglutinin (PHA). PBL from LFA-1 deficient
patients showed an impaired proliferative response to PHA (Table II).
Responses were 20% and 10% of normal at 2.5 µg/ml and 0.25 µg/ml
PHA, respectively. Interestingly, the responses by patient cells
were further diminished when anti-LFA-1 MAb was added to cultures.

Patient CTL lines were maintained in long term culture by stimulation every one to two weeks with irradiated JY cells in the
presence of T cell growth factor-containing medium. After three
weeks in culture, the efficiency of cytolysis by LFA-1 deficient
lymphocytes increased, but remained lower than that of normal lymphocytes from family members. Similar cytolytic efficiency persisted
for up to twenty weeks in continuous culture. FACS analysis showed
approximately 0.8% of normal expression of LFA-1 on CTL from patient
4 and < 0.1% of normal expression on CTL from patients 1 and 2
(Figure 1).

Table II. Proliferative Responses to PHA

	2.5 µg/ml	2.5 µg/ml, + anti-LFA-1	0.25 µg/ml	none
	^{3}H-thymidine incorporation ± SD (cpm x 10^{-3})			
Patient 2	28 ± 3	3.8 ± 0.2	1.5 ± 0.7	0.3 ± 0.05
Mother 2	101 ± 8	11.7 ± 2	9.1 ± 0.4	0.5 ± 0.01
Brother 2a	102 ± 2	2.9 ± 0.7	4.9 ± 2.1	0.5 ± 0.2
Brother 2b	138 ± 9	4.6 ± 0.1	10 ± 3.0	0.4 ± 0.1
Patient 4	23 ± 5	3.1 ± 0.1	0.6 ± 3.2	1.0 ± 1.0
Mother 4	75 ± 25	18.4 ± 5	13.9 ± 2.5	3.0 ± 2.4
Sister 4	108 ± 15	12.8 ± 2	9.2 ± 1.0	9.0 ± 13
Control	71 ± 14	5.5 ± 5	4.7 ± 4.9	1.1 ± 1.0

a. Proliferative responses to the indicated concentrations of PHA were measured on day 3 (5). Purified, TS1/18 F(ab')$_2$ anti-LFA-1 MAb (3 µg/ml) was added at the initiation of cultures.

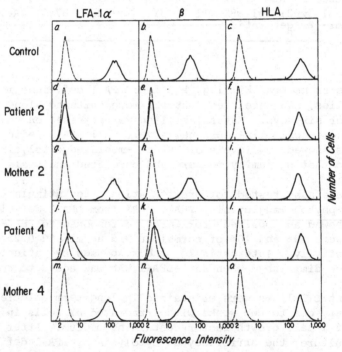

Fig. 1. Immunofluorescence Flow Cytometry of LFA-1 on Deficient and Normal CTL Lines. Long term CTL lines (four weeks) were labeled with MAb to the LFA-1 α subunit (a mixture of five MAb), to the LFA-1 β subunit (TS1/18), or to HLA (W6/32), then with fluorescin isothiocyanate-anti-mouse IgG, and analyzed on an Epics V cytometer (9).

314

CTL lines of patients, parents, and normal controls (Figure 1) were tested for their susceptibility to inhibition by anti-LFA-1 MAb. Effector and target cells were separately pretreated with anti-LFA-1 MAb and washed extensively prior to the ^{51}Cr release assay, and in one group anti-LFA-1 MAb was also included in the assay medium (Table III). Killing by healthy adult and parental CTL was inhibited by anti-LFA-1 MAb bound to the effector cell but not by MAb bound to the target cell as previously reported for normal CTL (5). Killing by patient 4 CTL was similarly inhibited by MAb bound to the effector. Thus, the small amount (0.8% of normal) of LFA-1 present on patient 4 is functionally important. Of note, in contrast to healthy CTL, killing by patient 4 CTL was also inhibited by MAb bound to the target cell.

Contrasting results were also found for the quantitatively more severely LFA-1 deficient CTL of patients 1 and 2. Killing by patient 2 CTL was poorly inhibited when anti-LFA-1 MAb was added to the assay, and pretreatment of killers or effectors gave equivocal or no blocking. CTL from patient 1 were inhibited when anti-LFA-1 was included in the assay. However, killing by patient 1 CTL was inhibited by MAb bound to the target cell and not by MAb bound to the effector cell. The findings with anti-JY CTL from patients 1 and 2 have been repeated many times; two representative experiments are shown in Table III.

The findings with patient 1 and 4 CTL suggest that LFA-1 on target cells can also contribute to the CTL-target cell interaction. It can be speculated that target cell LFA-1 also participates in normal CTL-mediated killing, but that its contribution to the interaction is negligible compared to that of effector cell LFA-1. The difference in anti-LFA-1 susceptibility between patient 1 and patient 2 is not understood at present. It may relate to different HLA disparities with JY as well as to differences in the LFA-1 mutation or level of expression.

Blocking by anti-LFA-1 MAb bound to the target cell might also be due to antibody bound by one combining site with target cell LFA-1 reacting through the second combining site with CTL LFA-1. Inhibition by this mechanism could be much more potent with patient CTL. Saturation of patient LFA-1 sites would occur with much less anti-LFA-1 bound per CTL, but might give equivalent inhibition of killing.

LYMPHOCYTE AGGREGATION IS INHIBITED BY ANTI-LFA-1

Another line of investigation provides independent evidence that LFA-1 on JY cells is functionally important, and supports a general role for LFA-1 in cell adhesion processes. Previous studies have demonstrated that phorbol esters induce adhesion in a wide variety of cell lines as well as in peripheral blood B and T lympho-

Table III. Inhibition of Cytolysis by Anti-LFA-1 MAb: Pre-treatment of Effectors or Targets[a]

Treatment	Experiment 1						Experiment 2	
	Control	Mom 1	Dad 1	Pat. 1	Pat. 2	Pat. 4	Pat. 1	Pat. 2
	% ^{51}Cr release from JY (at 2 different E:T ratios)							
None	61/49	64/45	64/48	49/35	66/69	52/28	52/29	48/32
Antibody in Assay	31/14	26/15	29/22	24/19	59/62	34/22	21/13	51/29
Effectors Pre-treated	46/36	37/27	43/35	47/42	54/45	25/19	55/26	42/32
Targets Pre-treated	61/48	61/39	63/47	28/19	85/68	23/22	29/21	56/41
Both Effectors and Targets Pre-treated	50/34	39/29	45/41	27/21	49/44	28/25	27/19	47/34

a. CTL-mediated killing expressed as % ^{51}Cr specific release was determined at effector:target ratios of 50:1 and 20:1 for patients and 25:1 and 10:1 for family members and the control. Effectors and target cells were separately pretreated with TS1/18 anti-LFA-1 MAb or mock pretreated with a control MAb, washed four times, then mixed together and assayed in the presence or absence of TS1/18 MAb as previously described (5). Assays were terminated after three to four hours, whenever 50% cytolysis was obtained at the higher E:T ratio.

Table IV. Effect of anti-LFA-1 MAb on PMA-Stimulated Aggregation of JY cells[a]

PMA	Additions	Exp. 1	Exp. 2
		Aggregated Cells (%)	
-	-	6	6.7
+	-	60	39.5
+	TS1/22 anti-LFA-1 α	0	1.3
+	TS1/18 anti-LFA-1 β	0	ND
+	TS1/18 + TS1/22	0	ND
+	TS2/18 (control)	62	ND
+	EGTA (5mM)	ND	0
+	EGTA (5mM) + Mg^{+2} (5mM)	ND	43.3

a. JY cells (3×10^6 in 300 µl of RPMI medium with 5 mM HEPES) were incubated alone, with PMA (50 ng/ml) or with PMA + MAb hybridoma supernatant (10 µl) at 37° C for 30 minutes with constant agitation. Aggregated and non-aggregated cells were counted in a hemocytometer.

cytes and monocytes (15-17). Similar divalent cation-dependent clustering occurs when autologous lymph node cells are cultured (18). LFA-1 seemed a likely candidate for mediating this adhesion process because of its wide distribution on leukocytes, its wide importance in functions requiring adhesion, its lack of antigen specificity, and its known participation in the divalent cation-dependent adhesion step in CTL-mediated killing. Therefore, the effect of LFA-1 on phorbol myristyl acetate- (PMA) mediated adhesion by JY cells was investigated (Table IV). Phorbol ester increased the percentage of aggregated JY cells from 6% to 40-60% (Table IV). Addition of MAb to the LFA-1 α or β subunit decreased aggregation to 0-1%. The decrease to below the level of spontaneous aggregation suggests anti-LFA-1 inhibits spontaneous as well as PMA-stimulated adherence, which has been confirmed in other experiments. The adhesion step is dependent on divalent cations, as shown by inhibition by EGTA, a strong Ca^{+2} and weak Mg^{+2} chelator, and the restoration of adhesion by addition of Mg^{+2} (Table IV). Previous studies had demonstrated that EDTA and EGTA inhibited (16,17). Addition of anti-LFA-1 MAb disrupted pre-formed aggregates (data not shown), in parallel with previous findings on CTL-target conjugates (13). These data suggest a strong similarity between phorbol ester-induced cell-cell aggregation and the LFA-1-dependent adhesion step in CTL-mediated killing (1,5,7,13), and suggest LFA-1 functions as an adhesion protein. Similar independent findings by Martz et. al. for spontaneous aggregation are reported elsewhere in this volume.

CONCLUSION

Patients with a genetic deficiency of LFA-1 demonstrate defects in antigen-specific killing, natural killing, and proliferative responses to lectins and alloantigens. These functional deficits conclusively demonstrate that LFA-1 is functionally important for lymphocyte cell interactions. The functional impairments of patient cells resemble those of anti-LFA-1 MAb-treated healthy control cells. This shows that MAb bound to LFA-1 inhibits LFA-1's normal physiological function, rather than activating some other mechanism such as a nonspecific "off-switch." The patients differed in the severity of their functional deficits, with the patient with the highest amount of cell surface LFA-1 showing the mildest effects on function. After repeated _in vitro_ stimulation, functional CTL lines could be established from all patients, although their cytolytic activity was below normal. Killing by CTL effectors of the two most deficient patients was resistant to inhibition by anti-LFA-1 MAb. This may suggest that LFA-1 is an auxiliary molecule which can boost the efficiency or avidity of CTL, but is not essential for function. However, of importance in these responses could be the small amounts of cell surface LFA-1 which appear present in even the most deficient patients, as shown by immunofluorescent cytometry and the effects of anti-LFA-1 MAb on proliferation to PHA.

The results with one patient demonstrated that LFA-1 on the target cell, as well as on the effector cell, can be functionally important. A bidirectional interaction may normally occur physiologically, with LFA-1 on the effector cell of the most importance as shown by blocking experiments. A bidirectional interaction mechanism was also supported by studies on phorbol ester-induced adhesion of JY cells. Anti-LFA-1 MAb inhibited aggregation of JY cells, a process which can be regarded as homotypic as opposed to the heterotypic adhesion between effector and target cells. The importance of LFA-1 in JY cell self-aggregation is in agreement with the findings that LFA-1 on JY cells can participate in adherence to CTL. LFA-1-dependent adhesion resembled CTL-target conjugate formation in divalent cation-dependence and reversibility with MAb. It is proposed that LFA-1 acts physiologically to promote adherence between leukocytes and other cells, thereby enhancing the efficiency or avidity of interactions mediated by other leukocyte surface receptors such as the antigen-receptor of T lymphocytes.

ACKNOWLEDGEMENT

Supported by NIH grants AI 05877, CA 31798, CA 34128, AM 35008, and Council for Tobacco Research Grant 1307A.

REFERENCES

1. D. Davignon, E. Martz, T. Reynolds, K. Kurzinger, and T. A.
   Springer, Monoclonal antibody to a novel lymphocyte function-
   associated antigen (LFA-1): Mechanism of blocking of T lymphocyte-mediated killing and effects on other T and B lymphocyte functions, J. Immunol., 127:590 (1981).
2. M. Pierres, C. Goridis, and P. Goldstein, Inhibition of murine
   T cell-mediated cytolysis and T cell proliferation by a rat
   monoclonal antibody immunoprecipitating two lymphoid cell
   surface polypeptides of 94,000 and 180,000 molecular weight,
   Eur. J. Immunol., 12:60 (1982).
3. F. Sanchez-Madrid, A. M. Krensky, C. F. Ware, E. Robbins, J. L.
   Strominger, S. J. Burakoff, and T. A. Springer, Three distinct
   antigens associated with human T lymphocyte-mediated cytolysis: LFA-1, LFA-2, and LFA-3, Proc. Natl. Acad. Sci. USA,
   79:7489 (1982).
4. J. E. K. Hildreth, F. M. Gotch, P. D. K. Hildreth, and A. M.
   McMichael, A human lymphocyte-associated antigen involved
   in cell-mediated lympholysis, Eur. J. Immunol., 13:202 (1983).
5. A. M. Krensky, F. Sanchez-Madrid, E. Robbins, J. Nagy, T. A.
   Springer, and S. J. Burakoff, The functional significance,
   distribution, and structure of LFA-1, LFA-2, and LFA-3: cell
   surface antigens associated with CTL-target interactions,
   J. Immunol., 131:611 (1983).
6. P. Bongrand, M. Pierres, and P. Goldstein, T-cell mediated
   cytolysis: on the strength of effector-target cell interaction, Eur. J. Immunol., 13:424 (1983).
7. A. M. Krensky, E. Robbins, T. A. Springer, and S. J. Burakoff,
   LFA-1, LFA-2 and LFA-3 antigens are involved in CTL-target
   conjugation, J. Immunol., 132:2180 (1984).
8. D. C. Anderson, F. C. Schmalsteig, S. Kohl, M. A. Arnaout, B. J.
   Hughes, M. F. Tosi, G. J. Buffone, B. R. Brinkley, W. D.
   Dickey, J. S. Abramson, T. A. Springer, L. A. Boxer, J. M.
   Hollers, and C. W. Smith, Abnormalities of polymorphonuclear
   leukocyte function associated with a heritable deficiency
   of high molecular weight surface glycoproteins (GP138):
   Common relationship to diminished cell adherence, J. Clin.
   Invest., 74:536 (1984).
9. T. A. Springer, W. S. Thompson, L. J. Miller, F. C. Schmalsteig,
   and D. C. Anderson, Inherited deficiency of the Mac-1, LFA-1,
   p150,95 glycoprotein family and its molecular basis, J. Exp.
   Med., in press.
10. D. C. Anderson, F. C. Schmalsteig, W. Shearer, K. Freeman, S.
    Kohl, C. W. Smith, and T. A. Springer, Abnormalities of PMN/
    Monocyte function and recurrent infection associated with a
    heritable deficiency of adhesive surface glycoproteins, Fed.
    Proc., in press.

11. M. A. Arnaout, N. Dana, J. Pitt, and R. F. Todd, III, Deficiency of two human leukocyte surface membrane glyco-proteins (Mol and LFA-1), Fed. Proc., in press.

12. S. Kohl, T. A. Springer, F. C. Schmalstieg, L. S. Loo, and D. C. Anderson, Defective natural killer cytotoxicity and polymorphonuclear leukocyte antibody-dependent cellular cytotoxicity in patients with LFA-1/OKM-1 deficiency, J. Immunol., in press.

13. T. A. Springer, D. Davignon, M. K. Ho, K. Kurzinger, E. Martz, and F. Sanchez-Madrid, LFA-1 and Lyt-2,3, molecules associated with T lymphocyte-mediated killing; and Mac-1, an LFA-1 homologue associated with complement receptor function, Immunol. Rev., 68:111 (1982).

14. P. Goldstein, C. Goridis, A. M. Schmitt-Verhulst, B. Hayot, A. Pierres, A. Van Agthoven, Y. Kaufmann, Z. Eshhar, and M. Pierres, Lymphoid cell surface interaction structures detected using cytolysis-inhibiting monoclonal antibodies, Immunol. Rev., 68:5 (1982).

15. M. Patarroyo, G. Yogeeswaran, P. Biberfeld, E. Klein, and G. Klein, Morphological changes, cell aggregation and cell membrane alterations caused by phorbol 12,13-dibutyrate in human blood lymphocytes, Int. J. Cancer, 30:707 (1982).

16. M. Patarroyo, P. Biberfeld, E. Klein, and G. Klein, Phorbol 12,13-dibutyrate (P(Bu2))-treated human blood mononuclear cells bind to each other Cell. Immunol., 75:144 (1983).

17. M. Patarroyo, M. Jondal, J. Gordon, and E. Klein, Characterization of the phorbol 12,13-dibuytrate (P(Bu2)) induced binding between human lymphocytes, Cell. Immunol., 81:373 (1983).

18. A. Hamann, D. Jablonski-Westrich, A. Raedler, and H.G. Thiele, Lymphocytes express specific antigen-independent contact interaction sites upon activation, Cell. Immunol., 86:14 (1984).

DISCUSSION

H. Spits: Did you look for expression of LFA-1 on PHA activated blasts of these patients?

T. Springer: Yes, absolutely. In fact, the S-35 methionine biosynthesis experiments were done partly with PHA blasts, and partly with EBV lines, and the PHA blasts are just as deficient as the patient's granulocytes. Also, I didn't show data for mononuclear cells, but they are also deficient. We don't see any increase on activated cells.

H. Spits: We have looked at similar patients. With PHA blasts LFA is coming up, but on EBV transformed B blasts they stay LFA-1 negative.

T. Springer: We would agree that the patient who has around 10% of the normal amounts on its granuloctes shows virtually nothing on its EBV lines. But our data did come from PHA blasts.

M. Sitkovsky: Can the beta chain from, let's say, Mac-1 be in association with the alpha chain from LFA-1 on monocytes? Something like a promiscuous beta chain. Can you expect that we will have always one beta chain?

T. Springer: When we've done crosslinking experiments, we can demonstrate that 100% of the molecules consist of non-covalently associated alpha and beta chains at any one moment.

M. Sitkovsky: When I do immunoprecipitation with anti-LFA-1 antibody, the alpha chain always is much darker than the beta chain. Do you think that the alpha chain has more tyrosine, or what? Or is more accessible to the iodine?

T. Springer: The sequence shows that LFA-1 has an internal tyrosine, whereas Mac-1 has an internal phenylalanine. I'm not sure that that single difference explains it but differences like that certainly might explain that phenomenon.

D. Hudig: Is there homology of the beta chain for other membrane molecules?

T. Springer: We have not been able to get any sequence information from the beta subunits. We think they're blocked. We did a computerized search of all known protein sequences, and it turns out that the LFA-1 alpha subunit shows between 28% and 42% homology to alpha interferon. There are over 8 different human interferons and 3 different rodent interferons sequenced and it shows homology to all of them. This is very statistically significant, but its a very surprising result because alpha interferon is a much smaller molecule and its a secreted mediator rather than a surface bound one.

P. Golstein: I think you presented a very fascinating set of results, especially the results on the impairment of cell adhesion in patients. I think you said that in these patients, adherance to substrates was impaired. The question is, how do you figure in molecular terms the role that LFA-1 may have in adherance to substrates.

T. Springer: That's a good question. By the way, we don't know whether it is LFA-1 or p150,95 or Mac-1 which is important. Don Anderson is doing antibody inhibition experiments, and they suggest that actually all of these molecules may be contributing to this adherance. The adherance is affected if you look at normal glass coverslips, serum-coated coverslips, fibronectin-coated coverslips, or albumin-coated latex beads. You always see a deficit. It might be that there are specific ligand-binding sites on these molecules, as well as nonspecific sites. They're very large molecules with certainly enough room for that. There must be some specific molecules to mediate adherance to substrates. I think these molecules are very important, but the mechanism is puzzling.

P. Golstein: Is there any need for thinking that there is somewhere a receptor for LFA-1?

T. Springer: The evidence is really not in on LFA-1, but Mac-1 clearly shows specificity for C3bi. There are reports from Peter Lachman and Gordon Ross that the C3bi receptor may be a lectin-like molecule. They see inhibition by sugars, however, we do not see inhibition by the same sugars in our hands.

W. Seaman: If you do sequential immunoprecipitation with your antibodies to alpha chain, or capping, are there other structures that use the beta chain?

T. Springer: That's how we picked up p150,95, with our anti-beta chain antibody. I couldn't rule out that there are other molecules present in much smaller amount which have the same beta subunit.

FUNCTIONAL INTERACTIONS OF LFA-1, T8 AND ALLOANTIGEN

SURFACE STRUCTURES IN T-CELL MEDIATED CYTOTOXICITY

Carl F. Ware and Jeanne L. Reade

Division of Biomedical Sciences, University of California

Riverside, California 92521-0121

INTRODUCTION

Monoclonal antibodies (MAb) have provided powerful tools for dissecting the complex cellular interactions involved in the lysis of target cells by immune cytotoxic T lymphocytes (CTL). Seven distinct surface-membrane structures have been implicated to function in the cytolytic process mediated by human effector cells by virtue of the ability of their MAb to inhibit cytolysis in the absence of complement (Table 1). All of these inhibitory MAb recognize cell surface structures present on non-immune mature lymphoid cells. The Ti, T3, T8 and T4 structures are unique to T cells and in the case for T8 and T4 define T-cell subpopulations that recognize antigen associated with Class I or Class II MHC glycoproteins, respectively (1-3). The clonotypic (Ti) surface structure and T3 appear to form the antigen binding recognition complex on the CTL surface (4) whereas the Lymphocyte Function Associated Antigen-2 (LFA-2) has been identified as the sheep red blood cell rosette receptor (5). In contrast, the LFA-1 molecule is present on both T and B lymphocytes and is structurally related to the OKM1/MAC-1 macrophage surface glycoprotein which is associated with complement receptor activity (CR3) (6,7). In contrast, the tissue distribution of LFA-3 is very broad including non-lymphoid cells (5).

Evidence is accumulating that MAb inhibition of cytolysis is through the specific blockade of a functionally relevant molecule and not by a nonspecific inactivation of the effector cell. This statement is derived in part from studies showing that MAb to several other CTL membrane proteins did not inhibit cytolytic function of murine CTL (8). Similar results have been seen with human CTL, for example Leu 1, anti-transferin receptor (4F2), anti-IL-2 receptor (49.9), and anti-HLA and other activation specific MAb (A1A5) did not inhibit cytolysis in vitro (C. Ware unpublished observations). It should be noted that MAb directed to MHC alloantigens on the target cell, but not the CTL, will block by interfering with antigen recognition.

Table 1

MOLECULAR COMPONENTS OF HUMAN AND MOUSE CYTOTOXIC T LYMPHOCYTES IDENTIFIED BY CYTOLYSIS INHIBITING MONOCLONAL ANTIBODIES

	MONOCLONAL ANTIBODY	DESIGNATION[2]	MOLECULAR WEIGHT[3] X10^3	SITE OF INHIBITION[4]	CELL DISTRIBUTION
HUMAN:	OKT3	T3	19	POST-RECOGNITION	ALL T CELLS
	OKT8; Leu 2a; B9	T8	30-33;43	RECOGNITION	SUBSET OF T CELLS
	OKT4	T4	55	RECOGNITION	SUBSET OF T CELLS
	TS1/18; SEVERAL OTHERS	LFA-1	177;95	RECOGNITION	ALL LYMPHOCYTES; T CELLS B CELLS
	TS1/8;9.6	LFA-2	49	RECOGNITION	90% OF PBL
	TS2/9	LFA-3	60	RECOGNITION	50% OF PBL
	Ti$_{1A}$; Ti$_{1B}$	Ti	49;43	?	CLONOTYPIC
MOUSE:	M5/24;53.6; SEVERAL OTHERS	Lyt-2,3	33;44	RECOGNITION	SUBSET OF T CELLS
	M7/14;441.8; H35-89.9	LFA-1	180;95	RECOGNITION	ALL LYMPHOCYTES; T CELLS B CELLS; 80% BONE MARROW
	384.5	Ti	?	?	CTL CLONE SPECIFIC, CLONOTYPIC

[1] Not included in this list are blocking antibodies directed at target cell MHC antigens.

[2] For reference only: no official designation has been agreed upon. LFA, lymphocyte function associated antigens.

[3] Obtained by immunoprecipitation of [125] I-labelled extracts and analysis under reducing conditions by SDS-PAGE.

[4] Phase of the CTL reaction blocked by the monoclonal antibody.

Initial results from several laboratories have indicated that mono-clonal antibodies to the LFA-1, 2, 3 and T8/T4 structures inhibit CTL function by blockade of the early Mg^{++}-dependent recognition/adhesion step as measured by the conjugate formation assay (9,11,23). Interestingly, anti-LFA-3 MAb appears to block by binding to the target cell whereas MAb to the other structures inhibit cytolysis by binding to the CTL (5). In the presence of anti-T3 MAb CTL-target conjugates still form but lysis was inhibited indicating that anti-T3 inhibits a post-recognition Ca^{++}-dependent step (10,11). Studies with polyclonal antisera produced against lectin activated human or murine lymphocytes have suggested additional CTL components may be involved in the later post adhesion lytic phase of the reaction (12-13).

The concept is emerging from these studies that the molecular events in the CTL reaction involves multiple components, perhaps in a cascade-like pathway or through multiple receptor-ligand interactions (14). From this general concept we have initiated studies to identify potential interactions between these function-associated surface components that may be required to initiate and deliver the lethal hit. As a first approach to this question we have examined the effects of combining MAb of different specificities on the CTL killing reaction in vitro with the possibility of observing synergistic, additive or independent action of combining two MAb. The effects of combining MAb would be expected to change either the magnitude of inhibition and/or the dose response curve. In the experiments presented here we have focused on the LFA-1 and T8 surface structures because both have been implicated to function during the early recognition/adhesion phase but are clearly distinct in molecular structure and in tissue distribution. In addition, a series of well-characterized monoclonal antibodies which recognize several distinct epitopes on the LFA-1 and T8 antigens are available (Table 2 and Ref 7,15,16).

Table 2

IMMUNOCHEMICAL PROPERTIES OF ANTI-HUMAN LFA-1 AND ANTI-T8
MONOCLONAL ANTIBODIES

ANTI-LFA-1	Ig SUBCLASS	EPITOPE REACTIVITY	LOCALIZATION OF EPITOPE	
TS1/18	γ_1 K	UNIQUE	β	(95,000 MR)
TS2/14	γ_1 K	UNIQUE	α	(177,000 MR)
TS1/11	γ_1 K	UNIQUE	α	
TS2/4	γ_1 K	SHARED (6,11,18,22)	?	
TS2/6	γ_1 K	SHARED (18,11)	α	
TS1/22	γ_1 K	SHARED (14,4,18,6,11)	α	

ANTI-T8				
B9.2	γ_3, K	SHARED (9,2,3,4,7,11)		
B9.3	γ_1, K	DISTINCT (ENHANCES 9,7 BINDING)		
B9.4	γ_{2b}, K	DISTINCT (ENHANCES 9,8 BINDING)		
B9.7	γ_{2A}, K	DISTINCT (ENHANCES 9,3 BINDING)		
B9.11	γ_1, K	SHARED (9,2,3,4,7,11)		

MATERIALS AND METHODS

Human effector cells were generated from peripheral blood mononuclear cells (PBL) in a one-way mixed lymphocyte reaction and expansion of reactive clones with T cell growth factor supplemented medium as previously described in detail (17). The target cell used to measure specific lysis was the JY B-lymphoblastoid cell line which shares the HLA-A2, B7 alloantigens with the original stimulator cells. Lysis was measured in a 2 to 4 hr 51-Chromium-release microcytotoxicity assay. The CTL lines used in this study (CTL-20, CTL-22 and CTL-25) were 7 to 12 weeks old and exhibited lysis of 40-70% of the JY target at an effector:target (E:T) ratio of 2:1 and less than 15% lysis of K562 (Natural Killer cell sensitive target line) at an E:T of 30:1. Surface marker analysis of these CTL lines by flow cytometry indicated that >97% were T8[+]; LFA-1[+]; T3[+]; T11[+] and less than 5% were reactive with the OKT4 MAb.

The anti-human LFA-1 and anti-T8 monoclonal antibodies, generously provided by Dr. T. Springer and Dr. B. Malissen, were used as culture supernatants that had been dialyzed against Hanks Balanced Salt Solution and buffered with 10 mM HEPES, pH 7.2. The immunochemical properties of these MAb are summarized in Table 2 and references 7, 15, 16 should be consulted for details. Quantitation of mouse MAb in culture supernatants was determined by a competitive radioimmunometric assay using the rat anti-mouse Kappa chain specific MAb, 187.1.10 and purified BBM.1 (IgG, K) specific MAb (18,19). The W6/32 MAb recognizes a monomorphic determinant on all Class I HLA-ABC molecules and was purified IgG from ascites diluted into culture supernatant (17,20).

RESULTS

Effect of Combining MAb to Different Epitopes on the LFA-1 or T8 Surface Structures: Independent action. Our earlier studies showed that monoclonal antibodies to different epitopes on Human LFA-1 exhibited considerable variability in their ability to block CTL activity (15) and indicated a complex relationship existed between the antigenic epitopes and functional (blocking) sites defined by these antibodies. This finding prompted us to investigate whether combining several anti-LFA-1 MAb into a pool (a novel way to develop a polyclonal antiserum!) to mask all available epitopes would lead to stronger inhibition of cytolysis. However, to our surprise, the anti-LFA-1 pool was no more efficient in blocking CTL function than the most effective individual MAb in either the magnitude of inhibition or the effective dose. This effect was independent of whether the MAb recognized the unique or shared epitopes on the LFA-1 molecule (Figure 1). This result indicated that the inhibitory action of these anti-LFA-1 MAb were acting at the same functional site and further suggested that the LFA-1 molecule was not obligatory for the CTL-22 line to mediate cytolysis.

In a similar type of experiment, several MAb of the B9 series (B9.3, 9.4 and 9.7) which recognize three distinct but overlapping epitopes on the T8 surface structure (16) were pooled and compared to the individual anti-T8 MAb for its ability to inhibit cytolysis (Figure 2). The data show that the pool of the B9 MAb was no more effective at blocking cytolysis than the most effective individual MAb. In fact, the anti-T8 pool exhibited considerable antagonistic effects (decreased inhibition) at concentrations of more than 1 ug/ml when compared to the inhibition seen with the B9.4 or B9.3 MAb alone. This observation is somewhat puzzling but may be related to the fingings that the B9.4, 9.3 or 9.7 MAb cause a significant increase in the binding of other anti-T8 MAb (Table 2 and (16)). These results indicate that antibodies reactive to different epitopes on the same molecule act in an independent fashion to inhibit cytolysis.

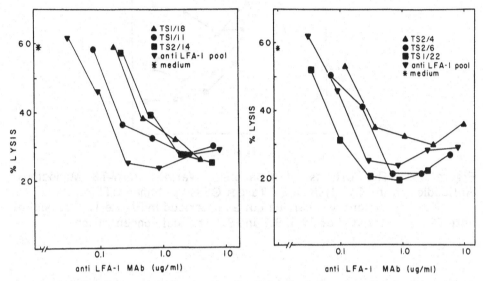

Figure 1. The Effect of Combining Various Anti-Human LFA-1 Monoclonal Antibodies on the Cytolysis of JY Cells by Human CTL.

The various anti-LFA-1 MAb (see Table 2 for details) or a pool of these MAb (TS1/18,22,11 and TS2/4,6) were serially diluted in medium. CTL-22 effector cells (6 x 10³) were added to each well and allowed a 10 min preincubation prior to the addition of 51-Cr-labelled JY target cells (HLA-A2,B7) (2 x 10³ cells). Incubation at 37°C was continued for 4 hr. at which time the microplates were harvested and the isotope released was quantitated in a gamma counter. The percentage of cytolysis was calculated according to the formula: (EXP-SR)/(T-SR) x 100, where SR = Spontaneous Release in absence of effectors, TR = Total Release of label in presence of detergent and EXP = Release of Label in presence of CTL. The standard deviation rarely exceeded 2-4% lysis. The antibody concentration in the anti-LFA-1 pool represents the antibody concentration of each individual MAb.

Left Panel: Titration of anti-LFA-1 MAb with unique (non-cross-blocking) epitopes.

Right Panel: Titration of anti-LFA-1 MAb with shared (cross-blocking) epitopes.

327

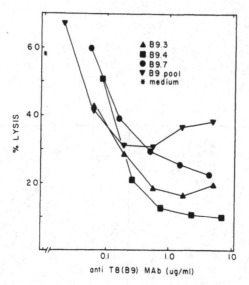

Figure 2. The Effects of Combining Various Anti-T8 Monoclonal Antibodies on the Cytolysis of JY Target Cells by Human CTL.

The experiment was carried out as described in Figure 1. The pool of anti-T8 MAb consisted of B9.3, 9.4 and 9.7 at equal concentrations.

Effect of Combining Anti-LFA-1 and Anti-T8 Antibodies: Additive and Synergistic Effects.   The next series of experiments were designed to investigate the effect of combining two MAb reactive with distinct molecular structures on CTL function. In this type of experiment one of the antibodies is titrated and then a constant amount of the other MAb, diluted to give a minimum level of inhibition, is added to create a mixture (i.e., a polyspecific antiserum).   When the anti-LFA-1 β chain specific MAb (TS1/18) was titrated in the presence of a constant amount of anti-T8 pool the magnitude of inhibition of killing seen at concentrations of TS1/18 of > .5 ug/ml was increased additively, whereas at lower concentrations (below .2 ug/ml) the inhibition was greater than that expected for a simple additive effect and is reflected in a lowered effective dose of the anti-LFA-1 MAb (Figure 3).   In contrast, the anti-LFA-1 α chain specific MAb (TS1/22) showed less than an additive effect in inhibiting killing when combined with the anti-T8 pool (Figure 4). A pool of the anti-T8 MAb was used in an attempt to avoid any possible epitope specific effects.   Titration of a pool of anti-LFA-1 MAb with a constant amount of the anti-T8 pool (Figure 5) yielded similar results to that seen with the TS1/18 MAb (Figure 3) where synergistic effects were observed at the lower concentrations of anti-LFA-1 MAb. Note also the magnitude of inhibition was increased to > 95% using pools of both anti-LFA-1 and anti-T8 antibodies, whereas the individual anti-LFA-1 MAb combined with the T8 pool maximally inhibited lysis 70 to 80%. These results indicated that the effects of combining anti-LFA-1 and T8 MAb on the inhibition of killing was dependent on the concentration and the epitope recognized by the anti-LFA-1 MAb. In additional experiments (data not shown) the other anti-LFA-1 MAb could be divided into two groups based on their ability to exhibit additive/synergistic effects with the anti-T8 pool. In group 1, the TS2/14, TS2/6, and TS2/4 MAb were similar to the TS1/18 MAb and group 2, were similar to TS1/22, and consisted of TS1/11 and TS1/12 anti-LFA-1 MAb.

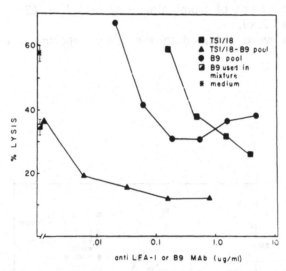

Figure 3. The Effect of Combining Anti-LFA-1 β Chain with Anti-T8 MAb on the Cytolysis of JY Target Cells by Human CTL. TS1/18 MAb was serially diluted in medium and mixed with a constant amount of a pool of anti-T8 MAb (20 ug/ml). CTL-22 cells were added to the MAb mixture with a 10 min preincubation at 22°C followed by 51-Cr-labeled JY targets (2:1 E:T). For comparison, the titration of the B9 pool is also shown. The level of inhibition obtained by the B9 pool alone can be seen by comparing with lysis in medium alone.

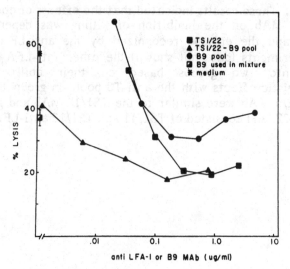

Figure 4. The Effect of Combining Anti-LFA-1 α Chain MAb (TS1/22) with the Anti-T8 Pool.

The data were obtained in the same experiment as described in Figure 3.

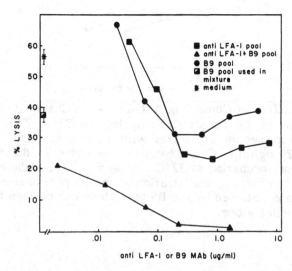

Figure 5. Inhibition of CTL Function by Combining a Pool of Anti-LFA-1 MAb with the Anti-T8 Pool.

The data were obtained in the same experiment as described in Figure 3.

<u>Effects Combining of anti-LFA-1 and anti-T8 MAb on the Kinetics of</u>
<u>Lysis and Surface Antigen Expression.</u> The strong inhibitory effects seen
when the anti-LFA-1 and T8 MAb were combined warranted additional
experiments to examine how these antibodies effected the CTL reaction
and expression of these surface antigens. We have previously shown that
the inhibitory effect of anti-LFA-1 (TS1/18) on the kinetics of lysis was
reversible and the blocking effects of the MAb was exhibited by decreasing
the initial rate of 51-Cr-release from CTL damaged target cells (15). As
shown in Figure 6, anti-T8 MAb exhibited a similar reversible effect on the
kinetics of lysis. However, combining anti-LFA-1 with anti-T8 MAb had a
very strong, essentially irreversible effect in inhibiting the rate of cytolysis. This result was observed even when incubation times were extended
to 6-8 hrs.

Another parameter we examined was the potential modulating effects that the anti-LFA-1 and anti-T8 MAb might have on the expression of
their surface antigens. The CTL-20 line was preincubated for 22 hr in the
presence of saturating amounts of either anti-LFA-1 (TS1/18), anti-T8
(B9.3), a combination of these two MAb or as a control in medium. The
cells were then washed and incubated with either anti-LFA-1 (TS1/11 or
TS1/18), anti-T8 (B9.3 or B9.7) or anti-HLA (W6/32) as a control. Quanti
tative analysis of the bound MAb was then measured using a ^{125}I-labeled
second antibody (187.1.10 MAb, a rat anti-mouse Kappa chain specific
antibody) under saturating conditions (Table 3). Relative to CTL in
medium alone, anti-T8 treated CTL showed a 39% loss in T8 expression
while LFA-1 expression was unchanged and HLA-ABC antigens were
slightly decreased (-17%). CTL pretreated with anti-LFA-1 exhibited a
slight increase in T8 and LFA-1 expression (10% and 16%, respectively),
while HLA was unchanged. However, a combination of anti-LFA-1 and
anti-T8 induced a significant change in LFA-1 expression (loss of 45%
relative to anti-LFA-1 treated CTL) whereas T8 and HLA remained
unchanged. In this experiment, the TS1/12 and B9.7 MAb were used as
independent markers for LFA-1 and T8 expression and showed identical
modulation profiles (data not shown).

<u>Synergistic Inhibition of CTL Killing by Combining anti-T8 and anti-</u>
<u>HLA-ABC Monoclonal Antibodies.</u> Several laboratories have demonstrated
a strong correlation with the expression of the T8 surface marker with CTL
that recognize Class I MHC alloantigens and the expression of the T4 T cell
surface marker with recognition of Class II MHC antigens (1-3). These
findings have led to the hypothesis that the T8 surface structure may
function as a receptor for a non-polymorphic region on the Class I MHC
molecule. It was of interest in the context of the approach taken here to
examine what the effect of combining anti-T8 and anti-HLA would be on
CTL killing. The prediction would be that if the T8 molecule functions as a
receptor for the HLA-ABC molecules on the target cell surface that a
combination of antibodies to these structures would act synergistically to
inhibit target cell lysis by Class I specific CTL. The CTL-22 line, specific
for HLA-A2,B7 alloantigens, was relatively sensitive to the blocking effect

of B9.4 (50% inhibition of lysis at 1-2 ug/ml) (Figure 7). A synergistic effect was observed when the B9.4 was tested for inhibition of killing in the presence of a constant amount W6/32 (anti-HLA-ABC MAb). At a non-inhibitory dose of W6/32 (10 ug/ml) the concentration of B9.4 required to inhibit lysis by 50% was decreased 10 to 15 fold. Reciprocal titrations of the anti-HLA-ABC with a constant amount of anti-T8 (B9.4 or B9.3) also showed a synergistic effect in blocking cytolysis (data not shown). These results provide additional evidence supporting the notion that T8 and HLA interact during the CTL reaction. In preliminary experiments using the CTL-25 line, which is not effectively inhibited by any of the anti-T8 MAb (less than 30% inhibition at > 5 ug/ml), the anti-T8 MAb did not show this marked shift in the dose response curve when combined with the W6/32 antibody suggesting that an interaction between HLA-ABC and T8 may not be essential for CTL-25 line to function.

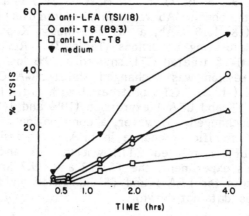

Figure 6. The Effect of Anti-LFA-1, Anti-T8 or a Combination of Anti-LFA-1/T8 MAb on the Kinetics of Cytolysis by Alloimmune Human CTL.
CTL-20 were incubated in 100 ul of medium or medium containing either anti-LFA-1 (TS1/18, 7 ug/ml), anti-T8 (B9.3, 6 ug/ml) or a combination of anti-LFA-1 and T8 (3.5 and 3 ug/ml, respectively) for 10 minutes at 37°C. 51-Cr-labeled JY target cells were then added (100 ul) (3:1 E:T ratio) and microplates were centrifuged to initiate contact and placed at 37°C. At the indicated times, the percentage of lysis was determined for each set.

Table 3

MODULATING EFFECTS OF ANTI-T8 AND LFA-1
MONOCLONAL ANTIBODIES ON CTL SURFACE ANTIGEN EXPRESSION.

SURFACE ANTIGEN EXPRESSION (SPECIFIC SITES/CELL):

MODULATING MAB	T8	LFA-1	HLA
CONTROL (NO MAB)	4.8×10^4	5.7×10^4	51×10^4
ANTI-T8 (B9.3)	2.9×10^4 (-39%)	5.6×10^4 (-2%)	4.2×10^4 (-17)
ANTI-LFA-1 (TS1/18)	5.3×10^4 (10%)	6.7×10^4 (16%)	53×10^4 (4%)
ANTI-LFA-1 + T8	2.6×10^4 (-45%)	4.1×10^4 (-29)	44×10^4 (-13)

CTL-20 (2×10^6 cells) were incubated in .5 ml of growth medium containing saturating levels of either anti-LFA-1 (TS1/18, 22 ug/ml), anti-T8 (B9.3, 27 ug/ml). A mixture of B9.3 and TS1/18, or medium for 22 hrs at 37°C. Each group was then washed 3 times in 1% BSA-BPS and aliquoted into microtiter wells containing 50 ul of either medium, anti-LFA-1, anti-T8 or anti-HLA (W6/32) at saturating concentrations. Cells were incubated for 1 hr on ice, followed by 3 washes with PBS-BSA. Quantitative analysis of antibody bound was measured using a ^{125}I-labelled second MAb, (187.1.10, a rat anti-mouse kappa chain specific antibody (specific activity of 1.53×10^6 cpm/ug protein)) under saturating conditions. Surface antigen expression, calculated as specific 187.1.10 sites/cell was determined for the MAb-treated cells by subtracting cpm bound in medium from cpm bound in the presence of the indicated MAb. The numbers in parenthesis represent the change in antigen expression relative to cells indubated in medium alone. The quantitative analysis are in good agreement with previously published determinations (15).

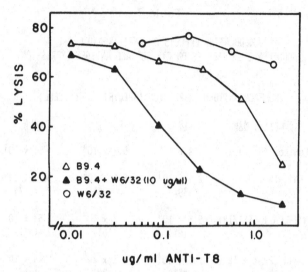

Figure 7. Synergistic Inhibition of CTL Function by Combining Anti-T8 with Anti-HLA-ABC Monoclonal Antibodies.

The CTL-22 cells were incubated (10 min) with serial dilutions of the B9.4 MAb alone or in combination with a constant amount of W6/32 (anti-HLA-ABC) (10 ug/ml), followed by the addition of 51-Cr-labelled J Y target cells (2:1 E:T ratio). The reaction was then incubated at 37°C for 4 hrs. For comparison the titration of W6/32 alone is shown but the concentration scale (x axis) should be multiplied by 10. Generally 75-100 ug/ml of W6/32 is required to inhibit CTL function 50-80% (see also reference 15).

DISCUSSION

The results presented here have investigated the effects of combining various cytolysis-inhibiting monoclonal antibodies on the cytolytic function of Class I allospecific human CTL. The LFA-1 and T8 surface structures were investigated as a model system to carry out these studies because of the availability of a series of well characterized MAb which recognize distinct epitopes on the LFA-1 or T8 structures (7,15,16) and because both structures appear to be involved in the early recognition/adhesion phase of the CTL lytic pathway in both the murine and human systems. The data reveal, depending on the combination of antibodies used, that synergistic, additive or independent (non-additive/synergistic) blocking effects were observed on the cytolytic action of human CTL.

Our initial hypothesis was that a combination of two antibodies exhibiting a synergistic effect in blocking CTL killing would imply a functional linkage between the two components, whereas an additive blocking effect would imply the two components were functioning separately in the cytolytic process. Synergistic action between two antibodies would be demonstrated by a greater than 2 to 4 fold decrease in the effective inhibitory concentration of one of the MAb and/or by a significant increase in the magnitude of the inhibition over that expected for a simple additive effect. Synergism and addition are used here in a very broad sense, in contrast to the meanings used in pharmacologic studies (21). Current models for the role of the T8 (Lyt-2,3) in the lytic process suggest that T8 participates as an auxiliary receptor for a non-polymorphic determinant(s) on the Class I MHC molecule to increase the apparent affinity of the CTL antigen-specific receptor, thus ensuring strong binding between the CTL and target cell membranes (22). CTL clones with relatively low affinity antigen-specific receptors would require the partici pation of the T8 structure and thus would be efficiently blocked by anti-T8 MAb. In view of this current model the data presented here showing that anti-T8 MAb combined with the W6/32 MAb, which recognizes a monomorphic determinant on all Class I HLA-ABC molecules, synergize to inhibit the cytolytic function of a Class I allospecific CTL line strongly supports the contention that the T8 surface molecule interacts with an HLA-Class I associated structure. However, one assumption made in this experiment is that the anti-HLA MAb exerted its inhibitory effect by binding to the target cell HLA-ABC antigens and not to the HLA-antigens expressed on the CTL. Although W6/32 when used by itself must be bound to the target cell to inhibit cytolysis, this has not been formally proven for the combination of the two MAb. We feel reasonably confident the anti-T8 MAb inhibited lysis by binding to the effector CTL since the target cell (B lymphoblastoid) does not express the T8 antigen. Experiments designed to test the validity of this assumption are in progress.

The results obtained when anti-LFA-1 and anti-T8 MAb were combined to inhibit CTL function were more complex and thus more difficult to interpret. The results suggest that there are two groups of anti-LFA-1 MAb, one group that acted in an additive fashion and one that exhibited a less than additive effect when combined with a constant amount of a pool of anti-T8 MAb. However, the TS1/18 MAb at low concentrations and a pool of the anti-LFA-1 MAb when combined with the anti-T8 pool inhibited lysis in a synergistic fashion, indicating that both additive or synergistic effects could be observed depending on the concentration of MAb used and that there is a significant contribution from the epitope specificities of these antibodies in determining whether additive or synergistic effects were observed.

In addition, in eight different experiments using three different CTL lines, we have noted some variability in the additive/synergistic effects when anti-LFA-1 and anti-T8 MAb were combined. This effect may be due in part to the clonal heterogeneity of the CTL lines used in this study. These CTL lines, although relatively antigen specific, are not cloned lines, and undoubtedly contained some high affinity and low affinity clones. The variability of the type of inhibition observed with the anti-LFA-1/T8 mixture is not an unexpected result since high affinity CTL which may not require the participation of the T8 structure to mediate cytolysis (as demonstrated by the lack of anti-T8 inhibition) would also be expected to be insensitive to the synergistic blocking effects of combining anti-T8 with anti-LFA-1. This notion is supported indirectly by preliminary results which indicate that a CTL line (CTL-25), which is largely insensitive to blocking by anti-T8 MAb, did not exhibit the synergistic susceptibility when anti-T8 and anti-HLA-ABC MAb were combined.

The reversible inhibition of CTL function mediated by the anti-LFA-1 or anti-T8 MAb (used by themselves) suggested that with increased reaction time sufficient low avidity contacts between the CTL and target cells could have occurred to promote target cell lysis, thus reversing the inhibitory effects of these MAb. However, anti-LFA-1 and anti-T8 in combination profoundly inhibited the rate of lysis, essentially irreversibly inhibiting CTL function. This suggested that either the LFA-1 or the T8 structures must be functionally active in order for the CTL to effectively engage the target cell. This conclusion is further supported by the findings that combining several of the anti-LFA-1 or anti-T8 MAb, which recognize distinct epitopes on these structures, did not increase the level of inhibition (independent action). These results are consistent with the model that both LFA-1 and T8 function as auxiliary receptors to strengthen the functional avidity of the antigen specific receptor. However, another possibility should be considered and that is when both antibodies bind simultaneous to their respective antigens on the CTL surface a negative signal is generated shutting off CTL function. This alternative explanation finds some support in Table 3 where a combination of the anti-LFA-1/T8 MAb resulted in a significant negative modulation of the LFA-1 surface antigen, whereas either MAb alone did not modulate the expression of LFA-1. Additional experiments will be required to analyze these possibilities.

What effect do combinations of other blocking or non-blocking MAb have on CTL function? Preliminary studies using the Leu 1 and A1A5 MAb (24) which by themselves do not inhibit CTL function also do not potentiate the blocking effects of anti-LFA-1 or anti-T8 MAb. However, anti-T11 and anti-T3 MAb showed significant enhancement of the inhibitory effects of anti-LFA-1. Further experiments are in progress extending these studies to the other CTL surface structures. In support of our hypothesis, a limited study by Krensky et al. (5) has provided evidence that a combination of anti-LFA-1 and anti-LFA-3 MAb, but not anti-LFA-1 and LFA-2, act synergistically to inhibit CTL function. This result has lead to the tempting speculation that LFA-1 and LFA-3 may form a receptor-ligand pair. Springer's group has presented some data showing for murine CTL that anti-Lyt2,3 and anti-LFA-1 exhibited additive effects when these antibodies were combined (14). However, the epitope diversity recognized by the rat anti-mouse LFA-1 is very limited (15) and thus the appropriate epitopes required to see synergy may not be represented.

The synergistic inhibitory effect of two MAb on CTL function implies a functional linkage between the two antigens but does not prove the existence of any physical link between the components. The approach we have taken here should be only viewed as a method to identify potential interactions between two components. Formal proof of a true molecular interaction between any of these components will require careful cross-linking and/or fluorescent-energy transfer studies. As can be seen in Figure 8, the potential for interactions between components on the CTL and target surface in receptor-ligand type interactions seem fairly certain because of the antigen-specificity of the CTL and the intimate contact required for killing to occur. In addition, lateral interactions between components either on the CTL or the target surface should also be considered which has recently been shown to occur for the Ti and T3 molecular structure (4). Indeed a prediction using the approach taken here would be that a combination of anti-T3 and anti-Ti MAb should act synergistically to inhibit cytolysis. The recent evidence that T4 may act as a receptor for Class II MHC molecules (23) suggests that anti-T4 and anti-HLA-Class II (anti-DR) MAb, when combined, should also block cytolysis in a synergistic fashion.

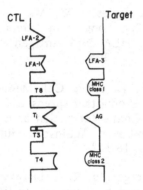

Figure 8. Schematic Representation of CTL and Target Cell Membrane Structures Involved in Cytolysis.

Putative interacting receptor-ligand pairs are placed across from each other. The bar between Ti and T3 denotes a functional and close physical (but noncovalent) linkage. The T4 and T8 structures do not reside on the same CTL.

The studies presented here also have practical implications for the use of anti-lymphocyte monoclonal antibodies as therapeutic agents, such as in the control of graft rejection, where a tailor-made mixture of anti-CTL MAb of the appropriate specificities may have significantly greater efficiency at controlling graft rejection than a single MAb. Our results also indicate that a mixture of MAb could also be used at much lower concentrations, perhaps avoiding problems associated with administration of xenogeneic antibodies such as the development of serum sickness disease.

ACKNOWLEDGMENTS

The authors would like to thank D. Haviland and P. Breton for help in preparing the manuscript. This work was supported by PHS Grant RO1 CA 35638 awarded by the National Cancer Institute, DHHS; by Grant RR05816 Biomedical Research Support Grant, DHHS and by the UCR Intramural Research Fund No. 07427.

REFERENCES

1. Swain, S.L. 1981. Significance of Lyt Phenotypes: Lyt2 Antibodies Block Activities of T Cells that Recognize Class 1 Major Histocompatibility Complex Antigens Regardless of Their Function. Proc. Natl. Acad. Sci. USA, 78:7101.

2. Krensky, A.M., C.S. Reiss, J.W. Mier, J.L Strominger and S.J. Burakoff. 1982. Long-term Human Cytolytic T-Cell Lines Allospecific for HLA-DR6 Antigen Are OKT4$^+$. Proc. Natl. Acad. Sci. USA, 79:2365.

3. Ball, E.J. and P. Stastny. 1982. Cell-Mediated Cytotoxicity Against HLA-D-Region Products Expressed in Monocytes and B Lymphocytes. IV. Characterization of Effector Cells Using Monoclonal Antibodies Against Human T-Cell Subsets. Immunogenetics, 16:157.

4   Meuer, S.C., K.A. Fitzgerald, R.E. Hussey, et al. 1983. Clonotypic Structures Involved in Antigen-Specific Human T Cell Function: Relationship to the T3 Molecular Complex. J. Exp. Med., 157:705.

5. Krensky, A.M., F. Sanchez-Madrid, E. Robbins, J. Nagy, T.A. Springer and S.J. Burakoff. 1983. The Functional Significance, Distribution, and Structure of LFA-1, LFA-2, and LFA-3: Cell Surface Antigens Associated with CTL-Target Interactions. J. Immunol., 131:611.

6. Sanchez-Madrid, F., A.M. Krensky, C.F. Ware, E. Robbins, J.L. Strominger, S.J. Burakoff, and T.A. Springer. 1982. Three Distinct Antigens Associated with Human T Lymphocyte-mediated Cytolysis: LFA-1, LFA-2, LFA-3. Proc. Natl. Acad. Sci., USA, 79:7489.

7. Sanchez-Madrid, F., J.A. Nagy, E. Robbins, P. Simon and T.A. Springer. 1983. Characterization of a Human Leukocyte Differentiation Antigen Family with Distinct Subunits and a Common Subunit: The Lymphocyte Function-Associated Antigen (LFA-1), the C3bi Complement Receptor (OKM1/Mac-1), and the p150,95 Molecule. J. Exp. Med., 158:1785.

8. Davignon, D., E. Martz, T. Reynolds, K. Kurzinger and T.A. Springer. 1981. Lymphocyte Function-Associated Antigen 1 (LFA-1): A Surface Antigen Distinct from Lyt-2,3 that Participates in T Lymphocyte-Mediated Killing. Proc. Natl. Acad. Sci. USA, 78:4535.

9. Krensky, A.M., E. Robbins, T.A. Springer and S.J. Burakoff. 1984. LFA-1, LFA-2, and LFA-3 Antigens Are Involved in CTL-Target Conjugation. J. Immunol., 132:2180.

10. Tsoukas, C.D., D.A. Carson, S. Fong and J.H. Vaughan. 1982. Molecular Interactions in Human T Cell-Mediated Cytotoxicity to EBV. II. Monoclonal Antibody OKT3 Inhibits a Post-Killer Target Recognition/Adhesion Step. J. Immunol., 129:1421.

11. Landegren, U., U. Ramstedt, I. Axberg, M. Ullberg, M. Jondal and H. Wigzell. 1982. Selective Inhibition of Human T Cell Cytotoxicity at Levels of Target Recognition or Initiation of Lysis by Monoclonal OKT3 and Leu-2a Antibodies. J. Exp. Med., 155:1579.

12. Ware, C.F., and G.A. Granger. 1981. Mechanisms of Lymphocyte Mediated Cytotoxicity. III. Characterization of the mechanism of inhibition of the human alloimmune cytotoxic reaction by the polyspecific anti-lymphotoxin serum in vitro. J. Immunol., 126:1934.

13. Ware, C.F., P.H. Chauvenet, P.S. Duffey, and G.A. Granger. 1981. Inhibition of the Lytic Phase of Murine T-cell Mediated Alloimmune Cytotoxicity by a Rat Anti-activated T-cell Antiserum. Cell. Immunol., 59:289.

14. Springer, T.A., D. Davignon, M.-K. Ho, K. Kurzinger, E. Martz and F. Sanchez-Madrid. 1982. LFA-1 and Lyt-2,3, Molecules Associated with T Lymphocyte-Mediated Killing; and Mac-1, an LFA-1 Homologue Associated with Complement Receptor Function. Immunological Reviews, 68:171.

15. Ware, C.F., F. Sanchez-Madrid, A.M. Krensky, S.J. Burakoff, J.L. Strominger and T.A. Springer. 1983. Human Lymphocyte Function Associated Antigen-1 (LFA-1): Identification of

Multiple Antigenic Epitopes and Their Relationship to CTL-Mediated Cytotoxicity. J. Immunol., 131:1182.

16. Malissen, B., N. Rebai, A. Liabeuf and C. Mawas. 1982. Human Cytotoxic T Cell Structures Associated with Expression of Cytolysis. I. Analysis at the Clonal Cell Level of the Cytolysis-Inhibiting Effect of 7 Monoclonal Antibodies. Eur. J. Immunol., 12:739.

17. Ware, C.F., M.S. Krangel, D. Pious, S.J. Burakoff and J.L. Strominger. 1983. Recognition of HLA-A2 Mutant and Variant Target Cells by an HLA-A2 Allospecific Human Cytotoxic T Lymphocyte Line. J. Immunol., 131:1312.

18. Yelton, D.E., C. Desaymard and M.D. Scharff. 1981. Use of Monclonal Anti-Mouse Immunoglobulin to Detect Mouse Antibodies. Hybridoma, 1:5.

19. Ware, C.F., J.L. Reade and L.C. Der. 1984. A Rat Anti-Mouse Kappa Chain Specific Monoclonal Antibody, 187.1.1.0: Purification, Immunochemical Properties and Its Utility as a General Second-Antibody Reagent. J. Immunol. Method., (submitted).

20. Brodsky, F.M. and P. Parham. 1982. Monomorphic Anti-HLA-A,B,C Monoclonal Antibodies Detecting Molecular Subunits and Combinatorial Determinants. J. Immunol., 128:129.

21. Sande, M.A. and G.L. Mandell. 1980. In: The Pharmacological Basis of Therapeutics. Gilman, A.G., L.S. Goodman and A. Gilman (Eds.). MacMillan and Co., New York, pp. 1170.

22. MacDonald, H.R., A.L. Glasebrook, C. Bron, A. Kelso and J.-C. Cerottini. 1982. Clonal Heterogeneity in the Functional Requirement for Lyt-2/3 Molecules on Cytolytic T Lymphocytes (CTL): Possible Implications for the Affinity of CTL Antigen Receptors. Immunological Rev., 68:89.

23. Biddison, W.E., P.E. Rao, M.A. Talle, G. Goldstein and S. Shaw. 1984. Possible Involvement of the T4 Molecule in T Cell Recognition of Class II HLA Antigens: Evidence from Studies of CTL-Target Cell Binding. J. Exp. Med., 159:783.

24. Hemler, M.E., C.F. Ware and J.L. Strominger. 1983. Characterization of a Novel Differentiation Antigen Complex Recognized by a Monoclonal Antibody (A-1A5): Unique Activation-Specific Molecular Forms on Stimulated T Cells. J. Immunol., 131:334.

DISCUSSION

T. Springer: I think its very interesting that you're seeing this kind of synergy with the antibodies directed against the different molecules. But, with all due respect, I'd like to disagree with your interpretation, that we should expect to see these molecules physically associated. I think all that the additive blocking shows is that both of those molecules participate in T cell[-mediated] killing. They could be separate recognition structures separately contributing to avidity, or they could actually be acting in steps, one step preceding the other step, both required for function. For example blocking 90% [at each step], with 10% going through and another 10% going through, you could see 1% going through in the final analysis.

C. Ware: Just to respond to that, I agree with you. I'm not trying to push the idea that there's an actual physical linkage involved. Especially in terms of additive effects, one could argue either way. But I think synergistic effects show that there's some kind of a functional interaction.

D. Sears: In reference to your modulation experiments, where you compare individual antibodies with pooled antibodies, do the individual monoclonals look like pooled monoclonals when you treat with second antiserum, rabbit anti-mouse immunoglobulin?

C. Ware: We haven't done that. I think that would be an interesting study.

T. Springer: In regard to possible associations between surface molecules, I'd like to mention results Mike Brenner presented at the Federation Meetings last week where he was using a monoclonal antibody against a constant region of the antigen receptor. He was cross-linking intact cells at neutral pH, and he did find cross-linking between T3 and the antigen receptor. He also immunoprecipitated with anti-LFA-1, and anti-LFA-2, and he found no physical association between those molecules and the antigen receptor.

C. Ware: Actually, I think you might expect that if you just look at a CTL that has not interacted with a target cell. I think the experiment to follow up what Mike did is to add antigen so the receptor is engaged in functional and physical interactions.

REQUIREMENT FOR LYT-2/3 MOLECULES ON ALLOSPECIFIC CYTOLYTIC T LYMPHOCYTE CLONES IS DEPENDENT UPON TARGET CELL ANTIGEN DENSITY

Richard Shimonkevitz, Jean-Charles Cerottini and
H. Robson MacDonald

Ludwig Institute for Cancer Research, Lausanne
Branch, Epalinges, Switzerland

INTRODUCTION

The Lyt-2/3 antigenic complex in the mouse (1) is expressed preferentially on cytolytic T lymphocytes (CTL) and appears to be involved in the recognition of target cells (2,3). In the course of investigating this phenomenon at the clonal level, we observed that individual CTL clones vary greatly in their requirement for Lyt-2/3 molecules in killing. Thus some CTL clones lose cytolytic activity when treated with monoclonal antibodies (MAbs) directed against Lyt-2/3 (4) or with doses of trypsin which selectively cleave the Lyt-2/3 antigenic determinant from the cell surface (5), whereas other clones are resistant to either treatment. Based on these findings, we (6) and others (7,8) have postulated that the role of the Lyt-2/3 molecules may be to facilitate and/or stabilize the interaction between CTL and their target cells. According to this model, the degree to which Lyt-2/3 molecules are required for effective CTL-target cell binding would be inversely related to the intrinsic affinity of the CTL antigen receptor (6).

At the present time, there is little direct evidence pertaining to the functional role of Lyt-2/3 molecules in the cytolytic process. In order to further test the hypothesis that they may be required to enhance low avidity interactions, we have derived a panel of alloreactive CTL clones which vary widely in their dependence upon Lyt-2/3 molecules for cytolysis. These clones were then tested for their ability to lyse thymoma cells in which the density of the appropriate target alloantigen (H-2K^d) could be quantitatively manipulated by exposure to Interferon-γ (IFN) or by pretreatment with monoclonal anti-H-2K^d

antibodies. The results indicate that there is clonal heterogeneity in the ability of CTL to lyse target cells expressing low levels of target H-2K alloantigens. Furthermore, this heterogeneity correlates with the degree of susceptibility of these clones to inhibition by anti-Lyt-2/3 MAbs.

DERIVATION OF H-2K^d SPECIFIC CTL CLONES

CTL clones were obtained either by micromanipulaton or by limiting dilution and maintained as described in detail elsewhere (9). For the present experiments, clones were derived from primed spleen cells from C57BL/6 mice immunized 2-6 months previously with P815 (DBA/2) mastocytoma cells and restimulated for 5 days with irradiated DBA/2 spleen cells in secondary mixed leukocyte cultures (MLC) (10). Clones specific for H-2K^d were selected on the basis of their ability to lyse IT-22 (H-2^q) mouse fibroblasts transfected with a H-2K^d genomic clone (kindly provided by Dr S. Kvist, EMBL, Heidelberg) (11).

EFFECT OF TARGET CELL ANTIGEN DENSITY ON LYSIS BY CTL CLONES

In order to determine whether the density of surface alloantigen expressed by the target cell influences CTL activity, we made use of our recent discovery that the BALB/c lymphoma ST-4.5 (12) can be stimulated by a factor(s) found in the supernatant of secondary MLC (MLC SN) to increase Class I surface antigen expression. Normally, ST-4.5 cells express very few surface K^d molecules (approximately 5-20% of the number expressed by P815 cells when compared by flow microfluorometry) and undetectable D^d or L^d antigens. After a 48 hour culture in medium supplemented with 10% MLC SN, K^d expression by ST-4.5 cells increased approximately five-fold and D^d by twenty-fold, while L^d remained undetectable (Fig. 1). This effect was apparently specific for H-2 Class I proteins as several other surface antigens (Thy-1, Lyt-2, L3T4 and I-A^d) did not increase after culture. Furthermore, in agreement with earlier reports (13), pure IFN prepared by recombinant DNA technology (a gift of Dr A. Zlotnik, DNAX, Palo Alto) was found to increase Class I expression in a comparable fashion to MLC SN.

The ability of 8 K^d-specific CTL clones to lyse normal and MLC SN-induced ST-4.5 cells was then compared. Table I indicates the effector to target (E:T) ratios required for 50% specific lysis of ^{51}Cr-labelled ST-4.5 targets, as well as control P815 targets, by each K^d-specific CTL clone. Several clones, for example 3,12 and 39, were incapable of efficiently lysing normal ST-4.5 cells but were highly active against ST-4.5 cells whose surface K^d antigen expression was increased after culture in MLC SN. We do not believe that these results reflect nonspecific

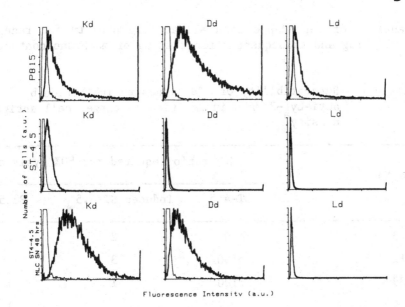

Fig. 1. Differential enhancement of expression of MHC Class I
antigens by ST-4.5 thymoma cells following culture in
MLC SN. ST-4.5 cells cultured for 48 hr in 10% (v/v)
MLC SN (or control ST-4.5 cells) were stained with MAbs
directed against K^d (S13-11, kindly provided by Dr S.
Tonkonogy, North Carolina State University), D^d (P48-7,
kindly provided by Dr J. Klein, Tübingen) or L^d
(28-14-85, kindly provided by Dr D. Sachs, NIH)
followed by fluoresceinated rabbit anti-mouse Ig. All
samples were analyzed on a FACS II flow cytometer gated
to exclude non-viable cells. P815 cells were included
as a positive control for L^d expression. Similar
enhancing effects were obtained with 100 units/ml of
recombinant IFN (not shown).

differences in the ability of the two targets to be cytolysed as
our preliminary studies indicated that both ST-4.5 and MLC
SN-induced ST-4.5 were similarly lysed by CTL populations in the
presence of phytohemagglutinin. These results do suggest that
there may exist a certain minimal threshold level of target cell
surface antigen required for some CTL to be demonstrably
cytolytic. Other CTL clones which could efficiently lyse normal
ST-4.5 targets (clones 4,66,78,81 and 92) behaved in a similar
fashion in that somewhat higher E:T ratios were required to
achieve 50% lysis of normal ST-4.5 cells as compared to MLC
SN-induced ST-4.5 or control P815 targets. It remains to be
determined whether the observed differences in cytolytic activity
exhibited by these CTL clones on the different targets reflects
heterogeneity in T cell receptor binding affinities for

alloantigen or dependence upon alloantigen density for receptor cross-linking and subsequent strengthening of membrane contacts.

Table 1. Susceptibility of CTL clones to inhibition by anti-Lyt-2 MAbs in relation to target cell antigen density[a]

Clone No	E:T ratio required for 50% lysis of		
	ST-4.5	Induced ST-4.5	P815
3	>100	2	2
12	>100	3	1
39	>100	1	1
4	2	2	1
66	6	3	1
78	3	1	1
81	6	3	3
92	3	0.3	0.3

[a] The indicated clones were assayed for cytolytic activity against ^{51}Cr-labeled P815, ST-4.5 or MLC SN-induced ST-4.5 target cells (see Fig. 1) at various E:T ratios. The ratio corresponding to 50% ^{51}Cr release is indicated.

INHIBITION OF CTL CLONES BY ANTI-LYT-2 MAb AS A FUNCTION OF TARGET CELL ANTIGEN DENSITY

The relationship between the level of alloantigen expression by the target cell and dependence upon Lyt-2/3 function in CTL-mediated cytolysis was investigated by assaying the ability of anti-Lyt-2 MAb to inhibit lysis of normal or induced ST-4.5 target cells. These assays were performed by pre-incubating titrated amounts of the MAb with K^d-specific CTL clones for 30 minutes prior to the addition of ^{51}Cr-labelled target cells. For each CTL clone, E:T ratios were chosen that provided 50-90% specific lysis in the absence of added antibody. The results of these assays, indicated in Table II, show that for 4 of 5 CTL clones (4,78,81 and 92) which lysed both normal and induced ST-4.5, a greater amount of anti-Lyt 2 MAb was required for 50% inhibition of lysis of the induced targets expressing relatively higher amounts of K^d antigen.

It should be noted that differences in susceptibility to anti-Lyt-2 inhibition varied widely from one clone to another (range of 1.5-fold to >48-fold). One clone (66) was particularly resistant to anti-Lyt-2 inhibition ; however, at the maximal concentration of MAb tested, inhibition of lysis of normal ST-4.5 was again superior to that observed on the induced targets (31% versus 6%).

Table 2. Susceptibility of CTL clones to inhibition by anti-Lyt-2 MAbs in relation to target cell antigen density[a]

Clone No	Susceptibility to anti-Lyt-2 MAb	
	ST-4.5	Induced ST-4.5
4	1:6400[b]	1:600
66	NI[c]	NI
78	1:4800	1:3200
81	1:4800	1:1600
92	1:9600	NI

[a] The 5 K^d-specific CTL clones capable of lysing normal ST-4.5 target cells (see Table 1) were assayed for cytolytic activity against normal or MLC SN-induced ST-4.5 cells in the presence or absence of various concentrations of anti-Lyt-2 MAb (53-6.7, kindly provided by Dr J. Ledbetter, Genetic Biosystems, Seattle). Control lysis in the absence of MAb ranged from 50-90%.
[b] Reciprocal of anti-Lyt-2 MAb dilution corresponding to 50% inhibition of cytolysis.
[c] Not inhibited at maximal MAb dilution tested (1:200).

These results directly demonstrate that the susceptibility of CTL clones to inhibition by anti-Lyt-2 MAb varies inversely with target cell alloantigen density. In this context, it should be noted that a similar conclusion was reached by Gromkowski et al. (14), who observed that lysis of target cells from which H-2 alloantigens had been enzymatically removed (by papain treatment) was more readily inhibited by anti-Lyt-2 MAbs than lysis of control target cells. The latter study is difficult to interpret in the sense that other putative target cell structures important for cytolysis may have been affected by the papain treatment. In the case of IFN-induced ST-4.5 cells, a similar caveat applies insofar as it cannot be excluded that the level of expression of such putative structures could be increased by the IFN treatment.

SYNERGISTIC INHIBITION OF CYTOLYSIS BY ANTI-LYT-2 AND ANTI-H-2-K^d MAbs

The data presented in the previous section suggest that the requirement for Lyt-2/3 molecules in CTL-mediated lysis varies according to the available density of target cell alloantigens. An alternative means of testing this hypothesis would be to assess the effect of anti-Lyt-2 MAbs on CTL clones in the presence or absence of MAbs directed against the target cell alloantigens (H-2K^d). Results obtained with 2 independently derived CTL clones (51 and 52) are shown in Fig. 2. It can be seen that the cytolytic activity of these clones is not significantly inhibited by either anti-Lyt-2 or anti-H-2-K^d MAbs; however, in the presence of a constant (non-inhibitory) amount of anti-Lyt-2 MAb, the 2 clones are inhibited in a dose-dependent fashion by anti-H-2K^d MAbs. Similar results were obtained by varying the anti-Lyt-2 MAb concentration in the presence of a fixed (non-inhibitory) amount of anti-H-2K^d (not shown).

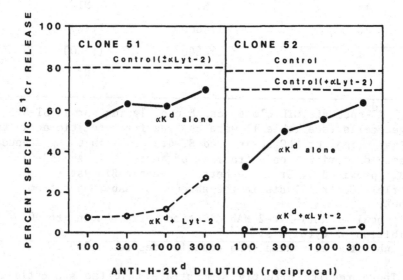

Fig. 2. Synergistic effect of anti-Lyt-2 and anti-H-2K^d MAbs on cytolysis by cloned CTL. C57BL/6 anti-H-2K^d clones 51 and 52 were assayed for cytolytic activity against ^{51}Cr-labeled P815 target cells in a 3 hr assay at a 2:1 E:T ratio. The indicated concentrations of anti-H-2K^d MAb were added in the presence (o---o) or absence (●---●) of a fixed amount (1:200 dilution of ascites fluid) of anti-Lyt-2 MAb. Control lysis values in the absence of anti-H-2K^d MAb (± anti-Lyt-2 MAb) are indicated by the dotted lines.

CONCLUDING REMARKS

The data presented in this communication demonstrate 2 important points concerning the role of target cell antigen density in allospecific CTL-mediated lysis

1) Target cells expressing low levels of alloantigen are lysed by some CTL clones but not others

2) The requirement for Lyt-2/3 molecules in cytolysis by a given CTL clone is increased when target cell antigen density is low.

As mentioned at the outset, it has been proposed by several groups that the main function of Lyt-2/3 molecular complex is to facilitate and/or stabilize the interaction between CTL and target cells (6-8). Such an effect could result from a direct interaction of Lyt-2/3 with a putative ligand present on the target cell (such as the Class I molecules themselves) and/or a functional association with a structure on the CTL membrane which is required for effective cell interaction (such as the specific antigen receptor). Although our data do not allow us to make a distinction between these (not mutually exclusive) hypotheses, they do indicate a greater complexity in CTL:target cell interactions than was previously envisaged. Thus individual CTL clones specific for a given alloantigen may or may not lyse a target cell depending upon the available density of antigen, and the degree to which Lyt-2/3 molecules play a role in this process is likewise antigen-density dependent. It is important to note that these conclusions are made in an operational sense using an artificial in vitro assay system to measure cytolysis ; nevertheless, it seems reasonable to speculate that antigen density (and/or availability) may represent a truly limiting factor in many CTL responses to physiological pathogens in vivo. In the latter context we have previously observed that in vivo immunization with alloantigens or viruses results in a selection for CTL whose function is relatively independent of Lyt-2/3 molecules (6). One explanation for this phenomenon would be to postulate that such CTL have become primed in an environment in which the concentration of available antigen is limiting.

ACKNOWLEDGMENTS

We wish to thank Rosemary Lees, Clotilde Horvath, Anne-Lise Peitrequin and Corinne Blanc for excellent technical assistance, and Josiane Duc for her invaluable help in the preparation of the manuscript.

REFERENCES

1. E.A. Boyse, M. Miyazawa, T. Aoki, and L.J. Old, Ly-A and
    Ly-B : two systems of lymphocyte isoantigens in the
    mouse, Proc. R. Soc. Lond. (Biol.) 170:175 (1968).
2. E. Nakayama, H. Shiku, E. Stockert, H.F. Oettgen, and L.J.
    Old, Cytotoxic T cells : Lyt phenotype and blocking of
    killing activity by Lyt antisera, Proc. natl. Acad. Sci
    76:1977 (1979).
3. N. Shinohara, and D.H. Sachs, Mouse alloantibodies capable
    of blocking cytotoxic T-cell function. I. Relationship
    between the antigen reactive with blocking antibodies
    and the Lyt-2 locus, J. exp. Med. 150:432 (1979).
4. H.R. MacDonald, N. Thiernesse, and J.-C. Cerottini,
    Inhibition of T cell-mediated cytolysis by monoclonal
    antibodies directed against Lyt-2 : heterogeneity of
    inhibition at the clonal level, J. Immunol. 126:1671
    (1981).
5. H.R. MacDonald, A.L. Glasebrook, and J.-C. Cerottini, Clonal
    heterogeneity in the functional requirement for Lyt-2/3
    molecules on cytolytic T lymphocytes : analysis by
    antibody blocking and selective trypsinization, J. exp.
    Med. 156:1711 (1982).
6. H.R. MacDonald, A.L. Glasebrook, C. Bron, A. Kelso, and
    J.-C. Cerottini, Clonal heterogeneity in the functional
    requirement for Lyt-2/3 molecules on cytolytic T
    lymphocytes (CTL) : Possible implications for the
    affinity of CTL antigen receptors, Immunol. Rev. 68:89
    (1982).
7. E. Martz, W. Heagy, and S.H. Gromkowski, The mechanism of
    CTL-mediated killing : monoclonal antibody analysis of
    the roles of killer and target cell membrane proteins,
    Immunol. Rev. 72:73 (1983).
8. S.L. Swain, T cell subsets and the recognition of MHC class,
    Immunol. Rev. 74:129 (1983).
9. H.R. MacDonald, J.-C. Cerottini, J.-E. Ryser, J.L.
    Maryanski, C. Taswell, M.B. Widmer, and K.T. Brunner,
    Quantitation and cloning of cytolytic T lymphocytes and
    their precursors, Immunol. Rev. 51:93 (1980).
10. J.-C. Cerottini, H.D. Engers, H.R. MacDonald, and K.T.
    Brunner, Generation of cytotoxic T lymphocytes in
    vitro. I. Response of normal and immune mouse spleen
    cells in mixed leukocyte culture, J. exp. Med. 140:703
    (1974).
11. B. Arnold, H.-G. Burgert, U. Hamann, G. Hämmerling, U. Kees,
    and S. Kvist, Cytolytic T cells recognize the two
    amino-terminal domains of H-2K antigens in tandem in
    influenza A infected cells, Cell 38:79 (1984).

12. D. Kemp, A. Harris, S. Cory, and J. Adams, Expression of the immunoglobulin Cu gene in mouse T and B lymphoid and myeloid cell lines, Proc. natl. Acad. Sci 77:2876 (1980).

13. D. Wallach, M. Fellows, and M. Revel, Preferential effect of ɣ interferon on the synthesis of HLA antigens and their mRNAs in human cells, Nature 299:833 (1982).

14. S.H. Gromkowski, W.E. Heagy, F. Sanchez-Madrid, T.A. Springer, and E. Martz, Blocking of CTL-mediated killing by monoclonal antibodies to LFA-1 and Lyt-2/3. I. Increased susceptibility to blocking after papain treatment of target cells, J. Immunol. 130:2546 (1983).

DISCUSSION

   T. Springer: This may be a semantic issue but I think we
should be very careful in interpreting the monoclonal antibody
blocking experiments. You have evidence that some of the CTL are
not affected by anti-Lyt-2. But I don't think that necessarily
means that Lyt-2 is not essential. It could be that there is
competition say between the antibody and the antigen, for Lyt-2,
and that the high avidity clones just compete more effectively for
antigen perhaps because the antigen receptor is bringing Lyt-2 into
closer proximity with the antigen.

   The other comment would be that trypsinization could be
removing the antigenic determinants recognized by these antibodies,
but not necessarily all the functional part of the molecule.

   H. R. MacDonald: With regard to the first point, I agree about
the semantics. In fact I think one of the things that we've shown
with these experiments, which is important to keep in mind, is that
in a clone which we would say on the basis of a single parameter
does not require Lyt-2 we in fact showed that that same clone will
require Lyt-2 if we change the conditions. If the conditions were
changed, possibly physiologically, in such a way that antigen were
limiting ... the same clone could either behave as if it needs
those molecules or as if it does not need those molecules depending
on the conditions.

   The second point is perfectly valid. As I indicated in my
presentation, all you can ever say in any experiment of this type
is that you have eliminated the antigenic determinants which are
recognized by the probe which you use to follow the molecules.
Whether there are residual proteolytic fragments of the Lyt-2,3
molecule around which could have some function is a very hard
question to address.

   M. Sitkovsky: What is the difference in immunoprecipitation
between clones L3 and C10 with your anti-Lyt-2,3 monoclonal
antibody?

   H. R. MacDonald: There's no difference we can detect either by
one or two-dimensionsional gel electrophoresis, but we haven't done
peptide mapping.

   M. Palladino: Have you tried blocking by monoclonal antibodies
in combinations of 2 and 3?

   H. R. MacDonald: Yes, we have done combinations of 2 and 3
over a wide range of concentrations, and with the antibodies we
have we see absolutely no synergistic effects.

C. Ware: I see synergism, at least in the human system with anti-T8 and anti-LFA-1. I'll be talking about that later.

M. Mescher: We've done some experiments recently looking at stimulation of the CTL response with affinity-purified H-2 in liposomes, where what appears to be occurring is that the precursors of the CTL recognize the H-2 on the liposomes directly and that provides the necessary signal. What we've found is that that interaction is still very sensitive to blocking by anti-Lyt-2,3, which I think would argue that if the Lyt-2,3 is acting with any kind of (inaudible) molecule its probably through non-polymorphic determinants.

H. R. MacDonald: I think everyone would agree that it must be through non-polymorphic determinants, but the question is does it react with the class I [MHC molecules] or not.

W. Seaman: Jeff Ledbetter and I did some experiments where we could selectively partially cleave Lyt-3, which is more susceptible to trypsin than Lyt-2. That way if you take off Lyt-3 and leave Lyt-2, what you do is remove the ability to block the CTL by anti-Lyt-3 but increase blocking by anti-Lyt-2. So the Lyt-3 component doesn't seem necessary.

H. R. MacDonald: Our results would be in contradiction to that. I didn't show the results, but in our quantitative trypsinization experiments, we lose activity at the same point where we lose expression of Lyt-3 determinants, before we lose Lyt-2. Its a difficult experiment to interpret.

FUNCTIONAL RELATIONSHIPS OF LYT-2 and LYT-3 EXPRESSION AND

T-CELL CYTOTOXICITY: A NEW MODEL SYSTEM

Michael A. Palladino, Jr.,[+] Gerald E. Ranges,[*]
Herbert F. Oettgen, and Lloyd J. Old

[+]Department of Pharmacological Sciences/Immunology
Genentech, Inc., 460 Point San Bruno Boulevard
South San Francisco, CA 94080
[*]Department of Medicine
University of Vermont College of Medicine
Burlington, VT 05405
Memorial Sloan Kettering Cancer Center
1275 York Avenue, New York, NY 10021

INTRODUCTION

Three systems of surface antigens, Lyt-1, Lyt-2 and Lyt-3, characterize cells of thymic origin in the mouse.[1] Lyt-1 antigens, coded by a locus with two alleles on chromosome 19, appear to be expressed on all classes of T-cells.[2] Lyt-2 and Lyt-3 antigens on the other hand, clearly distinguish subclasses of T-cells.[3,4] Cytotoxic and suppressor T-cells express Lyt-2 and Lyt-3, whereas helper T-cells generally lack these antigens. Lyt-2 and Lyt-3 are coded for by a single gene or closely linked genes on chromosome 6.[5]

The relationships between Lyt-2 and Lyt-3 expression and target cell lysis by cytolytic T-lymphocytes have been the object of intensive study over the past decade.[6-8] Blocking of T-cell mediated killing by antibodies to Lyt-2 or Lyt-3 suggested a role for these antigens in T-cell recognition. This view was enhanced by two observations: the reported close linkage between loci coding for the Lyt-3 antigen and immunoglobulin kappa light chain markers; and the demonstration that Lyt-2 and Lyt-3 negative variants of a cloned T-cell line lacked the ability to recognize target-specific allo-determinants but retained Con A mediated killing activity.[9,10] However, recent studies have described Lyt-2 and Lyt-3 positive T-cell clones that are resistant to Lyt-2 blocking and retain killing activity when the Lyt-2 antigens are stripped from the cell

355

surface by trypsin. These studies suggest Lyt-2 and Lyt-3 stabilizes the effector target cell complex rather than recognizes antigen.[6] Further information concerning the expression of Lyt-2 and Lyt-3 molecules and the mechanism by which antibodies to Lyt-2 and Lyt-3 block T-cell mediated killing will be presented in this report.

MATERIALS AND METHODS

Animals

BALB/c, C57BL/6 (B6) and (C57BL/6 x AKR)F_1 (AB6F_1) mice were obtained from the breeding colonies of Sloan-Kettering Institute. CD rats (Sprague-Dawley) were obtained from the Charles River Breeding Laboratories (Willington, MA).

Target Cells

YAC-1, a Maloney leukemia virus-induced T-cell lymphoma of A/SN origin was used. The Lyt phenotype of this tumor is Lyt-1+2,3⁻. The YAC-1 target cell was chosen because interpretation of the Lyt-blocking effects on the cytotoxic T-cells would not be complicated by the possible binding of the Lyt antisera to the target cells.

Table 1. Description of Lyt Antisera

Antiserum	Specificity Detected
B6-H-2^K anti-B6-H-2^K-CE-Lyt-2.1:DS	Lyt-2.1m*
(C3H/An x B6-Lyt-2.1)Fl anti-ERLD(B6)	Lyt-2.2m*
C58 anti-C58.CE-Lyt-3.2:DS$^+$	Lyt-3.2m*
Rat anti-mouse Lyt-2 clone 53-6.7	Lyt-2m*
(STS/A x B6-Ly5.2)Fl anti-ERLD (B6)	Ly-5.1m*
(CBA)/T6 x SJL) F_1 anti-C58	Lyt-3.1c**

*m, monoclonal.
**c, conventional.

Antisera

The Lyt antisera used in this study (Table 1) have been
described previously.[7]

Mixed Lymphocyte Cultures

Cytotoxic T-lymphocytes were generated in 24-well Linbro plates
(Flow Laboratories, McClean, VA) by adding 5×10^6 responding
spleen cells and 5×10^6 inactivated (1500R) BALB/c stimulator
cells per well in 2 ml of Eagle's minimum essential medium (MEM)
supplemented with 10% heat-inactivated fetal calf serum, 2 mM
L-glutamine, 1% nonessential amino acids, 100 U penicillin/ml,
100 ug of streptomycin/ml (complete MEM) and 5×10^{-5}M 2-mercapto-
ethanol.

Cytolytic T-Cell Assay

After five days of culture, the effector cells were harvested
and tested for cytolytic activity and the ability of Lyt-antisera
to block killing activity in a four-hour ^{51}Cr release assay.
Target cells were labeled with ^{51}Cr by incubating 10^6 cells
with 150 uCi of $Na_2{}^{51}CrO_4$ (New England Nuclear, Boston, MA) in
0.5 ml of complete MEM at 37°C for 45 min. After labeling, the
cells were washed three times in complete MEM and adjusted to a
concentration of 2×10^5 cells/ml. Fifty microliter effector
cell suspension (at varying concentrations), 50 ul target cell
suspension, and 50 ul of complete MEM were mixed in round bottom
microtiter plates and incubated at 37° for four hours.

Antibody Blocking Assay

Fifty microliter serially diluted antiserum (without the
addition of exogenous complement), 50 ul effector cells (5×10^4
to 1×10^5) and 50 ul target cells (1×10^4) were mixed and
incubated at 37°C for four hours.

Evaluation of Cytotoxicity Assays, Blocking Assays and Inhibition Assays

The supernatants were removed by Titertek (Flow Laboratories,
Rockville, MD) and assayed in a Packard Scintillation Counter
(Packard Instrument Co., Downers Grove, IL). Percent specific
lysis was calculated as follows: percent lysis = (A-B/C-B) x 100,
where A represents CPM of supernatants of effector cells and target
cells incubated together, B represents CPM of supernatants of
target cells incubated alone (spontaneous release), and C
represents CPM after lysis of target cells with NP-40, (maximum
radioactivity released from target cells). The results presented
in each table are representative of at least three experiments.

Production of Interleukin-2

Spleen cells from CD rats (10^6/ml) were cultured for 48 hours
in complete MEM + 5 x 10^{-5}M 2-mercaptoethanol and 5 ug/ml
concanavalin A (Con A, Miles Laboratories, Inc., Elkhart, IN).
After centrifugation for 10 minutes at 1000 rpm, the supernatant
was sterilized by passage through a 0.20u filter and stored at 4°C.
To prepare growth medium (GM), the IL-2 preparation was added to
complete MEM to a final concentration of 20-50 Units/ml.[11]

Culture of Cytotoxic T-Cells

Cytotoxic T-cells obtained as described above were seeded at
1 x 10^5 cells/well into 24-well Linbro tissue culture plates
(Flow Laboratories) containing 2 ml of GM (50 Units/ml). After
continuous growth and passage for at least one month in the Linbro
plates, the cells were grown in T-75 tissue culture flasks (Falcon
3024) containing 10 ml of GM (20 Units/ml). The cells were fed
with 5 ml of GM (20 Units/ml) every three days and passaged when
the cell concentration approximated 5 x 10^6/flask.

Cloning by Limiting Dilution

Cytotoxic T-cells were seeded at 0.5 cells/well in microtiter
plates (Falcon 3042) containing a feeder layer of irradiated (2000
rads) spleen macrophages in 200 ul GM (20 Units/ml). After ten to
14 days, clones from individual wells were placed in 24 well Linbro
plates for further expansion (one-two weeks) and testing. Clone
CTLL-BAB3 which showed enhanced killing activity for H-2^d determinants was retained for further studies.

RESULTS

Blocking of Killing Activity of AB6F$_1$ Cytotoxic T-Cells Requires
Antisera to Both Lyt-2/3 Alleles

Though several studies have reported in vitro blocking of
T-cell killing by anti Lyt-2 or Lyt-3 antibodies, relatively little
is known about the mechanism(s) of inhibition. Our first set of
experiments was designed to determine whether antisera to all Lyt-2
antigens expressed by a killer T-cell was necessary to inhibit
killing (Table 2).

MLC generated anti-H-2^d allospecific cytotoxic T-cells were
assessed for their killing activity and the ability of allele specific anti-Lyt-2.1 or anti-Lyt-2.2 sera to block killing activity. As
expected, B6 anti-H-2^d killer cell activity was blocked by anti-
Lyt-2.2 (Figure 1A) but not anti-Lyt-2.1, while AKR anti-H-2^d killer
cells were blocked by anti-Lyt-2.1 but not anti-Lyt-2.2 (Figure 1B).

Table 2. Presence of Lyt-2/3 Alleles
on Three Murine Strains

Murine Strain	Lyt-Alleles Expressed
B6	Lyt-2.2, Lyt-3.2
AKR	Lyt-2.1, Lyt-3.1
AB6F$_1$	Lyt-2.1, Lyt-2.2, Lyt-3.1, Lyt-3.2

However, in order to inhibit killing activity of AB6F$_1$ anti-H-2^d cells, it was necessary to include a monoclonal antibody directed at both the Lyt-2.1 and Lyt-2.2 determinants (Figure 1C). This Lyt-2 specific antibody also blocked killing activity in the other two systems (Figure 1A and 1B). The results with the AB6F$_1$ cytotoxic T-cells suggests that blocking most likely takes place at the cell surface, perhaps by steric hindrance rather than an internal phenomenon which switches off the cytotoxic mechanism after the binding of Lyt-2 antigens by antibody.

<u>Lyt 2 and Lyt 3 antigens do not show allelic exclusion.</u> The association of the genes coding for Lyt-2 and Lyt-3 with immuno-globulin light chain genes suggested that these molecules might be immunoglobulin in nature and might utilize the mechanisms of immunoglobulin synthesis in their role as the T-cell recognition unit.[10] If this were so, one might expect Lyt-2 and Lyt-3

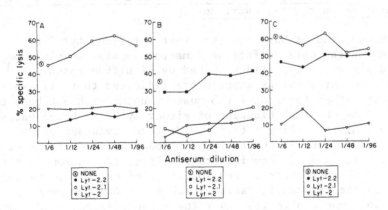

Figure 1. Blocking of T-cell mediated cytotoxicity by Lyt-2 and Lyt-2 allele specific antisera against B6 (A), AKR (B), and AB6F$_1$ (C) anti-BALB/c (anti-H-2^d) cytotoxic T-cells isolated from 5-day mixed lymphocyte cultures.

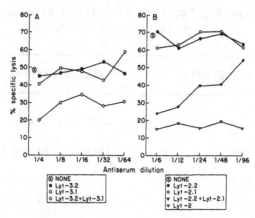

Figure 2. Lyt-2 and Lyt-3 molecules do not show allelic exclusion
on the surface of cytotoxic T-cell clone CTLL-BAB3
(AB6F$_1$ anti-BALB/c). Blocking of killing activity
was demonstrated only when antisera to both Lyt-3 (A)
or Lyt-2 (B) alleles was present during the assay.

antigens to show allelic exclusion at the single cell level in a
manner analogous to Ig expression on B cells. To examine this
hypothesis, we produced (AB6F$_1$) anti-H-2^d T-cell clones. One
clone, CTLL-BAB3, was isolated by limiting dilution at 0.5
cells/well and recloned at this same concentration to insure
clonality. If Lyt-2 and Lyt-3 expression was allelically excluded
only one of the alleles would be expressed on the T-cell surface
and blocking of killer activity would require antisera only to that
expressed allele. The data presented in Figures 2A and 2B show
this not to be the case, i.e. antisera to both alleles, whether
Lyt-2 or Lyt-3 were required to inhibit killing.

Genes for Lyt-2 and Lyt-3 are expressed in a cis, and not trans,
configuration on the cell surface

Previous studies have reported that Lyt-2 and Lyt-3 are
expressed on the cell surface as a macromolecular complex composed
of two different polypeptides linked by disulfide bonds.[12,13] The
results from our previous experiments indicated that all expressed
alleles of either Lyt-2 or Lyt-3 must be bound with antibody to
block killing and that blocking of either Lyt-2 or Lyt-3 was sufficient to inhibit killing activity. We took advantage of this observation to determine if the antigens encoded by the alleles of these
two loci were randomly combined to result in the macromolecular
complex or whether their expression was limited to combination with
alleles in the cis configuration. Table 3 shows the components of
the possible macromolecules under these two possible conditions of
expression.

Table 3. Components of Lyt-2 and Lyt-3 Surface
Macromolecule Complex on AB6F$_1$ Cells

If Randomly Expressed		If Restricted to cis Expression	
Lyt-2.1	Lyt-3.1	Lyt-2.1	Lyt-3.1
Lyt-2.1	Lyt-3.2	Lyt-2.2	Lyt-3.2
Lyt-2.2	Lyt-3.1		
Lyt-2.2	Lyt-3.2		

The sera combinations required to block killing by the F$_1$ cytotoxic cells indicate which of these situations prevails. If the antigens are randomly combined, then antisera to both alleles of Lyt-2 or Lyt-3 would be required to block killing. However, if cell surface antigen expression were restricted to combination with their cis partner, then antisera to one allele of Lyt-2 and the opposite allele of Lyt-3 would be sufficient to block killing.

We tested all possible combinations of anti-Lyt-2 and anti-Lyt-3 sera for their ability to block killing activity of either fresh MLC derived (AB6F$_1$) anti-H-2^d killer cell (Figure 3A) or the cloned line, CTLL-BAB3 (Figure 3B). In both situations, blocking was accomplished using antisera to one allele of Lyt-2 and the opposite allele of Lyt-3, indicating that the genes coding for these antigens are expressed on the cell surface in a cis manner. This restriction to cis expression is not determined by structural incompatabilites between the Lyt 2.1 and 3.2 polypeptides which might prevent their combination since the inbred B6 derived subline B6 (M) is phenotypically Lyt-2.1/Lyt-3.2 and killer activity of cytotoxic cells obtained from this strain is blocked by antisera to either one of these alleles (data not shown).

DISCUSSION

The salient findings of this study are: 1) Blocking of killing activity of AB6F$_1$ killer cells requires addition of Lyt antisera in a combination which blocks both alleles; 2) the expression of Lyt-2/Lyt-3 is not characterized by allelic exclusion; 3) Lyt-2 and Lyt-3 are expressed on the cell surface in a cis rather than trans manner.

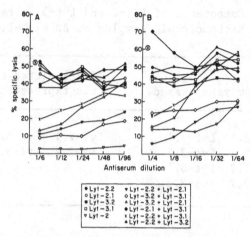

Figure 3. Genes for Lyt-2 and Lyt-3 are expressed in a cis configuration on the surface of AB6F$_1$ killer T-cells. Addition
of Lyt-2 and Lyt-3 antisera in all possible combinations
demonstrated that blocking of killing activity of cytotoxic T-cells isolated from 5 day mixed lymphocyte
cultures containing AB6F$_1$ spleen anti-BALB/c cytotoxic
T-cells (A) or CTLL-BAB3 (B) required antisera addition
in combinations which blocked both Lyt-2 or Lyt-3
alleles.

The fact that blocking by anti-Lyt-2 and/or anti-Lyt-3 requires
addition of the antisera in a specific combination suggests
blocking is a cell surface phenomenon rather than an internal
mechanism triggered by binding of the surface antigen. This interpretation is substantiated by the findings of Dialynas et al.[9] who
showed that a Lyt-2$^-$/Lyt-3$^-$ variant of a cloned T-cell could no
longer demonstrate target specific killing activity, though Con A-
mediated killing was unaffected. In addition, Fan et al.[14] have
given evidence to indicate that inhibition of killing by anti-
Lyt-2/Lyt-3 occurs by blocking of the binding between T-cells and
the target rather than during some postbinding step. None of these
data, however, indicate whether or not Lyt-2/Lyt-3 is part of the
T-cell receptor.

The close association between the Lyt-3 and kappa chain loci
could suggest that the Lyt and Ig loci products combine to form the
T-cell receptor. However our data along with those of Ledbetter
et al.[12] clearly demonstrate that unlike the situation of Ig
expression, Lyt-2 and Lyt-3 molecules are not allelically excluded.

Finally, the data from experiments where blocking of AB6F$_1$
killer T-cells was attempted with various combinations of allele

specific anti-Lyt-2 or anti-Lyt-3 sera indicate that these antigens are expressed only with their cis position partner. This result was not surprising in light of the observations that Lyt-2 and Lyt-3 are found on the cell surface in a macromolecular complex,[12,13] that the number of Lyt-3 molecules per cell was the same as for Lyt-2, and that while Lyt 2⁻ and Lyt 3⁻ variants have been found, no Lyt 2⁺/Lyt 3⁻ variants have. The cis nature of cell surface expression also suggests that Lyt-2 and Lyt-3 are two chains processed from the same precursor protein as has been shown for insulin and C4. However, studies by Rothenberg and Triglia do suggest that the loci for Lyt-2 do express unique gene products.[15] It will be of great interest to utilize molecular biology approaches to the study of these molecules as have been utilized for the study of the T-cell receptor.[16]

SUMMARY

We have developed H-2^d-specific cytotoxic T-cells from (AKR x B6)F$_1$ mice which express Lyt 2.1, 2.2, 3.1 and 3.2 determinants. Antisera specific for these determinants were used to block cytolytic activity of (AKR x B6) F$_1$-derived cytotoxic T-cells. Blocking of killer activity was demonstrated with Lyt 2.2 + 2.1, Lyt 3.2 + 3.1, Lyt 3.2 + 2.1, or Lyt 2.1 + 3.1, but not Lyt 2.1 + 3.1 or Lyt 2.2 + 3.2, or either antisera alone. The antibody-blocking effects were identical whether tested with 5-day MLC-generated cytotoxic T-cells or cloned H-2^d-specific T-cells. The results from these experiments indicate that: 1) blocking of cyto-toxicity by antisera to Lyt-2 and Lyt-3 is a cell surface phenomenon since sera to both alleles were necessary to inhibit cytotoxic activity; 2) the expression of Lyt-2 and Lyt-3 does not exhibit allelic exclusion; and 3) that Lyt-2 and Lyt-3 determinants are expressed on the cell surface in a cis, but not trans, configuration.

REFERENCES

1. E. A. Boyse, M. Miyazawa, T. Aoki, and L. J. Old, Ly-A and Ly-B: two systems of lymphocyte isoantigens in the mouse, Proc. R. Soc. Lond. (Biol) 170:175 (1968).
2. K. Itakura, J. J. Hutton, E. A. Boyse, and L. J. Old, Linkage groups of the theta and Ly-A loci, Nature 230:126 (1971).
3. H. Cantor and E. A. Boyse, Lymphocytes as models for the study of mammalian cellular differentiation, Immunol. Rev. 33:105 (1977).
4. H. Shiku, P. Kisielow, M. A. Bean, T. Takahashi, E. A. Boyse, H. F. Oettgen, and L. J. Old, Expression of T-cell differentiation antigens on effector cells in cell mediated cytotoxicity in vitro, J. Exp. Med. 141:227 (1975).

5. K. Itakura, J. J. Hutton, E. A. Boyse, and L. J. Old, Genetic linkage relationships of loci specifying differentiation alloantigens in the mouse, Transplantation 13:239 (1972).

6. H. R. MacDonald, A. L. Glasebrook, and J. C. Cerottini, Clonal heterogeneity in the functional requirement for Lyt-2 and Lyt-3 molecules on cytolytic T-lymphocytes: Analysis by antibody blocking and selective trypsinization, J. Exp. Med. 156:1711 (1982).

7. E. Nakayama, E. Shiku, E. Stockert, H. F. Oettgen, and L. J. Old, Cytotoxic T-cells: Lyt phenotype and blocking of killing activity by Lyt-antisera, Proc. Natl. Acad. Sci. 76:1977 (1979).

8. S. L. Swain, Significance of Lyt-phenotypes: Lyt-2 antibodies block activities of T-cells that recognize class 1 major histocompatibility complex antigens regardless of their function, Proc. Natl. Acad. Sci. 78:7101 (1981).

9. D. P. Dialynas, M. R. Loken, A. L. Glasebrook, and F. W. Fitch, Lyt-2⁻/3⁻ variants of a cloned cytolytic T-cell line lacks an antigen receptor functional in cytolysis, J. Exp. Med. 153:595 (1981).

10. P. D. Gottlieb, Genetic correlation of a mouse light chain variable region marker with a thymocyte surface antigen, J. Exp. Med. 140:1432 (1974).

11. M. A. Palladino, J. G. Ranges, M. P. Scheid, and H. F. Oettgen, Suppression of T-cell cytotoxicity by nu/nu spleen cells: Reversal by monosaccharides and Interleukin-2, J. Immunol. 130:2200 (1983).

12. J. A. Ledbetter, W. E. Seaman, T. T. Tsu, and L. A. Herzenberg, Lyt-2 and Lyt-3 antigens are on two different polypeptide subunits linked by disulfide bonds. Relationships of subunits to T-cell cytolytic activity, J. Exp. Med. 153:1503 (1981).

13. G. Jay, M. A. Palladino, G. Khoury, and L. J. Old, Mouse Lyt-2 antigen: Evidence for two heterodimers with a common subunit, Proc. Natl. Acad. Sci. 79:2654 (1982).

14. J. Fan, A. Ahmed, and B. Bonavida, Studies on the induction and expression of T cell-mediated immunity. X. Inhibition by Lyt 2, 3 antisera of cytotoxic T lymphocyte-mediated antigen-specific and non-specific cytotoxicity: evidence for the blocking of the binding between T lymphocytes and target cells and not the post-binding cytolytic steps, J. Immunol. 125:2444 (1980).

15. E. Rothenberg and D. Triglia, Lyt-2 glycoprotein is synthesized as a single molecular species, J. Exp. Med. 157:365 (1983).

16. S. M. Hendrick, E. A. Nielsen, J. Kavaler, D. I. Cohen, and M. M. Davis, Sequence relationships between putative T-cell receptor polypeptides and immunoglobulins, Nature 308:155 (1984).

THE ROLE OF THE T3 MOLECULAR COMPLEX

ON HUMAN T LYMPHOCYTE-MEDIATED CYTOTOXICITY

Constantine D. Tsoukas, Mary Valentine, Martin Lotz,
John H. Vaughan, and Dennis A. Carson

Department of Basic and Clinical Research
Scripps Clinic and Research Foundation
10666 North Torrey Pines Road
La Jolla, California 92037

INTRODUCTION

The mechanism via which cytotoxic T lymphocytes (CTL)[1]-lyse their target cells remains a mystery. The recent development of monoclonal antibodies that react with function-associated molecules on the surfaces of human or murine T cells has provided useful reagents for the delineation of the mechanism of CTL function. One such function-associated molecule is the T3 molecular complex present on the surfaces of all mature human T cells (1). Monoclonal antibodies to the T3 complex have diverse effects on T cell function including induction of proliferation of resting T cells (2,3), inhibition of CTL generation _in vitro_ (4), and inhibition of effector CTL

---

[1]**Abbreviations used in this paper:**

CTL, cytotoxic T lymphocyte; MLC, mixed lymphocyte culture; MHC, major histocompatibility complex; Con A, concanavalin A; PHA, phytohemagglutinin; PDLNL, post-dispersion lectin-dependent nonspecific lysis; WGA, wheat germ agglutinin; PMA, phorbol myristic acetate; IL2, interleukin 2; PBL, peripheral blood lymphocytes; LDL, lectin-dependent lysis; SRBC, sheep red blood cells; PBS, phosphate buffered saline; FACS, fluorescence activated cell sorter; EBV, Epstein-Barr virus; LU, lytic unit.

function in lytic assays (3,5-7). In the present report, we will discuss these properties of the monoclonal antibodies placing emphasis on the inhibition of CTL-mediated lysis of target cells.

BIOCHEMICAL CHARACTERISTICS OF THE T3 MOLECULAR COMPLEX

The T3 molecular complex is composed of a predominant 20 Kd glycoprotein as well as glycoproteins of 25-28 Kd, 37 Kd and 44 Kd (8-13). Metabolic labelling studies suggest that the 20 Kd glycoprotein becomes associated with the 25-28 Kd component during biosynthesis while its association with the 37 Kd and 44 Kd proteins takes place on the cell surface (10). Detection of all four glycoproteins depends on the particular anti-T3 antibody employed. For example, immunoprecipitation with monoclonal antibody OKT3 reveals all four components (10), while antibody Leu 4 precipitates only the 20 Kd and 25-28 Kd polypeptides (11). Immunoprecipitation studies have indicated that both antibodies react primarily with the 20 Kd glycoprotein (8-13). It is not clear, however, whether each one of the glycoproteins of the T3 complex possesses a determinant to which the antibodies bind. Alternatively, the antibodies may bind to one of the glycoproteins and co-precipitate the others along with it. Recent evidence supports the existence of a fifth member of the T3 complex, an unglycosylated 20 Kd species (12). The 20 Kd glycoprotein mentioned above has a polypeptide backbone of 14 Kd (12). The unglycosylated 20 Kd species can be specifically labelled with hydrophobic reagents, suggesting that this protein may contain transmembrane segments (12). However, the structural relationship between these two 20 Kd proteins and the other components of the T3 complex is not clearly understood.

MONOCLONAL ANTIBODIES REACTIVE WITH THE T3 MOLECULAR COMPLEX

Several monoclonal antibodies reactive with the T3 molecular complex have been described. These include OKT3 (1), anti-T3 (14), Leu 4 (15), UCHT-1 (16), and 64.1[2].

---

[2]C. Tsoukas et al. in preparation; and New England Nuclear technical bulletin.

TABLE I. Competitive Cross Inhibition of Monoclonal Antibodies to the T3 Molecular Complex

Preincubation	Percentage Positive Cells After Incubation With		
	Fl-G α M	Fl-OKT3	Fl-Leu 4
PBS	3.5	90.0	90.6
OKT3	91.5	2.1	14.0
Leu 4	90.8	3.1	4.0
64.1	94.9	84.8	83.9
Leu 5	96.3	84.7	90.7

Peripheral blood, SRBC receptor positive lymphocytes (T cells), were preincubated with various monoclonal antibodies or PBS. Following thorough washing the cultures were divided in three equal parts and cells were treated with fluorescein conjugated goat anti-mouse antiserum (Fl-G α M), or Fl-OKT3 or Fl-Leu 4 respectively. The cells were then analyzed on a FACS and the percentage fluorescent positive cells was determined. Treatment with Fl-GαM is a control for the binding of the monoclonal antibody to the lymphocytes. This control was necessary, since no Fl-64.1 was available to demonstrate self-crossblocking. Monoclonal antibody Leu 5 reacts with a T cell structure (SRBC receptor) distinct from the T3 complex.

Competitive cross-inhibition experiments have indicated that monoclonal antibody 64.1 reacts with an epitope distinct from the ones identified by antibodies OKT3 and Leu 4. Pre-incubation of human peripheral T cells with 64.1 does not affect the binding of antibodies OKT3 and Leu 4 (Table I). Although OKT3 and Leu 4 crossblocked each other, the data of Garson et al. (16) suggest that each of these two antibodies react with distinct epitopes, since Leu 4 reacts with Purkinje neurones but OKT3 does not. UCHT-1 also reacts with Purkinje neurons (16). Howard et al. (17) have reported that 70-90% of human thymocytes react with antibody Leu 4, while only 10% react with OKT3.

MONOCLONAL ANTIBODIES TO THE T3 COMPLEX INHIBIT THE GENERATION OF CTL

One of the biologic effects that anti-T3 monoclonal

TABLE II. Inhibition of CTL Generation by Monoclonal Antibodies
to the T3 Molecular Complex

Monoclonal Antibody	Concentration for 50% Inhibition of Control Cytotoxicity (pcg/ml)
OKT3	14
Leu 4	660
64.1	65

Cytotoxic T cells were generated in one way MLC of allogeneic PBL in the presence of various concentrations of purified monoclonal antibodies. Control cultures received either mouse myelomas of the same subclass as the antibodies (IgG1 or IgG2a) or medium. No significant differences were seen between the two types of controls. Cytotoxic activity was tested by the ^{51}Cr-release assay against EBV-infected B cell lymphoblasts of stimulator cell origin. Lytic units (LU) per 1×10^6 effector cells were calculated from the ^{51}Cr-specific release data. One LU was defined as the amount of effector lymphocytes causing 50% specific release of radioisotope. The control cultures of the experiment that is displayed above contained 18 LU/10^6 cells. From the LU content of cultures receiving various concentrations of monoclonal antibodies the 50% inhibition titers were calculated.

antibodies mediate is inhibition of CTL generation in MLC (4). Addition of picogram quantities of antibody to allogeneic MLC causes significant inhibition of cytotoxic activity (Table II). The three monoclonal antibodies tested varied in their ability to inhibit CTL generation over approximately 50-fold range of protein concentration. Although these differences may relate to the particular epitopes these antibodies recognize, they may also reflect differences in affinity or purity.

The mechanism of inhibition of CTL generation by the anti-T3 antibodies has not been elucidated. However, there are at least two possibilities. The T3 complex has been shown to exist in association with the T cell antigen receptor on the cell surface (18). Thus, when cytotoxic T cells are treated either with anti-T3 antibodies or anti-receptor antibodies, redistribution (patching, capping, endocytosis/shedding) of both the antigen receptor and the T3 complex occurs (18). This process is known as 'modulation'. It is, therefore, conceivable that addition of anti-T3 antibodies to MLC causes co-modulation of the antigen receptor of the responding cells which then become unresponsive due to lack of an antigen recognition structure. Another possibility which may not necessarily exclude the one above is the generation of suppressor T cells. This is supported by the data of Lau and Goldstein (19), who found that antibody OKT3 could indeed induce the generation of suppressor T cells.

MONOCLONAL ANTIBODIES TO THE T3 COMPLEX INHIBIT THE EFFECTOR FUNCTION OF CTL

Pretreatment of CTL with anti-T3 antibodies significantly reduces their ability to lyse their specific targets (Figure 1). This inhibitory effect is not dependent on any associative recognition structures (MHC Class I or II) on the target cell, as has been the case with other monoclonal antibodies that inhibit CTL function (i.e., OKT8, OKT4, Leu 2a)(20-23). The effect of anti-T3 antibodies is directly on the CTL as determined in assays where the target cells were B lymphoblasts which do not react with anti-T3 antibodies (7).

The ability of anti-T3 antibodies to inhibit CTL effector function differs in two important aspects from the other effects of these antibodies (i.e., induction of proliferation, inhibition of CTL generation, production of lymphokines). First, much higher concentrations of antibody are needed for inhibition of CTL effector function; for example 0.8 micrograms of antibody per ml were necessary to mediate fifty percent inhibition of CTL effector function (Figure 1), while only 14 picograms/ml were sufficient to mediate fifty percent inhibition of CTL generation (Table II). Second, inhibition of effector function can be also mediated by the enzymatic fragments (F(ab)'$_2$ and Fab) of the antibody (3,7), strongly suggesting that accessory cells and crossblocking of T3 molecules probably are not involved. In contrast, the other effects of anti-T3 antibodies on lymphocytes require the presence of monocytes and intact antibody molecules (2,3).

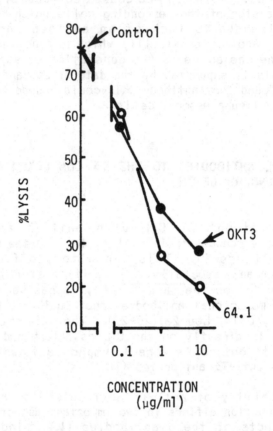

Figure 1: Inhibition of CTL effector function by monoclonal antibodies to the T3 molecular complex. CTL were generated against either allogeneic lymphocytes or autologous EBV-infected B lymphoblasts [for details see ref. (7)]. Effector cells were treated with various concentrations of monoclonal antibody OKT3 or 64.1 in the absence of complement. Control cultures were treated with either medium or myelomas of the appropriate subclass (IgG1 or IgG2a). No significant differences were seen between medium or myeloma treated CTL. The medium treated control cultures only are shown above. Lysis was assayed by the ^{51}Cr radioisotope release assay at effector:target of 30:1. The continuous presence of antibody during the assay was not necessary and washing the effector cells before addition of target cells gave identical results [for more details see ref. (7)].

TABLE III. Summary of the Effects of Monoclonal Antibodies OKT3 and Leu 2a on the Early Steps of the Lytic Process

Antibody	Recognition/Adhesion		Lethal Hit		Target Cell Lysis
	Before	After	Before	After	
	+				-
OKT3		+			-
			+		-
				+	+
	+				-
Leu 2a			+		+

CTL were generated against autologous EBV-infected B lymphoblasts. The monoclonal antibodies were added before or after the initiation of the indicated steps. The assay was then completed by dispersion in high molecular weight Dextran-containing medium and lysis assessed by ^{51}Cr-release [for details see reference (25)]. The (-) sign denotes no lysis of target cells, the (+) sign indicates lysis.

DELINEATION OF THE STEP(S) OF THE CYTOLYTIC PROCESS INHIBITED BY ANTI-T3 ANTIBODIES

The CTL-target interaction has been resolved into three operationally defined steps (24). The first, recognition/adhesion, which probably consists of two distinct steps not as yet operationally distinguishable, involves the recognition and binding of CTL to the specific target cells. This step requires Mg^{++} for its optimal completion, is very rapid, and can proceed at temperatures below 37°C although at a slower rate. Many monoclonal antibodies discussed elsewhere in this volume, have been shown to inhibit this step. The second step, 'lethal hit' or 'programming for lysis' involves the delivery of an assault to the target that results in non-reversible damage. The mechanism of the 'lethal hit' step is unknown. This step requires Ca^{++} and is more temperature dependent than the adhesion step. Finally, the third step is the killer-cell independent lysis which involves the final disintegration of the target. This step requires the longest period of time for its completion and is independent of divalent cations.

371

Monoclonal anti-T3 antibodies, inhibit cytolysis by interfering with a post-recognition/adhesion process, probably the 'lethal hit' step (25,26). Table III summarizes the effects that antibody OKT3 has on lysis when it is added at various times of the early steps of the lytic process. Another monoclonal antibody, Leu 2a, which reacts with a molecule on CTL distinct from T3, is included for comparison, as this antibody inhibits the recognition/adhesion step. It can be noted that antibody OKT3 inhibits lysis when added anytime before the initiation of the 'lethal hit'. These data are supported by microscopic observations of CTL-target conjugates after treatment with antibodies OKT3 and Leu 2a.

MECHANISM OF INHIBITION OF CTL-MEDIATED LYSIS BY ANTI-T3 ANTIBODIES

It was mentioned above that anti-T3 antibodies can cause the modulation of both the T3 complex and the antigen receptor. Since relatively high quantities of antibody are needed for inhibition of lysis, modulation and subsequent loss of the antigen receptor from the cell surface, could be cited as a possible mechanism. One would then expect inability of CTL to recognize and bind to target cells. This prediction, however, is not supported by the experimental data.

In the presence of agglutinating concentrations of several plant lectins such as Con A and PHA, CTL can lyse target cells nonspecifically (27,28). Experimental evidence indicates that agglutination by the lectins and bringing CTL and target in close contact is not sufficient for lysis (29,30). Therefore, lectins mediating nonspecific lysis must possess not only agglutinating properties, but also the ability to trigger the lytic process. This has been demonstrated by Parker and Martz with the post-dispersion lectin-dependent nonspecific lysis assay (PDLNL)(31). They found that at low concentrations some lectins such as WGA would allow 'non-lethal' adhesions. These 'non-lethal' adhesions could be developed to 'lethal' events by addition of another lectin, Con A. Con A was added in a viscous medium (high molecular weight Dextran) in order to prevent recirculation of CTL and new conjugate formation. These observations would suggest that Con A triggers the initiation of the 'lethal hit' step.

We have previously reported that inhibition of lysis mediated by monoclonal antibody OKT3 does not occur in the presence of mitogenic concentrations of Con A (25). These

findings indicate that treatment with the antibody does not
damage the lytic machinery in an irreversible manner.
Furthermore, based on the data of Parker and Martz (31) a
possible interpretation could be that the lectin triggers
the 'lethal hit' which has been inhibited by the presence
of OKT3 antibody. Since we could not exclude the
possibility of CTL recirculation and new conjugate
formation by Con A, we repeated the experiment using the
PDLNL assay where 'non-lethal' adhesions were formed
between alloreactive CTL treated with an antibody to the T3
complex (64.1) and their specific targets. As expected,
treatment with antibody and dispersion in dextran-medium
without Con A inhibited cytotoxicity (Figure 2). However,
when Con A was included in the dextran-medium, the cytotoxicity was restored to control values (Figure 2). In
contrast, dispersion in Con A-dextran-medium did not
restore the lytic activity of CTL that had been treated
with monoclonal antibody Leu 2a which unlike 64.1 inhibits
killer-target conjugate formation (Figure 2). These data
suggest that the T3 molecular complex might be involved in
the 'lethal hit' step.

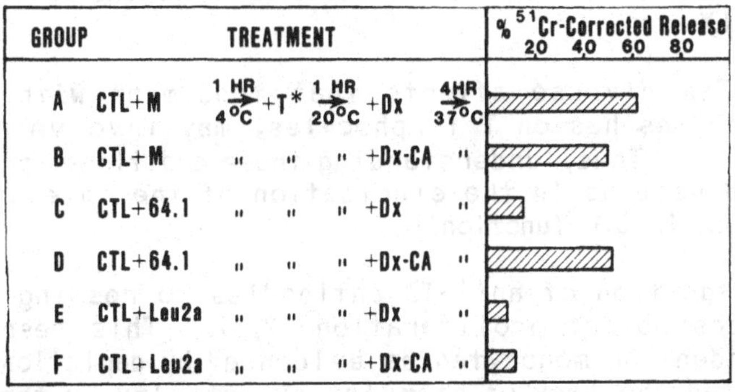

Figure 2: Antibodies to the T3 complex allow the formation
of 'non-lethal' conjugates, which can be resolved to lytic
events by mitogenic lectins. Alloreactive CTL were treated
with monoclonal antibody 64.1, or antibody Leu 2a, or
medium. The effectors were allowed to interact with their
radiolabelled targets under conditions that allow adhesion
formation, but not initiation of measurable 'lethal hit'
events (for details see ref. 25). Cultures were then
dispersed in dextran-medium with or without Con A and
allowed to incubate for an additional 4 hours at 37°C. The
percentage specific lysis was calculated from the released
radioactivity.

TABLE IV. Effect of Modulation of the T3 Molecular Complex on PHA Responsiveness

Treatment	^{3}H-Thymidine Incorporation (CPM)	% Decrease
OKT3	32,200	45%
Medium	58,642	---

Peripheral blood T lymphocytes were purified by SRBC rosetting and depleted of monocytes by carbonyl iron phagocytosis. The purity of these cells was assessed by reactivity with monoclonal antibody OKT3 (>99%) and esterase staining for monocytes (<0.1%). The T cells were treated at 4°C with antibody OKT3 or medium, followed by goat anti-mouse antiserum and then incubated for 1 hour - 37°C to modulate the T3 complex. After thorough washing the cells were cultured in the presence of optimal quantities of PHA and PMA. Proliferation was measured by ^{3}H-thymidine incorporation. (Valentine et al. in preparation).

OTHER EFFECTS MEDIATED BY ANTIBODIES TO THE T3 MOLECULAR COMPLEX

The diverse effects that treatment with anti-T3 antibodies has on T lymphocytes, may involve a common pathway. Thus, understanding these additional properties could help us in the elucidation of the role of the T3 complex in CTL function.

Addition of anti-T3 antibodies to resting T cells induces potent proliferation (2,3). This response is dependent on monocytes as evidenced by depletion studies (32) and the lack of stimulatory activity by the F(ab')$_2$ and Fab enzymatic fragments of the antibody [(3) and C. Tsoukas, unpublished]. In view of this property of anti-T3 antibodies, we tested the possibility that mitogenesis induced by lectins, such as PHA, is due to interaction with the T3 complex. Purified, resting T cells from the peripheral blood were depleted of monocytes and their T3 molecules modulated by sequential treatment with antibody OKT3 and an anti-mouse antiserum. These cells and untreated controls were then stimulated with a mitogenic concentration of PHA in the presence of PMA. Addition of PMA was necessary due to the lack of monocytes. The purity of T cells was established phenotypically by reaction with anti-T3 antibodies and esterase staining for monocytes. Functionally their purity was demonstrated by their lack of proliferation with antibody OKT3 alone. Modulation of the T3 complex was monitored by immunofluorescence which showed approximately 50% reduction in OKT3 binding at the time of addition of PHA in the culture. This clearance of the T3 complex resulted in 45% decrease in the PHA response (Table IV). These data suggest that a significant portion of PHA induced proliferation is mediated by a direct or indirect interaction with the T3 complex or that modulation of the T3 complex renders the T cells refractile to PHA stimulation.

Monocytes are necessary for the induction of T cell proliferation by anti-T3 antibodies (32). Presumably, monocytes release interleukin-1 which in turn induces the release of IL2 and the expression of IL2 receptors. Non-activated resting T cells do not respond to IL2 since they lack receptors for the lymphokine (33). We tested whether the monocyte requirement could be substituted by addition of exogenous IL2. Purified T cells were depleted of monocytes and incubated with monoclonal antibody 64.1 in the presence of various concentrations of purified IL2. We found that optimal proliferation of T cells depended on the presence of both IL2 and monoclonal antibody (Figure 3). The involvement of monocytes in this effect is very unlikely since no response is seen in the presence of antibody alone (Figure 3), and less than <0.1% esterase positive cells was present. The data of Meuer et al. have indicated that treatment of IL2 receptor positive T cell clones with antibodies to the antigen receptor also causes augmentation in the expression of IL2 receptors (34). In view of the association between the antigen receptor and the T3 complex on the cell surface (18), the above data suggest that the T3 molecular complex is involved in the induction of IL2 receptors in resting T cells.

Secretion of lymphokines is also induced upon treatment of T cells with anti-T3 antibodies. Interleukin 2 and gamma interferon are two of the lymphokines secreted (35-37). Although this effect is dependent on monocytes, Meuer et al. (34) have reported that incubation of T cell clones with anti-T3 antibodies fixed on a solid surface (Sepharose beads) can induce IL2 secretion in the absence of monocytes. This observation indicates that cross-linking of T3 molecules is required for lymphokine secretion.

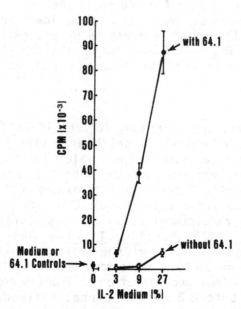

Figure 3: Monoclonal antibody 64.1 induces T lymphocytes to respond to IL2. Peripheral blood T lymphocytes were purified by SRBC rosetting and depleted of monocytes by carbonyl iron phagocytosis. The purity of the T cells was assessed as described in the legend of Table IV. The T cells, 2×10^5 per well of microtiter trays, were incubated in the presence or absence of monoclonal antibody 64.1 (50 ng/ml) and various concentrations of purified IL2 containing medium. Proliferation was assessed by ^{3}H-thymidine uptake after 3 days of culturing. The purified IL2 was obtained from Collaborative Research, Inc. (Lexington, Massachusetts). This product migrates as a single band in SDS gels (Collaborative Research Technical Bulletin). The activity of this IL2 preparation is completely neutralized by an anti-IL2 monoclonal antibody (data not shown). IL2 medium 27% corresponds to approximately 99 units of IL2 activity. One unit is the amount producing one half of the maximum plateau growth as determined with an IL2 dependent cell line.

Addition of several lectins, such as Con A and PHA to CTL cultures allows non-specific lysis of target cells (27,28). This phenomenon has been termed lectin dependent lysis (LDL). Treatment of PBL with monoclonal antibody OKT3 induces LDL (Table V). It is of interest that even in the absence of lectin during the lytic assay a small but significant amount of cytotoxicity was observed (Table V). It was mentioned above that anti-T3 antibodies are potent inhibitors of the generation of specific alloreactive CTL generated in primary MLC. It would be seemingly difficult to reconcile the CTL inhibitory property of the antibodies with their ability to generate LDL. Several possibilities could explain this phenomenon. Modulation of the T3-antigen receptor complex (18) is a possible mechanism for inhibition of specific alloreactivity. However, non-specific LDL might still be generated because lectins bypass the requirement for specific antigen recognition. Another possibility would be that the LDL is mediated by a cytotoxic population deriving from a distinct precursor pool. Finally, since the time kinetics of LDL generation are faster (3 days) than the induction of specific CTL (5-6 days) the LDL might escape inhibition by the suppressor cells that are induced in the same cultures (19). This phenomenon of simultaneous suppression of specific CTL and

TABLE V.   Induction of LDL by Monoclonal Antibody OKT3

Antibody Concentration (ng/ml)	Medium		Con A	
	L.U./10^6	L.U./Culture	L.U./10^6	L.U./Culture
100	.22	<0.6	33.3	90
10	.13	<0.3	66.7	160
1	.33	<0.7	22.2	49
0.1	.03	<0.08	0.2	<0.46
0	.03	<0.09	0.2	<0.46

Peripheral blood lymphocytes, 2×10^5/microtiter tray well, were incubated with various concentrations of monoclonal antibody OKT3 for 3 days. Cytolytic activity was assessed by the ^{51}Cr-release assay at various effector:target ratios with or without Con A (10 µg/ml). One L.U. is the amount of effector cells causing 50% specific release of radiolabel (Tsoukas et al. in preparation).

stimulation of LDL has been previously described in the murine system using Con A (38).

It was mentioned that treatment of antigen reactive T cell clones with antibodies to the T3 complex or the antigen receptor causes comodulation and subsequent clearance of these molecules from the surface of the cell. This could easily explain the inability of antigen reactive cells to proliferate in response to specific antigen when antibodies to T3 complex or the antigen receptor are present (18). In this context the observations of Zanders et al. (39) might be pertinent. These investigators found that addition of an appropriate concentration of influenza hemmagglutinin synthetic peptides to peptide reactive T cell clones, in the absence of monocytes, induced immunologic unresponsiveness. Of particular interest was the observation that the state of unresponsiveness correlated with the loss of T3 antigen in a peptide dose related fashion. One could hypothesize that presentation of free peptide to the T cells in the absence of accessory cells mediates co-modulation of the T3 complex and the antigen receptor in a manner similar to that seen with the monoclonal antibodies. This would suggest a novel mechanism of tolerance induction and further emphasize the importance of the T3 complex in antigen mediated T cell activation.

SUMMARY

The above overview of the experimental data clearly indicates that the T3 molecular complex is intimately involved in T cell activation. The precise role of the T3 complex in the activation process, however, is not clearly understood. The surface association of the T3 complex with the antigen receptor, along with the ability of antibodies to these molecules to render T cells receptive to IL2, reveal a possible mechanism by which specific antigen initiates T cell activation and growth. However, it would be difficult to reconcile this specific effect of anti-T3 antibodies with their effect on CTL function. Since the T3 complex is not a specific marker of any particular effector T cell population, but it is found on all T lymphocytes, we favor the hypothesis that the complex is involved in a more fundamental step of T cell activation, and we believe that triggering of the 'lethal hit', expression of IL2 receptors, and secretion of IL2 are mere manifestations of this basic process.

The natural ligand of the antigen receptor is

obviously the specific antigen. However, the natural
ligand of the T3 complex is unknown. Possibly, its natural
ligand is the antigen receptor itself after it has
interacted with antigen. A simple scenario, then of the
early events of T cell activation would include antigen
recognition and binding, followed by an interaction between
the antigen receptor and the T3 complex which then
activates or allows expression of specific pathways
depending on the particular effector population involved.
Thus, the inhibition of CTL function by anti-T3 antibodies
could be explained by interference with the antigen
receptor - T3 complex interaction following target cell
recognition. This interaction may be the event that
signals the initiation of the 'lethal hit' process.

ACKNOWLEDGMENTS

The present work was supported by NIH grants GM 23200,
AM 21175, RR 00833 and a grant from the Lilly Research
Laboratories.

The technical assistance of Theresa Wilcoxson, and
secretarial assistance of Shari Brewster, Frances Kral and
Jane Uhle is greatly appreciated.

This is publication number 3538BCR from the Research
Institute of Scripps Clinic, La Jolla, California.

REFERENCES

1.   Kung, P.C., Goldstein, G., Reinherz, E.L. and
     Schlossman, S.F. Monoclonal antibodies defining
     distinctive human T cell surface antigens. Science
     206:347-349 (1979).
2.   Van Wauwe, J.P., De Mey, J.R. and Goossens, J.G. OKT3:
     A monoclonal anti-human T lymphocyte antibody with
     potent mitogenic properties. J. Immunol. 124:2708-2713
     (1980).
3.   Chang, T.W., Kung, P.C., Gingras, S.P. and Goldstein,
     G. Does OKT3 monoclonal antibody react with an
     antigen-recognition structure on human T cells?. Proc.
     Natl. Acad. Sci. USA 78:1805-1808 (1981).
4.   Reinherz, E.L., Hussey, R.E. and Schlossman, S.F. A
     monoclonal antibody blocking human T cell function.
     Eur. J. Immunol. 10:758-762 (1980).

5. Biddison, W.E., Shearer, G.M. and Chang, T.W. Regulation of influenza virus-specific cytotoxic T cell responses by monoclonal antibody to a human T cell differentiation antigen. J. Immunol. 127:2236-2240 (1981).

6. Platsoucas, C.D. and Good, R.A. Inhibition of specific cell-mediated cytotoxicity by monoclonal antibodies to human T cell antigens. Proc. Natl. Acad. Sci. USA 78:4500-4504 (1981).

7. Tsoukas, C.D., Fox, R.I., Carson, D.A., Fong, S. and Vaughan, J.H. Molecular interactions in human T-cell-mediated cytotoxicity to Epstein-Barr virus. I. Blocking of effector cell function by monoclonal antibody OKT3. Cell. Immunol. 69:113-121 (1982).

8. Van Agthoven, A., Terhorst, C., Reinherz, E. and Schlossman, S. Characterization of T cell surface glycoproteins T1 and T3 present on all human peripheral T lymphocytes and functionally mature thymocytes. Eur. J. Immunol. 11:18-21 (1981).

9. Borst, J., Prendiville, M.A. and Terhorst, C. Complexity of the human T lymphocyte-specific cell surface antigen T3. J. Immunol. 128:1560-1565 (1982).

10. Borst, J., Alexander, S., Elder, J. and Terhorst, C. The T3 complex on human T lymphocytes involves four structurally distinct glycoproteins. J. Biol. Chem. 258:5135-5141 (1983).

11. Bergman, Y., Stewart, S.J., Levy, S. and Levy, R. Biosynthesis, glycosylation, and in vitro translation of the human T cell antigen Leu 4. J. Immunol. 131:1876-1881 (1983).

12. Borst, J., Prendiville, M.A. and Terhorst, C. The T3 complex on human thymus-derived lymphocytes contains two different subunits of 20KDa. Eur. J. Immunol. 13:576-580 (1983).

13. Rinnooy Kan, E.A., Wang, C.Y., Wang, L.C. and Evans, R.L. Nonconvalently bonded subunits of 22 and 28 Kd are rapidly internalized by T cells reacted with anti-Leu 4 antibody. J. Immunol. 131:536-539 (1983).

14. Reinherz, E.L., Meuer, S., Fitzgerald, K.A., Hussey, R.E., Levine, H. and Schlossman, S.F. Antigen recognition by human T lymphocytes is linked to surface expression of the T3 molecular complex. Cell 30:735-743 (1982).

15. Ledbetter, J.A., Evans, R.L., Lipinski, M., Cunningham-Rundles, C., Good, R.A. and Herzenberg, L.A. Evolutionary conservation of surface molecules that distinguish T lymphocyte helper/inducer and cytotoxic/suppressor subpopulations in mouse and man. J. Exp. Med. 153:310-323 (1981).

16. Garson, J.A., Beverley, P.C.L., Coakham, H.B. and Harper, E.I. Monoclonal antibodies against human T lymphocytes label Purkinje neurones of many species. Nature 298:375-377 (1982).

17. Howard, F.D., Ledbetter, J.A., Wong, J., Bieber, C.P., Stinson, E.B. and Herzenberg, L.A. A human T lymphocyte differentiation marker defined by monoclonal antibodies that block E-rosette formation. J. Immunol. 126:2117-2122 (1981).

18. Meuer, S.C., Fitzerald, K.A., Hussey, R.E., Hodgdon, J.C., Schlossman, S.F. and Reinherz, E.L. Clonotypic structures involved in antigen-specific human T cell function. Relationship to the T3 molecular complex. J. Exp. Med. 157:705-719 (1983).

19. Lau, C. and Goldstein, G. OKT3 induces suppressor cells for mixed lymphocyte and PHA mitogenic responses in human peripheral lymphocytes. Int. J. Immunopharmacol. 3:187-192 (1981).

20. Spits, H., Borst, J., Terhorst, C. and De Vries, J.E. The role of T cell differentiation markers in antigen-specific and lectin-dependent cellular cytotoxicity mediated by T8+ and T4+ human cytotoxic T cell clones directed at class I and class II MHC antigens. J. Immunol. 129:1563-1569 (1982).

21. Krensky, A.M., Reiss, C.S., Mier, J.W., Strominger, J.L. and Burakoff, S.J. Long-term human cytolytic T cell lines allospecific for HLA-DR6 antigen are OKT4+. Proc. Natl. Acad. Sci. USA 79:2365-2369 (1982).

22. Biddison, W.E., Rao, P.E., Talle, M.A., Goldstein, G. and Shaw, S. Possible involvement of the OKT4 molecule in T cell recognition of class II HLA antigens. Evidence from studies of cytotoxic T lymphocytes specific for SB antigens. J. Exp. Med. 156:1065-1076 (1982).

23. Meuer, S.C., Schlossman, S.F. and Reinherz, E.L. Clonal analysis of human cytotoxic T lymphocytes: T4+ and T8+ effector T cells recognize products of different major histocompatibility complex regions. Proc. Natl. Acad. Sci. USA 79:4395-4399 (1982).

24. Martz, E. Mechanism of specifric tumor cell lysis by alloimmune T lymphocytes: Resolution and characterization of discrete steps in the cellular interaction. Contemp. Top. Immunobiol. 7:301-361 (1977).

25. Tsoukas, C.D., Carson, D.A., Fong, S. and Vaughan, J.H. Molecular interactions in human T cell-mediated cytotoxicity to EBV. II. Monoclonal antibody OKT3 inhibits a post killer-target recognition/adhesion step. J. Immunol. 129:1421-1425 (1982).

26. Landegren, U., Ramstedt, U., Axberg, I., Ullberg, M., Jondal, M. and Wigzell, H. Selective inhibition of human T cell cytotoxicity at levels of target recognition of initiation of lysis by monoclonal OKT3 and Leu 2a antibodies. J. Exp. Med. 155:1579-1584 (1982).

27. Forman, J. and Moller, G. Generation of cytotoxic lymphocytes in mixed lymphocyte reactions. J. Exp. Med. 138:672-685 (1973).

28. Asherson, G.L., Ferluga, J. and Janossy, G. Non-specific cytotoxicity by T cells activated with plant mitogens in vitro and the requirement for plant agents during the killing reaction. Clin. Exp. Immunol. 15:573-589 (1973).

29. Golstein, P. and Smith, E.T. Mechanism of T cell-mediated cytolysis: the lethal hit stage. Contemp. Top. Immunobiol. 7:273-300 (1977).

30. Green, W.R., Ballas, Z.K. and Henney, C.S. Studies on the mechanism of lymphocyte-mediated cytolysis. XI. The role of lectin in lectin-dependent cell-mediated cytotoxicity. J. Immunol. 121:1566-1572 (1978).

31. Parker, W.L. and Martz, E. Lectin-induced non-lethal adhesions between cytolytic T lymphocytes and antigenically unrecognizable tumor cells and nonspecific 'triggering' of cytolysis. J. Immunol. 124:25-35 (1980).

32. Van Wauwe, J. and Goossens, J. Mitogenic actions of orthoclone OKT3 on human peripheral blood lymphocytes: effects of monocytes and serum components. Int. J. Immunopharmacol. 3:203-208 (1981).

33. Leonard, W.J., Depper, J.M., Uchiyama, T., Smith, K.A., Waldmann, T.A. and Greene, W.C. A monoclonal antibody that appears to recognize the receptor for human T cell growth factor; partial characterization of the receptor. Nature 300:267-269 (1982).

34. Meuer, S.C., Hussey, R.E., Cantrell, D.A., Hodgdon, J.C., Schlossman, S.F., Smith, K.A. and Reinherz, E.L. Triggering of the T3-Ti antigen-recptor complex results in clonal T cell proliferation through an interleukin 2-dependent autocrine pathway. Proc. Natl. Acad. Sci. USA 81:1509-1513 (1984).

35. Von Wussow, P., Platsoukas, C.D., Wiranowska-Stewart, M. and Stewart, W.E. Human gamma interferon production by leukocytes induced with monoclonal antibodies recognizing T cells. J. Immunol. 127:1197-1200 (1981).

382

36. Chang, T.W., Testa, D., Kung, P.C., Perry, L., Dreskin, H.J. and Goldstein, G. Cellular origin and interactions involved in gamma-interferon production induced by OKT3 monoclonal antibody. J. Immunol. 128:585-589 (1982).

37. Welte, K., Platzer, E., Wang, C.Y., Kan, E.A.R., Moore, M.A.S. and Mertelsmann, R. OKT8 antibody inhibits OKT3-induced IL2 production and proliferation in OKT8+ cells. J. Immunol. 131:2356-2361 (1983).

38. Tsoukas, C.D. and Martz, E. Simultaneous suppression of allogeneic cytolytic activity and stimulation of lectin-dependent cytolytic activity by Con A. Cell. Immunol. 40:103-116 (1978).

39. Zanders, E.D., Lamb, J.R., Feldmann, M., Green, N. and Beverley, P.C.L. Tolerance of T cell clones is associated with membrane antigen changes. Nature 303:625-627 (1983).

DISCUSSION

P. Golstein: This is an important experiment because, as was stressed before, anti-T3 would be the only monclonal antibody to inhibit past lethal hit. All this rests on the demonstration that this antibody does not inhibit conjugate formation, or does not reverse preformed conjugates. It may be relevant to tell a story about our anti-Lyt-2 antibody 27-9. This was very surprising to us: it was an anti-Lyt-2 antibody which did not inhibit conjugate formation, contrary to other anti-Lyt-2 antibodies which we had also. Then we came across an observation by Nurit Hollander: provided you do your experiments at 37° rather than at 20°, then you can demonstrate inhibition of conjugate formation by some antibodies. And indeed, 27-9, which did not inhibit conjugate formation at 20°, inhibited conjugate formation at 37°. But it still did not reverse preformed conjugates, even at 37°. Then we applied to these conjugates together with antibodies shearing forces of increasing strength. Finally the conjugates were dissociated, compared to those without antibodies. So for this antibody we could finally show that we have indeed affected conjugate formation -- I'm not saying that it affected recognition -- but we certainly could affect conjugate formation by using some tricks.

C. Tsoukas: After allowing these conjugates to form at 20°, and then allowing the antibody to bind at 4°, I applied rather harsh conditions to disperse in dextran-containing medium. So I think what I am measuring here is rather the strong conjugates. There might be some weak conjugates that break up in dextran when I vortex So there might be a subpopulation of weak conjugates, which are never detected in the assay, and which might be inhibited by this antibody.

T. Springer: OK, one last question.

B. Bonavida: Two questions (laughter) . . . two small questions. Number one: have you tried to pretreat the target cells with Con A prior to using them for your experiments with the antibody? Number two: have you looked at whether the antibody binds to the Con A-treated cells, or do you really inhibit the binding of antibody under those conditions?

C. Tsoukas: Two short answers: no, and no.

M. Mescher: We were interested in looking at the role of Lyt-2 and of alloantigen in maintaining conjugates once they were formed. The question was whether interaction with those molecules is important in maintaining adhesion, or whether adhesion might be a seconday event subsequent to triggering by interactions of those molecules. So we essentially set up conditions for a post-dispersion lysis kind of assay like Eric [Martz] worked out and then Constantine [Tsoukas] described. What we found was that using allogeneic CTL populations we could preform conjugates with targets and very easily demonstrate that those conjugates were reversable by anti-Lyt-2 and by some anti-H-2 antibodies against the target cell H-2 antigens. To confirm that, we looked at visual counts of conjugates. So I think that provides some evidence that both the Lyt-2 and the H-2 are involved not only in forming conjugates, but in the continued maintenance of the conjugates until the lethal hit occurred.

Also, we looked at a variety of different kinds of target cells. In that assay, you can get some sense of avidity of killer-target interaction by the spontaneous rate at which conjugates fall apart. Like Rob [MacDonald] and Eric [Martz] had described, there was an apparent inverse correlation between the avidity of the killer-target interaction, and the degree to which conjugates could be reversed by anti-Lyt-2 antibodies against the killer cell.

THE PLASMA MEMBRANE 'SKELETON' OF TUMOR AND LYMPHOID CELLS:

A ROLE IN CELL LYSIS?

Matthew F. Mescher and John R. Apgar

Department of Pathology
Harvard Medical School
25 Shattuck Street, Boston, Massachusetts 02115

INTRODUCTION

A detailed understanding of the structure and dynamics of
the surface membrane of cells is crucial to study of the mechanisms
of cell mediated cytotoxicity. The dynamics of the membrane
receptors, target cell antigens and accessory proteins almost
certainly affect the efficiency of establishing and maintaining
cell-cell contact and delivery of the transmembrane signal
resulting in triggering of the lytic mechanisms. Furthermore,
whether the primary event involved in target cell lysis is
formation of membrane lesions (pore formation) or transfer of a
lytic component (enzyme?) from the effector cell to the target,
the molecular requirements for these events will certainly depend
upon the structure and dynamics of the target cell plasma
membrane.

The plasma membrane is composed of the lipid bilayer, integral
membrane proteins and peripheral proteins associated with, but
not imbedded in the bilayer(1,2). The fluid mosaic model of
membrane structure, proposed by Singer and Nicolson in 1972 (1)
has provided the conceptual framework for current thinking about
the structure and dynamics of membrane proteins. In this model,
the membrane is viewed as a two-dimensional solution of oriented
proteins and lipids with the lipids forming the matrix of the
mosaic. With the exception of special cases of differentiated
structures, such as synapses, it was proposed that long-range
ordering of the proteins does not occur. Instead, the proteins
are viewed as dissolved, and free to diffuse, in the fluid lipid
bilayer. As information regarding the diffusion of cell surface
proteins and their redistribution upon crosslinking (capping) has

accumulated, the possibilities of interactions of membrane proteins with cytoskeletal components have become apparent, although the molecular basis of such interactions remains undetermined in most cases. Such peripheral interactions between transmembrane proteins and cytoskeletal elements do not alter the basic tenets of the fluid mosaic model of membrane structure.

The membrane of the erythrocyte is by far the most extensively studied eukaryotic plasma membrane. Associated with the cytoplasmic face of this membrane is a set of peripheral proteins including spectrin, actin, ankyrin and band 4.1 which interact to form a membrane skeleton (3,4). This skeleton provides mechanical stability to the membrane (5) and appears to influence cell surface protein mobility and lipid distribution in the bilayer (6,7). The spectrin-containing matrix can be readily isolated, since Triton extraction of the membranes solubilizes the lipid bilayer and most of the membrane proteins while leaving the skeleton, and associated proteins, insoluble.

Unlike red cells, nucleated cells have filamentous cytoskel-etal systems. It has been unclear, however, whether the plasma membranes of such cells have associated with them a membrane skel-eton distinct from the filamentous cytoskeletal systems. We had previously shown that a Triton X-100 insoluble protein matrix could be isolated from plasma membranes purified from murine lymphoid and tumor cells (8). The composition and properties of this matrix suggested that it might form a membrane skeleton similar in some respects to that of the red cell membrane skeleton. More recent work has provided morphological and biochemical evidence which strongly supports this suggestion (9,10). The membrane skeleton of lymphoid cells is clearly distinct from previously described cytoskeletal structures and differs from the red cell skeleton with respect to both the components of the skeleton and their interaction with the membrane bilayer and other membrane proteins. These findings are summarized below, followed by a discussion of the possible roles that this membrane skeleton structure might play in mechanisms of cell lysis.

THE PLASMA MEMBRANE MATRIX

Highly purified plasma membranes can be isolated from murine tumor and lymphoid cells by nitrogen cavitation to lyse the cells, followed by differential centrifugation and density gradient centrifugation to separate the subcellular components (11). The plasma membrane accounts for about 1.5% to 3% of the total protein of such cells and yields of 20 to 40% are obtained upon purification (11,12). The isolated membranes are predominantly in the form of closed vesicles ranging in size from about 0.1 to 1.2 um in diameter.

PLASMA MEMBRANES

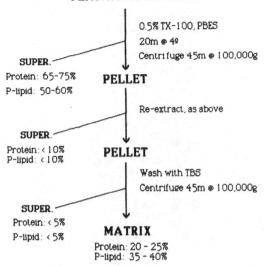

Fig. 1.   Isolation of the P815 membrane matrix by Triton X-100
extraction of purified plasma membranes. The protein and
phospholipid (P-lipid) recovered in the fractions is
expressed as percent of starting membrane material.
Values shown are ranges obtained for numerous preparations.

Treatment of plasma membranes with TX-100 using a detergent
to protein ratio of 5 to 1 or higher, followed by centrifugation
to pellet the insoluble material, results in solubilization of 75
to 80% of the total membrane protein and 60 to 65% of the membrane
phospholipid (Figure 1). The insoluble fraction does not result
simply from incomplete extraction, as retreatment of the pellet
with TX-100 or use of much higher detergent to protein ratios
does not result in significant further solubilization.

Examination of the polypeptide composition of the membranes
and TX-100 soluble and insoluble fractions by SDS-polyacrylamide
gel electrophoresis shows that the insoluble material consists of

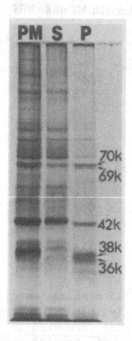

Fig. 2. Protein composition of P815 plasma membrane (PM), Triton
         soluble (S), and Triton insoluble matrix (P) fractions.
         Triton extraction was done as shown in Figure 1, the
         fractions electrophoresed on an SDS-polyacrylamide gel
         and protein visualized by staining with Coomassie blue.
         Samples contained 100 ug (PM), 75 ug (S) and 25 ug (P)
         protein. The molecular weights of the major membrane
         matrix components are indicated.

a discrete subset of the membrane polypeptides (Figure 2). The
major polypeptides of this fraction have molecular weights of 70k,
69k, 42k, 38k and 36k. 5'Nucleotidase, a glycosylated cell surface
enzyme, also remains associated with the insoluble membrane fraction.
The enzyme is present in low amounts and is not detected as a major
band on SDS gels. The physiological role of this enzyme is unclear,
but it has provided a convenient enzyme marker for the insoluble
fraction.

5'-Nucleotidase and the 70k, 69k, 38k and 36k proteins are
recovered almost exclusively in the insoluble fraction, while
proteins of about 42k are found in both the soluble and insoluble
fractions. Actin has previously been shown to be a component of
the plasma membrane of lymphoid cells (13) and limited-proteolysis
peptide mapping on SDS gels showed that the 42k protein in both

fractions is actin (8). Retreatment of the insoluble fraction with additional detergent does not result in further actin solubilization indicating that plasma membrane-associated actin is present in two different forms, based on its solubility properties. A small but reproducible difference in mobility on SDS gels is seen for the two forms of actin (Figure 2), suggesting that there might be a structural difference between the two forms (possibly post-translational modification).

Much of the work to characterize the TX-100 insoluble fraction has been done using plasma membranes isolated from P815 mastocytoma cells. Essentially identical findings were obtained when membranes from normal murine lymphocytes, lymphoid tumor cells and bovine lymphocytes were examined (8,10, and unpublished results). Davies et al. (14) have recently reported similar findings upon examination of membranes from human lymphoblastoid cells and pig lymphocytes. They showed the detergent insoluble fraction of these membranes to consist of 5'-nucleotidase and polypeptides with apparent molecular weights of 68k, 45k, 33k and 28k. In addition, there were prominent components of 200k in the pig and 120k in the human lymphocytes. Thus, these results are very similar to our findings with P815 and murine lymphoid cells, with the exception that we have not observed major components with molecular weights greater than 70k. It appears that a detergent-insoluble fraction consisting of a discrete set of proteins, including actin, is a feature common to most if not all lymphoid cells.

We have recently found that the TX-100 insoluble fraction includes major polypeptide components which are not detected by SDS-gel electrophoresis despite the fact that they have relatively low molecular weights. Occurence of additional components was realized when it was found that EGTA treatment of the insoluble fraction resulted in release of all of the 70k, 69k, 38k and 36k proteins while solubilizing only about 15% of the total protein in the fraction (C. Ming Show, Senior Thesis, Harvard College (1982)). SDS-gel electrophoresis of the EGTA insoluble material showed only actin, but comparison to known amounts of actin standards run on the same gels indicated that the actin could account for only about 5% of the protein in this fraction. Using Sepharose CL-4B and size exclusion chromatography by HPLC in the presence of SDS we have found that the EGTA insoluble material consists largely of two polypeptides of about 20k and 40k molecular weights (15, and Apgar and Mescher, manuscript in preparation). Preliminary evidence indicates that the 20k protein can aggregate even in the presence of SDS and 2-mercaptoethanol, and that the 40k protein may be a dimeric form of 20k. The aggregation properties of these proteins may account for their failure to enter SDS gels, despite their low molecular weight. This novel membrane protein(s) accounts for about 15% of the total plasma membrane protein and about 75 to 80% of the TX-100 insoluble fraction.

Table 1. Phospholipid (P-lipid) Composition of Plasma Membranes and the TX-100 Insoluble Membrane Matrix

P-lipid	Membrane (% of total P-lipid)	Matrix (% of membrane P-lipid recovered with matrix)
PE	30 + 5	14%
PC	30 + 5	33%
SM	17 + 1	89%
PS	17 + 2	13%
X1	3 + 2	100%
X2	1 + 1	40%
X3	0.6	100%

Values shown are the averages of four separate determinations done on three separate membrane and matrix preparations.

Abbreviations are: PE, phosphatidylethanolamine; PC, phosphatidylcholine; SM, sphingomyelin; PS, phosphatidylserine. X1-X3 are minor, unidentified phospholipids.

Some of the plasma membrane phospholipid also remains associated with the detergent insoluble fraction (Figure 1, ref. 10). As in the case of the proteins, the associated phospholipids represent a subset of the total membrane lipid. Most of the phosphatidylethanolamine and phosphatidylserine are extracted by TX-100, while almost all of the sphingomyelin and about one-third of the phosphatidylcholine remain in the insoluble fraction (along with some minor unidentified lipids) (Table 1). Re-extraction of the insoluble material with additional TX-100, even at very high detergent to protein ratios, does not remove this bound lipid. Davies et al. (14) have similarily found that sphingomyelin remains selectively associated with the detergent insoluble fraction of membranes from human and pig lymphoid cells.

Occurence of a discrete set of membrane proteins and phospholipids in the detergent insoluble fraction suggested that this material might represent a protein matrix persisting as intact structures following removal of most of the membrane lipid and protein, as opposed to simply being insoluble protein and/or lipid aggregates. Sucrose density gradient centrifugation of the insoluble fraction demonstrated that all of the components comigrated on the gradient, thus providing support for this suggestion (8,10). When the detergent insoluble material was examined by thin-section electron microscopy, it was found to

consist of discrete structures, with much of the material having
the appearance of closed structures of about the same size
distribution as the plasma membrane vesicles it derived from (8).
Little or no lipid bilayer was evident in these structures. Thus,
the evidence very strongly suggests that a discrete set of the
plasma membrane proteins and lipids interact to form an extended
matrix which persists as an intact macrostructure following removal
of the lipid bilayer and most of the membrane proteins.

The EGTA soluble proteins (70k, 69k, 38k and 36k) and actin
are localized to the cytoplasmic face of the membrane, as demonstrated by vectorial labeling by lactoperoxidase-catalyzed
iodination (8). The properties of the EGTA soluble proteins
indicate that they are peripheral membrane proteins (15). The
relative amounts of the various proteins present, and the persistence of insoluble structures following EGTA treatment to remove
the 70k, 69k, 38k and 36k proteins strongly suggest that the novel
20k and 40k proteins are the structural components responsible for
stability of the extended matrix structure.

THE MATRIX AS A MEMBRANE SKELETON

While the properties of the detergent insoluble matrix of the
plasma membrane suggested that it might serve as a membrane skeleton,
study of purified membranes could not rule out the possibility that
the matrix was localized to only some regions of the cell surface
membrane. Yields obtained upon purification of plasma membranes
from lymphoid cells are 20 to 40%, thus raising the possibility
that the isolated membrane and associated matrix represented a
specialized fraction of the surface membrane. We therefore examined
detergent extraction of whole P815 cells.

Treatment of intact P815 cells with 0.5% TX-100 under the same
conditions used for isolation of the matrix from purified membranes
resulted in 90 to 100% recovery of structures having a relatively
intact nucleus, an empty cytoplasmic space and a continuous layer
of material at the periphery (9). Using light microscopy with
phase contrast optics, these 'Triton shells' had the appearance of
a nucleus contained within an otherwise empty bag. Large amounts
of amorphous appearing material were associated with the peripheral
layer of the shells. When nucleases (RNAase and DNAase) were
included during Triton extraction of the shells much cleaner
preparations were obtained. The peripheral layer of these shells
was difficult to see using phase contrast microscopy but was readily
apparent when the preparations were examined using Nomarski optics
and a video enhancement system (Figure 3). Treatment of isolated
nuclei with TX-100 under the same conditions did not result in
structures having the same appearance as the Triton shells. The
nuclear remnant remained but no peripheral, bag-like structure

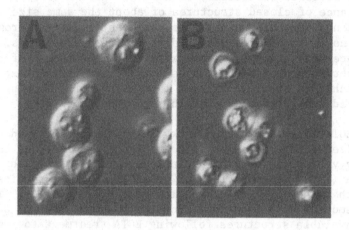

Fig. 3. Photomicrographs of P815 cells (left panel) and Triton shells (right panel). Triton shells were prepared by extracting P815 cells with 0.5% TX-100 in PBES for 20 m at 4^0. Samples were then diluted with extraction buffer, fixed in 1% gluteraldehyde for 20 m at 4^0 and examined using Nomarski optics with a Zeiss UEM. Videomicrographs were stored on videotape with a contrast enhancement camera (Dage-MTI) and subsequently photographed from the monitor.

was seen. Thus, the peripheral TX-100 insoluble structure of the Triton shells does not derive from the nucleus.

Examination of the Triton shells by thin-section electron microscopy confirmed the observations made at the light level and showed little or no lipid bilayer structure remaining associated with the peripheral layer (9). In all cases the nuclear remnant was seen to be surrounded by a continuous peripheral layer. The stability of this peripheral layer of the shells was dependent on protein, as demonstrated by disappearance of this layer upon protease treatment of the shells. P815 cells have little organized filamentous cytoskeletal structure and such structures were not seen in the cytoplasmic space of the Triton shells. Further evidence that the peripheral layer was independent of the filamentous cytoskeleton was provided by the demonstration that pretreatment of the cells with cytochalasin, colchicine or both, followed by TX-100 extraction yielded Triton shells having the same appearance as those prepared in the absence of the cytoskeleton perturbants.

These observations strongly suggested that the plasma membrane matrix was continuous over the cell periphery and persisted as an intact macrostructure following TX-100 extraction of the cells. Biochemical characterization of the Triton shells provided further support for this conclusion (10). The Triton extraction used to prepare shells is the same as that routinely used to solubilize cell surface transmembrane proteins (e.g. H-2 antigens and surface Ig) and was shown to result in solubilization of 85% or more of the cell surface proteins labeled by lactoperoxidase-catalyzed iodination. At the same time, 5'-nucleotidase, the cell surface glycoprotein which remains associated with the membrane matrix, was quantitatively recovered in the Triton shells. Comparison of the Triton shells and isolated plasma membranes by SDS-gel electrophoresis revealed the presence in the shells of proteins having the same mobilities as those of the membrane matrix. Additional proteins are present in the shell, most of them appearing to be of nuclear origin. The relative staining intensities of the 70k, 69k, 42, 38k, and 36k bands in shell and membrane samples derived from the same number of starting cells indicated that the membrane matrix was quantitatively recovered with the shells. This was true for the actin (42k) band, as well as the others, further indicating that the peripheral layer of the shells is independent of the filamentous cytoskeletal system.

Thus, the evidence obtained so far clearly demonstrates that there is a protein matrix associated with isolated plasma membranes and very strongly suggests that this matrix forms a membrane skeleton which is continuous at the cell periphery and independent of either the filamentous cytoskeletal system, the lipid bilayer or most of the membrane proteins for its persistence as a stable macrostructure. While we have not yet directly demonstrated the identity of the matrix and the peripheral layer seen in Triton shells, alternatives to this appear very unlikely. The biochemical evidence clearly shows the matrix components to be present in the shells, so an alternative interpretation would have to suggest that the matrix is not seen by microscopy and furthermore that there is another, previously undescribed, Triton insoluble structure which is continuous at the cell periphery but which is not isolated along with the plasma membrane. Antibodies specific for the isolated matrix components are being prepared and should provide the means for directly demonstrating the identity of the peripheral layer and the matrix.

DISCUSSION

The studies described above have provided very strong evidence for the presence of an extended protein matrix intimately associated with the plasma membranes of murine tumor and murine and bovine lymphoid cells (8-10,15). A very similar matrix appears to be present in association with pig lymphocytes and human lymphoblastoid cells (14). Thus, it appears likely that a protein matrix structure will be a feature common to the plasma membrane of all lymphoid cells. A similar structure may also occur in other nucleated cells. Some studies of cytoskeleton preparations from adherent cells (such as fibroblasts) have noted that the filamentous cytoskeleton is covered by a lamina which appears to derive from the plasma membrane and includes some cell surface proteins (16-19). Furthermore, Owens et al. (20) have recently shown that an antibody specific for the 68k matrix protein from pig lymphocyte membranes crossreacts with a component of a lamina-like network of detergent extracted fibroblasts.

While the membrane matrix of lymphoid cells bears some similarities to the Triton insoluble spectrin matrix of erythrocyte membranes, it clearly differs in many respects. Proteins cross-reactive with antibodies to the red cell skeleton components have been shown to occur in many cell types (21-23) but such proteins do not appear to be components of the lymphocyte membrane matrix. We have found that P815 cells possess proteins cross-reactive with antibodies made against spectrin, ankyrin and band 4.1 but none of these copurify with the plasma membrane (unpublished results). Furthermore, the size and properties of the lymphocyte matrix proteins clearly differ from those related to the red cell skeleton components. It also appears likely that the nature of the association of the matrix skeleton with the membrane bilayer differs between red cells and lymphoid cells. The structural components of the red cell skeleton include spectrin, actin and associated proteins, all of which are peripheral proteins and interact with the membrane via ankyrin attachment to band 3, a transmembrane protein (3,4). In contrast, the structural components of the P815 membrane matrix, the 20k and 40k proteins, have properties consistent with their being integral membrane proteins (15 and unpublished results). If confirmed, this would indicate that the membrane skeleton of these cells is truly a component of the membrane structure rather than a peripherally associated structure as is the red cell skeleton.

The nature of the tumor and lymphoid cell plasma membrane skeleton, and analogy to the red cell skeleton, suggest a number of possibilities for its role(s) in cellular function. It would appear likely that this extended network of interacting protein provides the membrane with greater mechanical stability than could be obtained with the lipid bilayer and integral membrane proteins. The matrix may also influence the properties of the lipid bilayer, if the strong association between the matrix and sphingomyelin (which accounts for 17% of the membrane phospholipid) reflects the situation in the native membrane. There is evidence for a role of the spectrin matrix of red cells in maintaining the lipid assymetry in these membranes (7).

The location and nature of the matrix would also suggest it as a candidate for mediating interactions between cell surface proteins and the filamentous cytoskeleton, interactions which might affect the mobility and redistribution of the surface proteins as well as the shape and motility of the cell and processes of endo- and exocytosis. Clearly interactions of this type may have important effects on cell-cell interaction and transmembrane signalling leading to cell mediated lysis of a target. Recent studies of cytolytic T lymphocyte (CTL)-mediated lysis have presented an increasingly complex picture of these events. Formation of the functional CTL-target cell conjugate appears to require not only the antigen specific receptor on the CTL and the antigen on the target but also a number of accessory molecules on the CTL and possibly on the target surface. Cell shape changes resulting in extensive interdigitation of the opposing membranes have also been noted and there is now considerable evidence to indicate that release of granule-encapsulated material by the CTL is involved in lysis of the target. These aspects of CTL-target interaction are discussed in detail elsewhere in this volume. Thus, a complex series of events must occur prior to actual lysis of the target cell, all of them involving components of the plasma membrane and their interactions with the machinery inside the CTL.

Consideration of the membrane skeleton is also likely to be relevant to attempts to understand the mechanisms of lysis of the target cell. The occurence of long range protein interactions to provide a mechanically stable structure presents a very different picture of the membrane than that of a lipid bilayer matrix with proteins simply dissolved in it. Complement mediated lysis of liposome and erythrocyte membranes is a 'one hit' process while complement lysis of nucleated cells displays multi-hit characteristics (24). A variety of repair mechanisms have been suggested to account for this greater resistance, and some evidence for such mechanisms has been obtained (25). The membrane skeleton may, however, contribute to the greater resistance and might allow for repair mechanisms to operate before irreversible membrane damage has occured.

Liposomes, lacking a membrane skeleton, and red cells, having a very different kind of membrane skeleton, may provide a poor model for understanding the action of complement on the membrane of nucleated cells. We have found that matrix-containing liposomes can be formed by isolating the matrix from P815 membranes, mixing it with lipids in the presence of deoxycholate and dialyzing to remove the detergent (26,27). The lipid preferentially associates with the matrix to form a bilayer, and transmembrane proteins such as H-2 antigen can be incorporated into the liposome if they are added to the initial mixture prior to dialysis. Comparison of complement-mediated lysis of such liposomes to that of liposomes prepared using the same lipids and transmembrane proteins but lacking the matrix, may provide a means of assessing a possible role of the membrane skeleton in conferring resistance to the nucleated cell membrane.

As discussed elsewhere in this volume, cell-mediated lysis may involve transfer of granular contents from the effector to the target cell resulting in the formation of pores in the target cell membrane, similar in some respects to the pore structures resulting from complement attack. Whether formation of such pores accounts for the ultimate lysis of the target cell is unclear. Alternatively, the pores might provide sites for insertion of other effector cell components (enzymes?) into the target cells and the action of these components result in the damage leading to lysis. Some support for this possibility is provided by the observations that the morphological changes occuring in the target cell during cell-mediated lysis are very different from those seen during complement mediated lysis (28) and that destabilization of the nucleus can be detected prior to any indication of osmotic damage to the targat (discussed elsewhere in this volume). If lysis does involve insertion of a lytic component into the cell then a possible site of action is the membrane skeleton, with the component acting to destabilize the matrix interactions required for stability of the skeletal structure. In this regard, preliminary results (unpublished) indicate that the major structural proteins of the matrix (the 20k and 40k proteins) can exist in phosphorylated forms. If phosphorylation of these proteins plays a role in determining their interactions (for which there is as yet no evidence) then delivery by the effector cell of an enzyme(s) which altered phosphorylation levels and destabilized the skeleton could be a primary or contributory mechanism leading to target cell lysis.

While discussion of the possible roles of the plasma membrane skeleton in cell-mediated lysis must clearly be speculative at this time, such speculation appears warranted. The plasma membranes of both the effector and target cells are intimately involved in all stages of the lytic process and the skeleton constitutes a major component of this membrane, likely to have a variety of effects on the structural stability of the membrane and the dynamics of its other components.

ACKNOWLEDGEMENTS

This work was supported by NIH Grant CA-30381. John R. Apgar was supported by a Postdoctoral Fellowship from the Leukemia Society of America, Inc.

REFERENCES

1. S.J. Singer and G.L. Nicolson, The fluid mosaic model of the
    structure of cell membranes, Science. 175:720 (1972).
2. M.S. Bretscher and M.C. Raff, Mammalian plasma membranes,
    Nature. 258:43 (1975).
3. S.E. Lux, Dissecting the red cell membrane skeleton, Nature.
    281:426 (1979).
4. D. Branton, C.M. Cohen and J. Tyler, Interaction of cyto-
    skeletal proteins on the human erythrocyte membrane, Cell.
    24:24 (1981).
5. Y. Lange, R.A. Hadesman and T.L. Steck, Role of the reticulum
    in the stability and shape of the isolated human erythrocyte
    membrane, J. Cell Biol. 92:714 (1982).
6. D. Shotton, B. Burke and D. Branton, Molecular structure of
    spectrin, J. Mol. Biol. 131:303 (1979).
7. P. Williamson, J. Bateman, K. Kozarsky, K. Mattocks,
    N. Hermanowicz, H.R. Choe and R.A. Shlegel, Involvement of
    spectrin in the maintenance of phase-state asymmetry in the
    erythrocyte membrane, Cell. 30:725 (1982).
8. M.F. Mescher, M.J.L. Jose and S.P. Balk, Actin-containing
    matrix associated with the plasma membrane of murine tumor
    and lymphoid cells, Nature. 289:139 (1981).
9. S.H. Herrmann, J.R. Apgar, J.M. Robinson and M.F. Mescher,
    Plasma membrane skeleton of murine tumor cells. I. Prepara-
    tion and morphology of Triton shells, submitted for publication.
10. M.F. Mescher, J.R. Apgar and J.M. Robinson, Plasma membrane
    skeleton of murine tumor cells. II. Composition of isolated
    membrane skeleton and Triton shells, submitted for publication.
11. F. Lemonnier, M. Mescher, L. Sherman and S. Burakoff, The
    induction of cytolytic T lymphocytes with purified plasma
    membranes, J. Immunol. 120:1114 (1978).
12. M.J. Crumpton and D. Snary, Preparation and properties of
    lymphocyte plasma membrane, Contemp. Top. Mol. Immunol.
    3:27 (1974).
13. B.H. Barber and M.J. Crumpton, Actin associated with purified
    lymphocyte plasma membrane, FEBS Letters. 66:215 (1976).
14. A.A. Davies, N.M. Wigglesworth, D. Allan, R.J. Owens and
    M.J. Crumpton, Nonidet P-40 extraction of lymphocyte plasma
    membrane, Biochem. J. 219:301 (1984).
15. J.R. Apgar and M.F. Mescher, Plasma membrane matrix of murine
    tumor cells, Fed. Proc. 43:2016 (1984).
16. A. Ben-Ze'ev, A. Duerr, F. Solomon and S. Penman, The outer
    boundry of the cytoskeleton: A lamina derived from plasma
    membrane proteins, Cell. 17:859 (1979).
17. A.B. Fulton, J. Prives, S.R. Farmer and S. Penman, Develop-
    mental reorganization of the skeletal framework and its
    surface lamina in fusing muscle cells, J. Cell. Biol. 91:103
    (1981).
18. C.H. Streuli, B. Patel and D.R. Critchley, The cholera toxin

receptor ganglioside GM 1 remains associated with Triton X-100 cytoskeletons of BALB/c-3T3 cells, Exp. Cell. Res. 136:247 (1981).

19. V-P. Lehto, T. Vartio, R.A. Badley and I. Virtanen, Characterization of detergent-resistant surface lamina in cultured human fibroblasts. Exp. Cell Res. 143:287 (1983).

20. R.J. Owens, C.J. Gallagher and M.J. Crumpton, Cellular distribution of P68, a new calcium-binding protein from lymphocytes. EMBO J. 3:in press.

21. V. Bennett, Immunoreactive forms of human erythrocyte ankyrin are present in diverse cells and tissues, Nature. 281:597 (1979).

22. B. Geiger, Proteins related to the red cell cytoskeleton in non-erythroid cells, Trends Biochem. Sci. 7:388 (1982).

23. E. Lazarides and W.J. Nelson, Expression of spectrin in nonerythroid cells, Cell. 31:505 (1982).

24. C.L. Koski, L.E. Ramm, C.H. Hammer, M.M. Mayer and M.L. Shin, Cytolysis of nucleated cells by complement: Cell death displays multi-hit characteristics, Proc. Natl. Acad. Sci. USA. 80:3816 (1983).

25. S.H. Ohanian and S.I. Schlager, Humoral immune killing of nucleated cells: Mechanisms of complement-mediated attack and target cell defense, CRC Crit. Rev. Immunol. 1:165 (1981).

26. S.H. Herrmann and M.F. Mescher, Secondary cytolytic T lymphocyte stimulation by purified H-2K^k in liposomes, Proc. Natl. Acad. Sci. USA. 78:2488 (1981).

27. S.H. Herrmann and M.F. Mescher, Lymphocyte recognition of H-2 antigen in liposomes, J. Supramol. Struct. and Cell. Biochem. 16:121 (1981).

28. C.J. Sanderson, Morphological aspects of lymphocyte mediated cytotoxicity, in: "Mechanisms of Cell Mediated Cytotoxicity," W.R. Clark and P. Golstein, eds., Plenum Press, New York (1982).

p215 AND p24: TWO MEMBRANE-ASSOCIATED PROTEINS EXPRESSED ON CLONED

CYTOLYTIC T-CELLS BUT NOT ON CLONED HELPER T-CELLS

Maurice K. Gately[1], Michael D. Dick, Tomiya Masuno,
Richard M. McCarron, and Beatrice Macchi

Surgical Neurology Branch, National Institute of
Neurological and Communicative Disorders and Stroke,
National Institutes of Health, Bethesda, Maryland 20205

INTRODUCTION

It has been shown that the mechanism by which cytolytic T lymphocytes (CTL)[2] lyse target cells can be divided into three successive steps (reviewed in 1): (i) binding of CTL to target cells
(adhesion formation), (ii) the action of CTL upon target cells to
cause the targets to become irreversibly committed to lyse (programming for lysis, also called the lethal hit), and (iii) actual
target cell lysis which occurs independent of continued contact
between target cells and CTL. However, the molecular mechanisms by
which these processes occur are poorly understood. Studies with
monoclonal antibodies which can inhibit lysis in the absence of
complement have permitted identification of several molecules which
appear to play a role in the cytolytic mechanism (reviewed in 2-6).
These include Lyt 2 and its human homologues (2-5), LFA-1 (2-5), T3
(7, 8), and clonotypic molecules which likely represent the T cell

---

[1]Present address: Department of Immunopharmacology, Hoffmann-La
Roche, Inc. Nutley, N.J. 07110

[2]Abbreviations used: CTL, cytolytic T lymphocytes; CHAPS, 3-[(3-
cholamidopropyl)dimethylammonio]-1-propanesulfate; Con A, concanavalin A; IL-2, interleukin 2; MLC, mixed leukocyte culture; NK,
natural killer; PMA, phorbol myristic acetate; SaCI, Staphylococcus
aureus Cowan strain I; SDS-PAGE, polyacrylamide gel electrophoresis
run in 0.1% sodium dodecyl sulfate; T_C, cytolytic T cells; T_H,
helper T cells; TCA, trichloroacetic acid.

receptor (9, 10). Lyt 2 and LFA-1 appear to play a role in the binding of CTL to target cells (3, 5) whereas T3 may serve as a triggering link between the antigen-specific receptor and the lethal hit (6). No molecules have yet been identified which have been shown unambiguously to be involved in the actual delivery of the lethal hit.

The recent demonstration by Harris et al. (11) that liposomes containing membrane components from CTL clones could be used to transfer lytic activity to noncytolytic T and B cell lines suggests that the molecule(s) that mediates specific cytolytic activity resides in or is associated with the cell membranes of CTL. It was, therefore, of interest to compare the membrane-associated proteins of cytolytic and noncytolytic T lymphocytes to determine whether any proteins could be identified which are unique to CTL and thus might play a role in the lytic function of these cells. When we compared the ^{35}S-labeled proteins in membrane fractions from cloned lines of alloreactive murine cytolytic (T_C) and helper (T_H) T lymphocytes, two proteins were found which were associated with each of three T_C lines examined but none of four T_H lines. One of these, p215, was a variant of T200 of higher molecular weight than T200 on T_H. The other, p24, appeared to be a previously unidentified protein unique to T_C.

MATERIALS AND METHODS

Generation and maintenance of cloned T cell lines.

Cloned T cell lines were derived by limiting dilution cloning of in vitro sensitized cells as described by Glasebrook and Fitch (12) with minor modifications (13). Primary clonings were performed at a multiplicity of 1 cell per well, and cloned lines were subcloned at a multiplicity of 0.25 cells per well. Established lines were passed in the presence of irradiated DBA/2 splenocytes as feeder cells and lectin-depleted supernatant from cultures of Con A-activated rat splenocytes as a source of interleukin 2 (IL 2) (13).

Characterization of cloned T cell lines

The cytolytic activity of cloned T cells was measured in 4 hr ^{51}Cr release assays as previously described (13). Percent specific ^{51}Cr release was calculated as $(e - c)/(100-c)$ where e represents the percentage of ^{51}Cr released in cultures containing both effector and target cells and c the percentage of ^{51}Cr released in control cultures containing target cells alone.

Cloned T cells were induced to secrete IL 2 by incubation with Con A in the absence of feeder cells as previously described (13). Culture supernatants were assayed for IL 2 content by determining their ability to support the proliferation of IL 2-dependent CT-6 cells as described (13). The reciprocal of the supernatant dilution which caused 50% maximum ^{3}H-thymidine incorporation was defined to be the IL 2 titer, expressed in units/ml.

Radiolabeling of cells with ^{35}S-methionine

Cloned T cells to be labeled with ^{35}S-methionine were suspended at a concentration of 8×10^4 cells/ml without feeder cells in methionine-free medium (14) with 10% IL 2-containing supernatant (either supernatant from cultures of PMA-activated EL4 thymoma or lectin-depleted supernatant from cultures of Con A-activated rat spleen cells, as described in 13). The IL 2-containing supernatants were prepared in tissue culture medium with methionine and thus served as a source of unlabeled methionine, which was essential to the viability of the cloned T cells. After incubation of the cell suspensions for 24 hr at 37°C, sufficient ^{35}S-methionine was added to each culture to give a final concentration of 7.5 µCi/ml. The cultures were incubated at 37°C for a further 14 to 16 hr, at the end of which time the ^{35}S-labeled cells were harvested, centrifuged on Ficoll-Hypaque to remove any dead cells, and washed three times with tissue culture medium. The amount of radioisotope incorporated into trichloroacetic acid (TCA)-precipitable material was measured as described (14).

Isolation of membrane fractions

Low density (plasma membrane-enriched) and high density (endoplasmic reticulum-enriched) membrane fractions were isolated from ^{35}S-labeled cells as previously described in detail (14). In brief, radiolabeled cells mixed with a 50-fold excess of unlabeled EL4 cells as carrier were equilibrated with 30% glycerol in culture medium and then lysed in ice cold hypotonic buffer solution containing 10 mM Tris buffer, pH 7.6, 1 mM $CaCl_2$, 2 mM $MgCl_2$, and 2 mM phenylmethylsulfonyl fluoride. The suspensions were subjected to a series of centrifugations as outlined in Table 1. The contents of the membrane fractions obtained by this procedure were characterized by measurement of 5'-nucleotidase activity (14) and by electron microscopy. The low and high density membrane fractions were collected separately from the sucrose gradients, resuspended in 10 mm Tris buffer, pH 7.2, and centrifuged for 30 min at 38,000 rpm in a Beckman type 40 rotor. The resulting membrane pellets were dissolved in loading buffer for SDS-polyacrylamide gel electrophoresis (SDS-PAGE) or resuspended in borate-buffered saline for immunoprecipitation studies.

Table 1

Fractionation of ^{35}S-Labeled Cells by Hypotonic Lysis
and Differential Centrifugation

Step #	Procedure	Fraction	Contents of Fraction	% Recovery of ^{35}S
1	^{35}S-labeled cells & unlabeled EL4		Cell suspension	100
2	Equilibrate cells with 30% glycerol; spin at 500 x g, 5 min	Pellet	Glycerol-loaded cells	94-98
3	Lyse cells in hypotonic buffer; spin at 3600 x g, 5 min; wash pellet x 2 and combine supernatants	Low speed supernatant	Cytosol + membranes	46-60
		Low speed pellet	Nuclei + mitochondria	18-35
4	Spin low speed supernatant at 22,000 x g, 30 min.	High speed supernatant	Cytosol	31-43
		High speed pellet	Cell membranes	9-14
5	Suspend high speed pellet in 37% sucrose in Tris buffer. Overlay with 25% sucrose. Spin at 45,000 x g, 12-20 hr	Interfacial band	Low density membranes	0.2-1.5
		Pellet	High density membranes	3.6-9.3

Membrane proteins were fractionated by SDS-PAGE in the presence of 2-mercaptoethanol as previously described (14). The stacking gel contained 3% acrylamide and the running gel consisted of a linear gradient from 7.5% to 17.5% acrylamide. ^{14}C-methylated protein standards were myosin (200kD), phosphorylase B (92kD), bovine serum albumin (68kD), ovalbumin (45kD), carbonic anhydrase (30kD), α-chymotrypsinogen (25kD), β-lactoglobulin (18kD), cytochrome C (12kD), and bovine trypsin inhibitor (6kD).

Immunoprecipitation studies

[35]S-labeled membrane pellets to be used in immunoprecipitation studies were suspended in borate-buffered saline, pH 8.0, with 20 mm iodoacetamide and 20 mM CHAPS detergent (Calbiochem). The mixtures were incubated on ice for 60 min and then centrifuged at 100,000 g for 30 min at 4°C in a Beckman airfuge. The supernatants, which contained solubilized membrane proteins, were harvested and precleared by incubation with protein A-bearing Staphylococcus aureus, Cowan I strain (SaCI) (Calbiochem) for 45 min on ice followed by a second incubation with SaCI which had been precoated with affinity-purified rabbit anti-rat IgG (Cappel). After removal of the SaCI by centrifugation, the supernatant was divided into aliquots for treatment with monoclonal antibodies or an equivalent amount of control mouse ascites. The monoclonal antibodies used in these studies were rat antibodies to murine antigens: M1/9 (anti-T200), M17/4 (anti-LFA-1), 53.6 (anti-Lyt 2), and M5/49 (anti-Thy 1). These antibodies were generously donated by Dr. Eric Martz, University of Massachusetts. Mixtures of precleared supernatant and monoclonal antibodies or control ascites were incubated for 1 hr on ice. To each mixture was then added SaCI which had been coated with rabbit anti-rat IgG, and the resulting mixtures were incubated for a further 90 min on ice. The mixtures were then centrifuged at 4000 g for 5 min at 4°C, and the SaCI pellets were washed extensively. The final pellets were suspended in loading buffer for SDS-PAGE, and the suspensions were heated in a boiling water bath for 3 min. The SaCI were spun down, and the supernatants containing eluted proteins were collected and analyzed by SDS-PAGE.

PROPERTIES OF ^{35}S-LABELED CLONED T CELL LINES

The functional characterization of the alloreactive cloned T cell lines used in these studies has been previously described in detail (13). In brief, the T_C lines used in this work were helper-dependent T_C lines which mediated both specific and lectin-dependent cytolysis but did not proliferate in response to alloantigen or secrete IL 2 in response to Con A. T_H lines, on the other hand, mediated neither specific nor lectin-dependent cytolysis; however these lines proliferated in response to alloantigen, secreted IL 2 in response to Con A, and supported the growth of functional T_C in the presence of alloantigen without added IL 2 (13).

Labeling of T cell lines with ^{35}S-methionine as described in Materials and Methods resulted in incorporation of 2.5 to 10.5 cpm of TCA-precipitable ^{35}S per cell (Table 2). It was important to

Table 2

Properties of ^{35}S-Labeled Cell Populations[a]

Cells	^{35}S-Met incorporated: cpm/cell	% Specific ^{51}Cr release from:[b]		IL-2 released: units/ml	
		P815	EL4	−Con A	+Con A
2° MLC	1.4	57	1	<0.1	0.2
24/15 (T_C)	8.5	20	2	0.2	0.2
E/2 (T_C)	6.8	45	0	0.1	0.1
28/B (T_H)	5.7	−1	3	<0.1	2.8
B4/1 (T_H)	2.5	0	−1	<0.1	10.1

[a]The results in this table are from the same experiment as the electrophoretic profiles in Fig. 1.

[b]Each value is the mean of triplicate determinations at an effector/target ratio of 2/1.

determine whether cell lines which had been radiolabeled in this manner retained functional activity. Therefore, each population of ^{35}S-labeled cells was tested for its ability to mediate specific lysis of allogeneic P815 mastocytoma cells and for its ability to secrete IL 2 in response to Con A. As shown in Table 2, the ^{35}S-labeled T_C cells in these experiments retained their ability to cause specific cytolysis of allogeneic targets, and the ^{35}S-labeled T_H cells retained their ability to secrete IL 2 when incubated with Con A. Thus the 16 hour labeling procedure used in these experiments left the cells functionally intact.

COMPARISON OF MEMBRANE-ASSOCIATED PROTEINS OF CLONED T_C AND T_H

When the electrophoretic profiles of ^{35}S-labeled proteins in the low density (plasma membrane-enriched) (Fig. 1) and high density (endoplasmic reticulum-enriched) (not shown) membrane fractions from the T_C and T_H lines were compared, most of the ^{35}S-labeled bands were present in the electrophoretic profiles from both the T_C and the T_H lines. In four separate experiments in which membrane-associated proteins from a total of three T_C lines and four T_H lines were examined, only two bands could be identified which were consistently found in the membrane fractions from each of the three T_C lines but none of the four T_H lines. One of these, p215, migrated as a broad

406

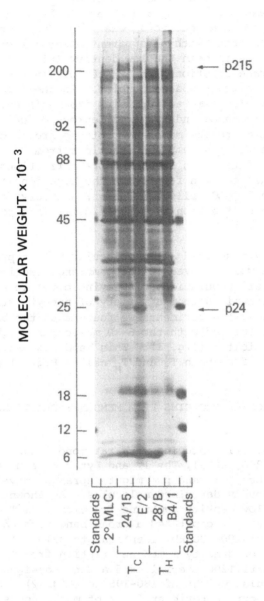

Fig. 1. SDS-PAGE of low density (plasma membrane-enriched) membrane fractions from ^{35}S-labeled cell populations. Samples were reduced in 2-mercaptoethanol prior to electrophoresis. The number of cpm of ^{35}S applied to each well was constant. Similar results were observed with membrane fractions from two additional T_H lines and one additional T_C line.

band with an apparent molecular weight of 200-220 kD. The T_H clone 28/B (Fig. 1) displayed no bands in the corresponding region of the gel whereas in membrane fractions from other T_H clones, such as B4/1 in Fig. 1, p215 was replaced by a doublet of sharp bands. The other protein which appeared unique to T_C was p24. This protein usually migrated as a sharp band with an apparent molecular weight of 24 kD and was readily seen in both the low density (Fig. 1) and high density (not shown) membrane fractions from T_C cells. In some experiments, p24 migrated as a closely spaced doublet. In the experiment shown in Fig. 1, ^{35}S-labeled membrane proteins from unfractionated lymphoid cells harvested from a secondary mixed leukocyte culture (MLC) were examined in addition to the membrane proteins from cloned T_H and T_C. p215 could be seen in the membrane fractions from 2^O MLC cells although it was fainter than in the membrane fractions from T_C lines. Likewise, p24 could be seen faintly in the high density membrane fraction from the 2^O MLC cells (not shown) and very faintly in the low density membrane fraction from these cells (not picked up by the photograph in Fig. 1).

We previously described a low molecular weight protein, which we called T11, which was observed in the membrane fractions from MLC- and Con A-activated cell populations displaying cytolyic activity but not in the membrane fractions from a variety of noncytolytic cell populations. In the present experiments we found that the band formerly designated T11 comigrated with the 6 kD molecular weight standard bovine trypsin inhibitor (Fig. 1). This band was prominent in the membrane fractions from both T_C and T_H cells (Fig. 1) and thus was not unique to T_C.

IMMUNOPRECIPITATION OF PROTEINS FROM MEMBRANE FRACTIONS OF CLONED T_C AND T_H

Immunoprecipitation studies with rat monoclonal antibodies to murine antigens T200, LFA-1, Thy 1, and Lyt 2 were undertaken in order to determine whether p215 and p24 might represent novel molecules or variants of previously described molecules. As shown in Fig. 2, treatment of the low density membrane fraction from T_C clone E/2 with monoclonal anti-T200 precipitated a broad band with an apparent molecular weight of 200-220 kD, identical to p215. In contrast, treatment of the low density membrane fraction from T_H clone 27/C with monoclonal anti-T200 precipitated a band, designated p185, with an apparent molecular weight of 180-195 kD (Fig. 2). Further comparison of the electrophoretic profiles of membrane-associated proteins from T_C and T_H (see Fig. 1) revealed that each of the T_H clones studied in these experiments possessed a band with a mobility identical to that of p185, migrating immediately behind the band identified by immunoprecipitation (Fig. 2) as LFA-1$_\alpha$. None of the T_C clones possessed a band of comparable mobility. Thus it appears that p215 and p185 represent variants of T200 on T_C and T_H clone cells, respectively.

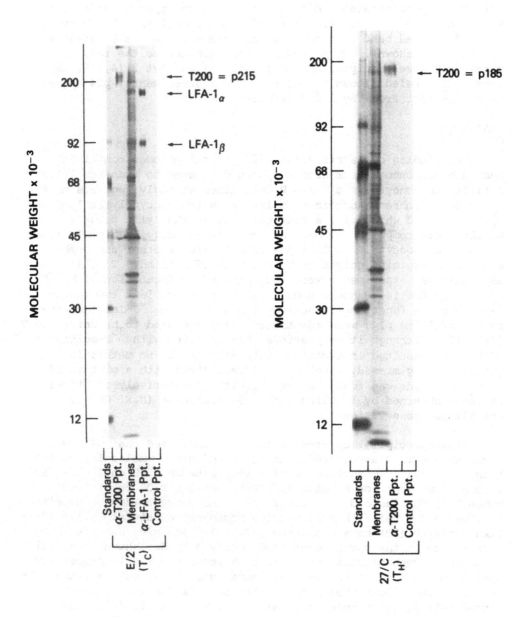

Fig. 2.　Immunoprecipitation of T200 from the low density membrane
fractions of T_C clone E/2 (<u>left</u>) and T_H clone 27/C (<u>right</u>).
CHAPS extracts of the membrane fractions were treated with
rat monoclonal antibodies to T200 or LFA-1 or with control
ascites and then with SaCI coated with rabbit anti-rat IgG.
Precipitates were analyzed by SDS-PAGE under reducing conditions. A sample of the whole extract of the low density
membrane fraction was run in each experiment in the track
labeled "Membranes".

Treatment of membrane fractions from T_C clone E/2 with monoclonal anti-Thy 1 precipitated a diffuse band with an apparent molecular weight of 24-32 kD, and treatment with monoclonal anti-Lyt 2 precipitated a broad band with an apparent molecular weight of 35-43 kD (results not shown). These results were similar to the results of others who have precipitated Thy 1 (15, 16) and Lyt 2 (4, 15, 16) from ^{125}I-labeled cloned T_C cells. In our experiments, p24 appeared to be distinct from Thy 1 and Lyt 2.

DISCUSSION

The finding of Harris et al. (11) that liposomes containing membrane components from cloned T_C could be used to transfer lytic activity to noncytolytic T and B cell lines strongly suggests that T_C possess membrane-associated molecules which noncytolytic lymphocytes lack and which play a critical role in the lytic mechanism. We therefore compared the membrane-associated proteins from T_C lines to those of noncytolytic T_H lines to determine whether any membrane associated proteins unique to T_C could be identified. T cell lines used in these experiments were radiolabeled by incubation with ^{35}S-methionine for 14-16 hours under conditions which left the radiolabeled cells functionally active (Table 2). Two ^{35}S-labeled proteins, p215 and p24, were identified which appeared to be unique to T_C (Fig. 1). Although it is possible that labeling with ^{35}S-methionine might have resulted in proteins containing few or no methionine residues being missed, labeling of T cell lines with a mixture of ^{14}C-amino acids was found to give results qualitatively identical to those obtained by labeling with ^{35}S-methionine (M.K. Gately, unpublished observations).

Immunoprecipitation studies (Fig. 2) indicated that p215 was a variant of T200 associated with T_C and of higher molecular weight than T200 on T_H. Structural differences between T200 on T cells and a related molecule on B cells (17, 18), between T200 on different human T lymphoblastoid cell lines (17), and between T200 on specific T_C lines and T cell lines displaying nonspecific natural killer (NK)-like activity (19) have been reported. p215 and p185 bear striking resemblance to the variants of T200 observed by Morishima et al. (17) on human T lymphoblastoid cell lines; however the T cell subset lineage of the cell lines examined by those authors was not reported. In comparing the electrophoretic profiles of ^{125}I-labeled T_C and T_H cloned cell lines, Sarmiento et al. (20), Bach et al. (21), and MacDonald et al. (22) all observed differences in the 200 kD range. It seems likely that these differences were due, at least in part, to variations in T200. What role, if any, T200 plays in the mechanism of T cell-mediated cytolysis is unclear. Monoclonal antibodies to T200 in the absence of complement have been reported to block NK- but not CTL-mediated cytolysis (18, 23, 24). Nevertheless, indirect evidence suggesting a possible role for T200 in CTL-mediated lysis has been reported (25, 26).

The second protein, p24, which appeared to be unique to T_C was shown by immunoprecipitation studies to be distinct from Thy 1 and Lyt 2. Sitkovsky et al. (27) recently identified a 23 kD protein as one of nine Con A-binding proteins on cloned T_C lines. Since preincubation of CTL with Con A resulted in loss of cytolytic activity (27), the authors suggested that one or more of the Con A-binding proteins, which also included T200, might play a role in the lytic mechanism. Whether the 23 kD molecule identified by those authors is the same molecule we have called p24 is unknown. Many additional questions regarding p24 are also unresolved. We do not know whether p24 is an integral membrane protein or merely remains associated with the membrane fractions during our isolation procedure. Since all analyses of membrane proteins in these experiments were done by SDS-PAGE using reducing conditions, we do not know whether p24 is associated, either covalently or noncovalently, with other macro-molecules in intact cells. Most importantly, we do not know whether p24 plays any role in the mechanism of CTL-mediated cytolysis. The production of an antiserum to p24 will be required to assess the functional significance of this molecule.

SUMMARY

Cloned lines of murine alloreactive cytolytic and helper T cells were derived from secondary mixed leukocyte cultures. Cells from three T_C lines and four T_H lines were internally labeled with ^{35}S-methionine and then disrupted by hypotonic lysis. Low density (plasma membrane-enriched) and high density (endoplasmic reticulum-enriched) membrane fractions were isolated from each cloned cell line and analyzed by SDS-PAGE under reducing conditions. Two proteins were identified which were associated with membrane fractions from each of the T_C lines but none of the T_H lines. One of these, p215, migrated as a broad band with an apparent molecular weight of 200-220 kD. The other, p24, migrated as a sharp band or closely spaced doublet with an apparent molecular weight of 24 kD. Immunoprecipitation studies using monoclonal antibodies to T200, LFA-1, Thy 1, and Lyt 2 revealed that p215 was a variant of T200 found on T_C lines but not on T_H lines. Treatment of solubilized membrane proteins from T_H lines with anti-T200 precipitated a 180-195 kD protein band seen on each of the T_H lines but none of the T_C. In contrast, p24 was not precipitated by any of these monoclonal antibodies. It appears that p24 represents a previously unidentified protein which is unique to T_C and thus deserving of further study as to its functional significance.

ACKNOWLEDGMENTS

The authors are grateful to Ms. Martha Johnson for her technical assistance in performing these experiments and to Ms. Mary Moore for her assistance in preparing the manuscript. We thank Dr. Eric Martz for supplying the monoclonal antibodies used in this work.

REFERENCES

1. Martz, E. 1977. Mechanism of specific tumor cell lysis by alloimmune T lymphocytes: resolution and characterization of discrete steps in the cellular interaction. Contemp. Top. Immunobiol. 7:301

2. Sarmiento, M., D.P. Dialynas, D.W. Lancki, et al. 1982. Cloned T lymphocytes and monoclonal antibodies as probes for cell surface molecules active in T cell-mediated cytolysis. Immunol. Rev. 68:135.

3. Golstein, P., C. Goridis, A.-M. Schmitt-Verhulst, et al. 1982. Lymphoid cell surface interaction structures detected using cytolysis-inhibiting monoclonal antibodies. Immunol. Rev. 68:5.

4. MacDonald, H.R., A.L. Glasebrook, C. Bron, A. Kelso, and J.-C. Cerottini. 1982. Clonal heterogeneity in the functional requirement for Lyt-2/3 molecules on cytolytic T lymphocytes (CTL): possible implications for the affinity of CTL antigen receptors. Immunol. Rev. 68:95.

5. Springer, T.A., D. Davignon, M.-K. Ho, K. Kurzinger, E. Martz, and F. Sanchez-Madrid. 1982. LFA-1 and Lyt-2,3 molecules associated with T lymphocyte-mediated killing; and Mac-1, an LFA-1 homologue associated with complement receptor function. Immunol. Rev. 68:171.

6. Martz, E., W. Heagy, and S.H. Gromkowski. 1983. The mechanism of CTL-mediated killing: monoclonal antibody analysis of the roles of killer and target-cell membrane proteins. Immunol. Rev. 72:73.

7. Chang, T.W., P.C. Kung, S.P. Gingras, and G. Goldstein. 1981. Does OKT3 monoclonal antibody react with an antigen-recognition structure on human T cells? Proc. Natl. Acad. Sci. USA 78:1805.

8. Platsoucas, C.D., and R.A. Good 1981. Inhibition of specific cell-mediated cytotoxicity by monoclonal antibodies to human T cell antigens. Proc. Natl. Acad. Sci. USA 78:4500.

9. Meuer, S.C., K.A. Fitzgerald, R.E. Hussey, J.C. Hodgdon, S.F. Schlossman, and E.L. Reinherz. 1983. Clonotypic structures involved in antigen-specific human T cell function. Relationship to the T3 molecular complex. J. Exp. Med. 157:705.

10. Lancki, D.W., M.I. Lorber, M.R. Loken, and F.W. Fitch. 1983. A clone-specific monoclonal antibody that inhibits cytolysis of a cytolytic T cell clone. J. Exp. Med. 157-921.

11. Harris, D.T., H.R. MacDonald, and J.-C. Cerottini. 1984. Direct transfer of antigen-specific cytolytic activity to noncytolytic cells upon fusion with liposomes derived from cytolytic T cell clones. J. Exp. Med. 159:261.

12. Glasebrook, A.L., and F.W. Fitch. 1980. Alloreactive cloned T cell lines. I. Interactions between cloned amplifier and cytolytic T cell lines. J. Exp. Med. 151:876.

13. Dick, M.D., W.R. Benjamin, T. Masuno, J.J. Farrar, and M.K. Gately. 1984. Differential effects of positive and negative proliferative stimuli on murine cytolytic and helper T-cell clones. Cell. Immunol. 86:118.

14. Gately, M.K., and E. Martz. 1981. T11: a new protein marker on activated murine T lymphocytes. J. Immunol. 126:709.

15. Sarmiento, M., A.L. Glasebrook, and F.W. Fitch. 1980. IgG or IgM monoclonal antibodies reactive with different determinants on the molecular complex bearing Lyt 2 antigen block T cell-mediated cytolysis in the absence of complement. J. Immunol. 125:2665.

16. Luescher, B., H.Y. Naim, H.R. MacDonald, and C. Bron. 1984. The mouse Lyt-2/3 antigen complex. I. Mode of association of the subunits with the membrane. Mol. Immunol. 21:329.

17. Morishima, Y., S. Ogata, N.H. Collins, B. Dupont, and K.O. Lloyd. 1982. Carbohydrate differences in human high molecular weight antigens of B- and T-cell lines. Immunogenetics 15:529.

18. Sarmiento, M., M.R.. Loken, I.S. Trowbridge, R.L. Coffman, and F.W. Fitch. 1982. High molecular weight lymphocyte surface proteins are structurally related and are expressed on different cell populations at different times during lymphocyte maturation and differentiation. J. Immunol. 128:1676.

19. Brooks, C.G., D.L. Urdal, and C.S. Henney. 1983. Lymphokine-driven "differentiation" of cytotoxic T cell clones into cells with NK-like specificity: correlations with display of membrane macromolecules. Immunol. Rev. 72:43.

20. Sarmiento, M., A.L. Glasebrook, and F.W. Fitch. 1980. Cell surface polypeptides of murine T-cell clones expressing cytolytic or amplifier activity. Proc. Natl. Acad. Sci. USA 77:1111.

21. Bach, F.H., B.J. Alter, M.B. Widmer, M. Segall, and B. Dunlap. 1981. Cloned cytotoxic and non-cytotoxic lymphocytes in mouse and man: their reactivities and a large cell surface membrane protein (LMP) differentiation marker system. Immunol. Rev. 54:5.

22. MacDonald, H.R., R.P. Sekaly, O. Kanagawa, et al. 1982. Cytolytic T lymphocyte clones. Immunobiol. 161:84.

23. Seaman, W.E., N. Talal, L.A. Herzenberg, L.A. Herzenberg, and J.A. Ledbetter. 1981. Surface antigens on mouse natural killer cells: use of monoclonal antibodies to inhibit or to enrich cytotoxic activity. J. Immunol, 127:982.

24. Newman, W., L.D. Fast, and L.M. Rose. 1983. Blockade of NK cell lysis is a property of monoclonal antibodies that bind to distinct regions of T-200. J. Immunol. 131:1742.

25. Redelman, D., and D. Hudig. 1982. T200-like molecules are involved in cell-mediated lysis by rabbit, human, and mouse effector cells Immunobiol. 163:147 (Abs.).

26. Pasternack, M.S., M.V. Sitkovsky, and H.N. Eisen. 1983. The site of action of N-α-tosyl-L-lysyl-chloromethyl-ketone (TLCK) on cloned cytotoxic T lymphocytes. J. Immunol. 131:2477.

27. Sitkovsky, M.V., M.S. Pasternack, J.P. Lugo, J.R. Klein, and H.N. Eisen. 1984. Isolation and partial characterization of concanavalin A receptors on cloned cytotoxic T lymphocytes. Proc. Natl. Acad. Sci. USA 81:1519.

MECHANISM OF T-DEPENDENT CYTOTOXICITY: ROLE OF PAPAIN-SENSITIVE NON CLASS I MHC TARGET MOLECULES AND EXPRESSION OF TARGET ANTIGEN FOR CYTOTOXICITY

Benjamin Bonavida, Hanna Ostergaard, and Jonathan Katz

Department of Microbiology and Immunology
UCLA School of Medicine
Los Angeles, CA

INTRODUCTION

Cell mediated cytotoxicity (CMC) has been shown to play a major role in resistance to viral infections, tumor rejection and allograft rejection. The mechanism by which the cytotoxic phenomenon operates has been the subject of many investigations, but still remains elusive. Several approaches have been used, such as chemical inhibitors which allow for the dissection of lysis into three steps, namely, binding and/or recognition, programming for lysis, and the killer cell independent lysis stage (1). Other approaches have made use of blocking antibodies which allow for the characterization of surface molecules involved in lysis (2). These studies suggest that lysis is a complex phenomenon requiring several interactions between the lymphocyte and the target cell before lysis is achieved. The nature of these interactions and the biochemical nature of the molecules involved has been studied in part. For instance, it is clear that H2 antigens on target cells are recognized by the CTL receptor. Likewise, several molecular species on CTL have also been implicated in cytolysis such as Lyt23 and the LFA family of molecules (3-5).

Our previous studies have attempted to characterize membrane structures, present on either the effector or target cell membrane, that are involved in lysis. We have developed an approach using lectin- or oxidative-dependent cellular cytotoxicity systems in which CTL lyse targets in an antigen non-specific fashion (6-10). The premise for this approach is that the lectin bypasses the initial recognition event and proceeds to the subsequent steps necessary for lysis. However, this premise has not been verified experimentally, and has in fact been questioned in recent work by Berke et al. (11, 12). These investigators have implicated the role of H2 and the CTL

(1) GLUING

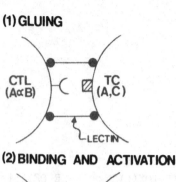

(2) BINDING AND ACTIVATION

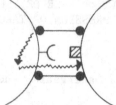

(3) MODIFICATION OF H-2 OR HL-A

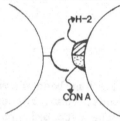

**(4) BINDING AND EXPRESSION OF TARGET ANTIGEN
FOR CYTOTOXICITY (TAC)**

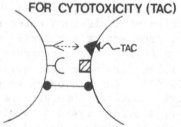

Figure 1. Models proposed for LDCC or ODCC.

receptor in LDCC by suggesting that the lectin modifies H2 and the modified molecule is involved in T cell recognition. Although this model is supported by several lines of evidence, other models have been proposed (Figure 1). One model suggests that lectin mimics the receptor and activates the effector cell to mediate lysis while the target cell is passive. Another model suggests that the lectin modifies the target cell so that the cell expresses structures recognized by the CTL and these structures are involved in lysis.

The present study investigates the role of lectin on target cells and the nature of target cell structures involved in lysis. Two sets of experiments were carried out, namely, the examination of the role played by non-class I MHC target antigens in CMC, and the active role of target cells in ODCC and LDCC. These experiments emphasize the role of target cell surface membrane structures in CMC.

MATERIALS AND METHODS

Effector Cells

Effector cells, human PBL, and the LGL fraction were prepared as previously described (10,13). Mouse CTL were prepared by immunizing C57Bl/6 mice intraperitoneally with allogeneic P815 tumor cells. Nine to 11 days later the peritoneal exudate lymphocytes were obtained and purified on a nylon wool column. The Raji cell line and the HLA class I negative Daudi cell line were grown in suspension in RPMI containing 10% FCS supplemented with antibiotics and L-glutamine. EL4 and P815 tumors were maintained in ascitic forms in C57Bl/6 and BBA/2 mice respectively.

Assays

The chromium release assay and the single cell assay were used as previously described (13). The LDCC assay was performed as previously described (14). For the ODCC assay, the cells were washed three times with PBS and brought to $10X20^6$/ml. These cells were incubated with the appropriate concentration of sodium periodate for 25 minutes on ice, after which the cells were washed three times with 10% FCS in HBSS. The viability of these cells was greater than 85% (2).

Papain Digestion

Various concentrations of papain (Worthington Biochemicals) in HBSS supplemented with 0.02 M cysteine (Sigma) and 0.2 mg/ml deoxyribonuclease (Sigma) was added to radiolabeled target cells (1-20X 10^6/ml) and incubated for 30 minutes at 37°. The treated cells were washed twice in HBSS and resuspended in 10% FCS RPMI medium and kept on ice until used.

Immunofluorescence

Monoclonal antibodies directed against HLA class I and class II

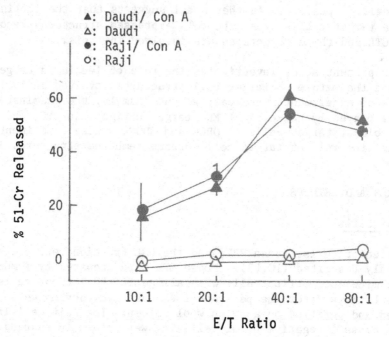

Figure 2. Daudi (Class I MHC negative) serves as target in LDCC.

Table 1. Frequency of Binders and Killers for Daudi and
Raji Target Cells

Target	ConA (20 ug/ml)	% Binders	% Target Cell killed[a]
Daudi	–	18.0±1.7	6.5±4.7
	+	31.8±0.6	40.0±3.1
Raji	–	24.6±4.5	17.1±3.5
	+	27.9±2.1	35.3±1.2

[a]This percentage represents the frequency of killer cells in
the conjugates.

antigens were the generous gift of Doctors Ron Billing and Sidney
Bolub at UCLA. $5X10^5$ cells were pelleted and resuspended in various
dilutions of antibody or control ascites and incubated on ice for 30
minutes. To each tube, one milliliter of FCS was added and the tube
centrifuged at 3,000g for 10 minutes and the supernatant decanted.
The pellet was resuspended in 0.02% azide PBS and washed 2 times.
The pellet was resuspended in 1:16 dilution of FITC goat anti-mouse
immunoglobulin (FC specific, Cappel Laboratories) and incubated in
the dark on ice for 30 minutes. The cells were washed two times and
viewed under a fluorescence microscope. For labeling of effector
cells bound to target cells, the conjugates were formed first and
then treated as above for fluorescence.

RESULTS

I. Papain Sensitive HLA Negative Membrane Target Structures
Involved in Cytotoxicity

To delineate the role of non-HLA target cell antigens in cytotoxicity, we chose Daudi target cells which are genetically deficient
in beta 2 microglobulin synthesis and therefore do not express class
I MHC products (15). The results were compared to those obtained
using HLA+ Raji target cells (16). Our first experiment was designed
to determine whether Daudi serves as a target in LDC using human
peripheral blood lymphocytes as effector cells. The results shown in
Figure 2 clearly demonstrate that both Daudi and Raji serve as target
cells in LDCC, and the cytotoxic activity is dependent on the effector to target cell ratio used. These results also show that class I
MHC products are not required for LDCC.

Several aspects of this finding were examined. The frequency of
binders and killers in the single cell assay was comparable for both
Daudi and Raji (Table 1). These results suggest that the same population of effector cells is involved for the lysis of both targets.

Furthermore, the cells mediating LDCC were characterized as T
cells by direct immunofluorescence and by fluorescence directed at
the level of the conjugate (Table 2). Thus, T cells mediate lysis of
HLA class I negative cells and HLA class I positive target cells.

Previous studies have reported that target cells treated with
papain render the cells insusceptible to lysis (17,18). This has
been interpreted to indicate that class I MHC antigens are involved
since they are papain sensitive. We performed experiments to determine whether target cells express non-class I MHC and papain sensitive molecules that are also involved in lysis. Daudi and Raji were
treated with various concentrations of papain and tested for cytotoxicity. As shown in Table 3, papain treatment significantly
inhibited LDCC. These results demonstrate that papain removes non-

Table 2. The T Cell Nature of Effector Cells Mediating
Binding and Killing of Daudi and Raji Targets

| Antibody | % Cells Fluorescent[a] | | |
| | Total | Conjugates | |
		Daudi	Raji
OKT3	82.4	77.0	74.0
-	1.2%		

[a]Indirect immunofluorescence was done using monoclonal antibody and FITC goat anti-mouse IgG (FC specific) as described
in Materials & Methods.
[b]Percentage of effector cell (nylon wool purified) that
stained with the antibody.

Table 3. Inhibition of LDCC Following Papain Treatment of
Target Cells

| Expt. | Papain[a] (ug/ml) | % ^{51}Cr Release[b] (Inhibition) | |
		Daudi	Raji
1	0.0	66	35
	0.5	35 (47)	31 (12)
	1.0	28 (57)	28 (20)
	2.5	30 (55)	17 (51)
2	0.0	87	80
	0.5	45 (48)	72 (10)
	1.0	33 (62)	59 (28)
	2.5	32 (63)	42 (48)

[a]Radiolabeled target cells were treated with various concentrations of papain with MEM for 20 min. at 37°, washed 3
times, and used for the CMC assay.
[b]LDCC was done in the presence of ConA (20 ug/ml).

HLA class I target cell structures necessary for lysis.

To further corroborate this notion, we examined the kinetics of recovery of papain treated target cells is LDCC. Treated cells were allowed to incubate for various periods of time, and then used in the LDCC assay. LDCC activity recovered within a short period of time, comparable to the recovery of papain treated HLA+ cells (Figure 3). These results demonstrate that aside from HLA antigens other papain sensitive target structures are involved in lysis and follow the same kinetics of recovery as class I HLA antigens.

Since Daudi is a B cell and expresses class II MHC antigens, we investigated the role of these antigens in LDCC. Treatment of cells with papain did not remove class II antigens and therefore suggested that the papain sensitive molecules are not class II MHC products.

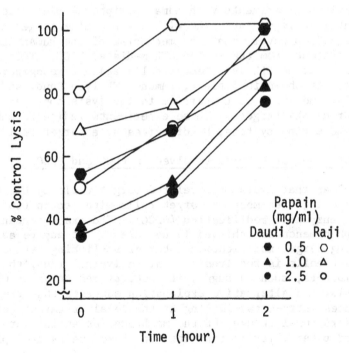

Figure 3. Recovery of Daudi susceptibility to lysis following papain treatment.

Table 4. Daudi Serves as Target for LDCC with Murine CTL

Target	% ^{51}Cr Release (E:T 40:1)[a]	
	No ConA	ConA (10 ug/ml)
Daudi	2.4	54.6
Raji	1.0	44.6
P815X2	74.7	

[a]The effector CTL were derived by allosensitization of murine C57 Bl/6 mice with P815X2 tumor cells.

The previous experiments with human peripheral blood clearly indicate that T cells mediate LDCC with HLA negative target cells. It may be argued, however, that the mechanism of the human LDCC system is different from the murine CTL mediated LDCC. This was examined using murine CTL as effector cells against xenogeneic human target cells. As shown in Table 4, immune CTL lyse Daudi and Raji significantly, and lysis is comparable to the lysis obtained with the syngeneic murine EL4 targets. These experiments indicate that in both human and murine systems, Daudi serves as a target cell in LDCC.

II. Target Membrane Structures Involved in LDCC and ODCC

It is clear that lysis of unrelated target cells by CTL can be achieved following treatment of target cells with lectin (LDCC) or by chemical and enzymatic modification (ODCC). The exact mechanism by which this phenomenon is achieved is not clear. It may be assumed that following target modification inter-cross-linking between effector and target cells is required to achieve lysis. Thus, the addition of inhibitors, such as sugars in LDCC, or reduction of ODCC inhibits lysis. An alternative explanation suggests that the modification produces intra-cross-linking at the level of target cells, leading to structural changes of the membranes essential for cytolysis. A third possibility is that both of these events take place in LDCC.

To investigate these possibilities, we made use of two previous findings in our laboratory, namely, periodate treated targets are not lysed by borohydride treatment in ODCC, and neuraminidase treatment of target cells is required for SBA to be effective in LDCC, even though conjugate formation is obtained in the absence of enzymatic

Table 5. Periodate Treated Target Cells are not Lysed in the Presence of SBA when the Cells are Reduced with KBH_4 <u>Immediately</u> After $NaIO_4$ Treatment

Lectin	$NaIO_4$ (mM)	% ^{51}Cr Release[a]		
		−	KBH_4 (2mM)	KBH_4 (5mM)
None	0	2.4	1.9	0.6
	5	26.2	11.6	3.1
ConA	0	29.2	28.2	28.3
(20ug/ml)	5	24.0	25.6	23.6
SBA	0	1.8	3.0	6.8
(20ug/ml)	5	16.0	0.2	0.7

[a]The effector to target ratio was 10:1 using allosensitized CTL.

treatment (10). We reasoned that if one signal were to be involved in membrane target modification and another were to provide for binding, lysis could be achieved when both modifications were made. Each modification taken alone, however, would not be sufficient to initiate lysis.

The results in Table 5 show that periodate-treated and borohydride-reduced target cells are not lysed in the presence of SBA. The reduced target, however, serves as a target if ConA is added. These results demonstrate that reduction of periodate treated cells does not make the cells resistant to lysis, but that a second signal provided by SBA is sufficient to render the cells susceptible to lysis. Alternatively, it is possible that intra-cross-linking by periodate on the target cell requires time, and that the addition of borohydride immediately after oxidation may prevent this event. We examined this possibility using target cells treated with periodate and allowed to incubate at 37° for 1 hour. The cells were then reduced with borohydride, and SBA was added. Under these conditions, significant lysis was achieved (Table 6). These results demonstrate that the target cells undergo modification. Thus, two signals may be involved: One provided by SBA, and the other by the periodate modification.

We then tested whether the signal provided by SBA is achieved by other lectins or agglutimating agents. It was found that other lectins which cannot mediate LDCC by themselves, such as SBA and WGA, were effective when modified by periodate and borohydride (Table 7).

Table 6. Target Cells are Lysed in the Presence of SBA when the IO_4 Treated Cells are Incubated at 37° for 1 Hour Before KBH_4 Treatment

Lectin	$NaIO_4$	-	% ^{51}Cr Release KBH_4 (2mM)	KBH_4 (5mM)
None	0	0.2	0.8	1.8
	5	19.7	8.9	4.1
SBA	0	6.7	4.9	4.6
(20ug/ml)	5	19.5	18.3	19.7
ConA	0	21.0	19.7	18.9
(20ug/ml)	5	14.9	16.9	15.7

Table 7. Target Cells are Lysed in the Presence of Lectin But Not Poly-L-lysine when the Target Cells are Incubated at 37° for 1 Hour Between $NaIO_4$ and KBH_4 Treatments

Lectin[a]	$NaIO_4$ (mM)	-	% ^{51}Cr Release KBH_4 (5mM)	KBH_4 (10mM)
None	0	3.0	1.3	2.9
	5	17.5	1.0	0.7
SBA	0	2.4	2.5	2.1
	5	18.8	27.9	16.3
PNA	0	2.6	6.6	6.3
	5	17.2	18.9	16.1
WGA	0	5.3	8.6	9.8
	5	19.6	27.8	16.6
PLL	0	3.4	5.1	6.9
(5ug/ml)	5	19.5	3.1	4.6

[a]Final concentration was 20 ug/ml.

However, the agglutimating agent PLL was not effective. It is not clear whether the interaction provided by PLL is similar to that provided by lectins. These experiments indicate the role of two signals in LDCC and ODCC, one involving target modification and the other involving binding and possibly activation of lymphocytes.

The exact nature of the membrane perturbation induced by IO_4 is not clear, however, the results support the data shown in the previous section indicating that target cell modification is required for lysis.

DISCUSSION

Evidence is presented which demonstrates, by two independent systems, the role of target membrane structures involved in cell mediated cytotoxicity. The first line of evidence demonstrates that target cells which are genetically deficient in class I MHC antigens can serve as targets in LDCC. In addition, non-HLA papain sensitive structures are shown to be involved in CMC. The second line of evidence shows that periodate-treated and borohydride-modified target cells serve as targets in the presence of SBA. This suggests that chemical modification allows the expression of target cell structures which are involved in cytotoxicity. These two lines of data emphasize the role of non-MHC target structures in lysis, and corroborate the suggestion that multiple target cell-effector cell interactions take place during the process of cytolysis.

The present studies with Daudi targets indicate that cytotoxicity can take place in the absence of class I MHC expression. This is reminiscent of other studies using H2 negative cells (19,20). However, recent studies have proposed that the lectin modifies class I MHC, and that the T cell receptor recognizes the modified target antigen in LDCC, thus leading to lysis. These hypotheses are supported by various lines of evidence, namely: blocking of LDCC by anti-H2 antibody, abrogation of LDCC by papain treatment, and poor lysis by H2-target cells (11,12).

Our studies with papain are consistent with those reported by Gromkowsky et al. who used a different experimental design describing the role of target antigens in cytotoxicity using monoclonal blocking antibodies (21). These same investigators have shown that non-class I MHC trypsin-sensitive structures are also involved in cytotoxicity (22). All of these studies stress the role of target membrane structures, which are not related to the MHC, in lysis. The exact biochemical nature of these structures is not yet known.

The role of target cell structures in lysis was also investigated based on the hypothesis that during effector-target interactions, in SCMC, LDCC or ODCC, the target undergoes perturbation or modification which is essential for lysis. This perturbation is brought upon by the initial interaction mediated by the T cell receptor or the lectin. Thus, lectin may have a multiple role in LDCC in that it modulates the target cell, provides bridging, and may also activate the CTL. Our studies provide evidence that the target cell is modified following treatment by periodate and borohydride, provided the cells are incubated first for 1h after IO_4 treatment and lysis takes place in the presence of SBA. These studies are consistent with intra-cross-linking which takes place on the target cells and leads to target modification. The addition of borohydride may stabilize the cross-linking obtained.

The role of SBA in the cytotoxic reaction may facilitate the interaction between the effector cell and target cells, and may also facilitate the triggering of the effector cell. Our results with poly-L-lysine indicate that agglutination alone may not be sufficient for lysis to take place. The failure of the PLL to mediate lysis may be due to its failure to interact with the appropriate ligand, or to the fact that PLL does not provide the appropriate trigger of the CTL required for lysis.

In conclusion, the mechanism of LDCC and ODCC has been the subject of various investigations. Several models have been proposed which are schematically diagrammed in Figure 1. Our studies are consistent with model 4 in which the lectin provides at least two signals, one on the target cells and one on the effector cells. The characterization of the structures involved may be accomplished either by chemical means or by using antibody-mediated blocking experiments. Such studies may further define the role of lectin in LDCC, as well as the nature of the target cell membrane molecules involved in lysis.

ACKNOWLEDGEMENT

This work was supported by CA 35791 from the National Cancer Institute and in part by the Cancer Research Coordinating Committee (Berkeley, CA).

REFERENCES

1. E. Martz, Mechanism of specific tumor cell lysis by alloimmune T lymphocytes. Resolution and characterization of discrete steps in the cellular interaction. Contemp. Topics Immunobiol. 7:301 (1977).
2. J. Fan and B. Bonavida, Studies on the induction and expression of T-cell mediated immunity XIV. Role of Lyt-2 antigens of CTL and H2 antigens of target cells on antigen non-specific oxidation dependent cellular cytotoxicity (ODCC) mediated by

sodium periodate oxidation of either effector or target
cells. J. Immunol. 131:1426 (1983).

3. B. Bonavida, T. P. Bradley, J. Fan, R. Effros, J. R. Hiserodt,
and H. Wexler, Molecular interactions in T-cell mediated
cytotoxicity. Immunol. Rev. 72:119 (1983).

4. E. Martz, W. Heagy, and S. H. Gromkowski, The mechanism of CTL-
mediated killing: monoclonal antibody analysis of the roles
of killer and target cell membrane proteins. Immunol. Rev.
72:73 (1983).

5. T. A. Springer, D. Davignon, M. Y. Ho, K. Kurzinger, E. Martz,
and F. Sanchez-Madrid, LFA-1 and Lyt-2,3 molecules associated with T lymphocyte-mediated killing: and Mac-1, and
LFA-1 homologue associated with complement receptor function. Immunol. Rev. 68:171 (1982).

6. M. J. Bevan and M. Cohn, Cytotoxic effects of antigen- and
mitogen-induced T cells on various targets. J. Immunol.
114:559 (1975).

7. A. Novogrodsky, Induction of lymphocyte cytotoxicity by modification of the effector or target cells with periodate or
with neuraminidase and galactose oxidase. J. Immunol.
114:1089 (1975).

8. B. Bonavida and T. P. Bradley, Studies on the induction and
expression of T-cell mediated immunity. V. Lectin-induced
nonspecific cell-mediated cytotoxicity by alloimmune lymphocytes. Transplantation 21:94 (1976).

9. B. Bonavida, A. Robins, and A. Saxon, Lectin-dependent cellular
cytotoxicity in man. Transplantation 23:261 (1977).

10. T. P. Bradley and B. Bonavida, Mechanism of cell-mediated cytotoxicity at the single cell level. V. The importance of
target cell structures in cytotoxic T-lymphocyte mediated
antigen non-specific lectin-dependent cellular cytotoxicity. J. Immunol. 129:2352 (1982).

11. G. Berke, H. E. Mcvey, and W. R. Clark, T-lymphocyte mediated
cytoloysis. I. One common mechanism for target recognition
in specific and lectin-dependent cytolysis. J. Immunol.
127:776 (1982).

12. G. Berke, V. Hu, E. Mcvey, and W. R. Clark, T-lymphocyte-
mediated cytolysis. II. Role of target cell histocompatibility antigens in recognition and lysis. J. Immunol. 127:782
(1981).

13. T. P. Bradley and B. Bonavida, Mechanism of cell-mediated cytotoxicity at the single cell level. IV. Natural killing and
antibody dependent cellular cytotoxicity can be mediated by
the same human effector cell as determined by the two target
conjugate assay. J. Immunol. 129:2260 (1982).

14. T. P. Bradley and B. Bonavida, Mechanism of cell-mediated cytotoxicity at the single cell level. VII. Trigger of the
lethal hit event is distinct for NK/K and LDCC effector
cells as measured in the two target conjugate assay. Cell.
Immunol. 83:199 (1984).

15. G. Klein, P. Terasaki, R. Billing, Somatic cell hybrids between human lymphoma lines. III. Surface markers. Int. J. Cancer 19:66 (1977).

16. M. Jondal, C. Spina, and S. Targan, Human spontaneous killer cells selective for tumor-derived target cells. Nature 272:62 (1978).

17. K. Thoma, H. D. Engers, J. -C. Cerottini, and K. T. Brunner, Enzymatic removal of H2 alloantigens from the surface of P815-X2 mouse tumor cells. Eur. J. Immunol. 6:257 (1976).

18. R. F. Todd, Lymphocyte-mediated cytolysis of allogeneic tumor cells in vitro. III. Enzyme sensitivity of target cell antigens. Cell Immunol. 20:287 (1975).

19. M. J. Bevan and R. Hyman, The ability of H2+ and H2- cell lines to induce or be lysed by cytotoxic T cells. Immunogenetics 4:7 (1977).

20. T. Hunig, Monoclonal anti-Lyt2.2 antibody blocks lectin-dependent cellular cytotoxicity of H2 negative target cells. J. Exp. Med. 159:551 (1984).

21. S. H. Gromkowski, W. Heagy, F. Sanchez-Madrid, T. A. Springer, and E. Martz, Blocking of CTL-mediated killing by monoclonal antibodies to LFA-1 and Lyt-2,3. I. Increased susceptibility to blocking after papain treatment of target cells. J. Immunol. 130:2546 (1983).

22. S. H. Gromkowski, W. Heagy, and E. Martz, Blocking of CTL-mediated killing by monoclonal antibodies to LFA-1 and Lyt-2,3. II. Evidence that trypsin pretreatment of target cells removes a non-H2 molecule important in killing. (Submitted for publication.)

CELL-CELL CONTACT PROTEINS IN ANTIGEN-SPECIFIC AND ANTIGEN-NONSPECIFIC CELLULAR CYTOTOXICITY

Michail V. Sitkovsky[1], Martin A. Schwartz[2], and
Herman N. Eisen[1]

[1]Department of Biology and Center for Cancer Research
Massachusetts Institute of Technology, Cambridge, MA 02139

[2]Department of Physiology, Harvard Medical School
Boston, MA 02115

The lysis of target cells (TCs) by cytotoxic T lymphocytes (CTLs) is probably mediated by proteins in the CTL plasma membrane. While the physiology of CTL-TC interactions has been described in detail (1-3), little is known about the molecular organization of the CTL surface membrane in the contact area of CTL-TC conjugates. The ability of certain alloantisera and monoclonal antibodies to inhibit CTL-mediated cytotoxicity in the absence of complement has served to identify functionally important CTL cell surface molecules: Lyt-2 (4,5) and lymphocyte function-associated antigens (LFA) (6,7). A similar approach has suggested that Lyt 5, also called T200, participates in the lytic mechanism of natural killer (NK) cells (8).

The use of monoclonal antibodies to identify functionally important cell surface antigens in the contact area of CTL-TC conjugates ("contact proteins") has certain limitations. A given antigen may not be an effective immunogen and, even if it is, it is not always clear that inhibition of CTL activity by antibodies is the result of an interaction with one of the "contact proteins".

In this study we describe an alternative approach, based on the use of a photosensitive, heterobifunctional, cleavable crosslinking reagent (XL) to detect and isolate "contact proteins" from CTLs in CTL-TC conjugates. In this procedure molecules of XL are delivered to the CTL contact area by a protein carrier bound to the surface of the target cells. The use of Con A as a protein carrier and affinity purified antibodies to Con A allowed us to isolate a set of "contact proteins" which includes proteins with Mr (in Kd) of

210, 190, 180, 155, 120, 105, 80, 47, and two minor components with Mr 38 and 33 Kd. The same set of contact proteins is also involved in antigen-nonspecific, lectin-mediated cytotoxicity. Use of the crosslinking reagent allowed us to show that nonspecific, lectin-dependent cytotoxicity is not mediated by bridging between CTLs and Con A-pretreated target cells.

ABBREVIATIONS

CTL, cytotoxic T lymphocyte; LFA-1, lymphocyte function-associated antigen-1; Con A, Concanavalin A; α-MM, α-methylmannoside; ^{51}Cr-TC, Na$_2$^{51}CrO$_4$-labeled EL4 cells; Con A-TC, Con A-pretreated TC; Con A-CTL, Con A-pretreated CTL; LDCC, lectin-dependent cellular cytotoxicity; E/T ratio, the number of effector cells divided by the number of target cells; K medium, supplemented culture medium for CTL assay; MHC, major histocompatibility complex; XL, crosslinking reagent N-succinimidyl-6(4'-azido-2'-nitrophenylamino) hexanoate; XL·Con A, Con A coupled to crosslinker; BSA, bovine serum albumin; *Con A, ^{125}I-radiolabeled Con A; Ag, antigen; PBS, phosphate buffered saline; mAb, monoclonal antibody; TC, target cell; CFM, conjugate formation medium; FCS, fetal calf serum; DTT, dithio-threitol.

MATERIALS AND METHODS

Cloned CTL lines, maintenance of the tumor target cells, pro-cedures for the pretreatment of the cells with Con A, for the iso-lation of high affinity Con A-binding glycoproteins, and for prepa-ration of the labeled Con A, estimation of ^{125}I-Con A binding to the cells, cell surface radiolabeling, and ^{51}Cr-release assay for cyto-toxicity were described in (9,10).

Coupling of Con A to the Crosslinking Reagent

The heterobifunctional, photoreactive, cleavable crosslinking reagent 3-[(2-nitro-4-azidophenyl)-2-aminoethyldithio]-N-succinimidyl propionate (XL) was synthesized and purified as described (11). The crosslinker was stored in toluene and was evaporated to dryness under a stream of nitrogen. The residue was dissolved in 15 μl of dimethylformamide. This was mixed with 300 μl of protein at 1 mg/ml. A ten to twenty time excess of XL was used. To protect the binding properties of the lectin from inactivaiton, 100 mM of haptenic sugar (α-MM) was included in the reaction. The Con A derivative (XL·Con A) was separated from unreacted XL on a Bio-Gel P2 column equilibrated with PBS. The protein was eluted in the exclusion volume and the amount of purified protein coupled to XL was estimated using a Bio-Rad protein assay. In separate experi-ments, we have shown that XL·Con A retains the mitogenic and binding properties of unmodified lectin and equally well mediates LDCC.

Pretreatment of Cells with Con A or XL·Con A

Cells (P815 or EL4) were suspended in 1 to 2 ml of CFM or RPMI 1640 with 0.1% BSA at 10^6 cells/ml in 50 ml conical tubes precoated with BSA. XL·Con A or Con A dissolved in PBS was then added to achieve the desired Con A concentration, and the cells were incubated for 90 minutes on ice at 22^oC or 37^oC; 10 to 20 ml of fresh, cold CFM were then added and the cells were harvested by centrifugation at 300 x g for 5 minutes. After four additional washes in CFM, Con A-TC or XL·Con A-TC were resuspended in CFM to 10^7 cells/ml and mixed with radiolabeled CTLs.

Conjugate Formation and Photolysis

The procedure for specific conjugate formation was adopted from (12,13). To prevent disulfide exchange between molecules of XL and -SH containing proteins in FCS, cells were resuspended in CFM which was composed of RPMI 1640 and 10% alkylated FCS (treated with 22 mM iodoacetic acid for 30 minutes at 37° C and extensively dialyzed). 200 µl of XL·Con A-TC (10^7/ml) were mixed with 200 µl of radiolabeled CTLs (10^7/ml); nonspecific conjugates were dispersed by standardized shearing forces and the cell suspensions were placed into the well of the 24 well "Costar" plate. All manipulations were made in the dark using a dim light. Photolysis of the cell suspensions on ice was carried out in the UV using a long wave, 100 watt mercury arc lamp with a maximum output at 365 nm and a cutoff at 320 nm. (XL absorbs continuously throughout the near UV). The crosslinking reaction was initiated by irradiation of the cells from a distance of 6 inches for 3 minutes.

Immunoprecipitation

After UV irradiation, washed cell pellets were solubilized on ice with extraction buffer according to (10) in the presence of 10 mM iodoacetic acid. Radiolabeled material chemically crosslinked to Con A was immunoprecipitated by affinity purified rabbit antibody to Con A and Protein A-bearing Staphylococcus Aureus.

RESULTS AND DISCUSSION

Design of the Experiment

The experimental appraoch developed here is based on the use of photosensitive, heterobifunctional, cleavable crosslinking reagents. According to the design, XL is coupled covalently to the protein carrier (e.g., Con A) in the dark (step 1) and TCs are

coated with XL·Con A under conditions whereby XL·Con A molecules
are distributed uniformly (in small clusters) over the TC surface
(step 2). Functionally active cloned CTLs with radiolabeled surface
proteins are mixed with XL·Con A coated TCs to form specific conjugates. Upon exposure of the CTL-TC conjugates to UV light, the
photoactivated moiety of XL·Con A on the TCs form covalent bonds
with radiolabeled surface proteins in the contact area of the CTL
surface (step 3). Covalent links also form with Con A itself and
with neighboring proteins on the TC surface, but these proteins are
not radiolabeled. After solubilization of the CTL-TC conjugates
with detergents (step 4) the crosslinked, radiolabeled CTL "contact
proteins" are isolated with affinity purified anti-Con A Ab and
thus separated from other radiolabeled CTL surface proteins which
are not crosslinked (step 5). Reductive cleavage (step 6) of the
susceptible S-S bond in the XL molecule in the immunoprecipitated
complex will then yield radioactive "contact proteins" (step 7)
which can be resolved and revealed by SDS PAGE and autoradiography.

Protein Carrier

The choice of a protein carrier for XL is crucial in this
approach. The ideal protein carrier must have the following characteristics: i) it should be randomly distributed over the TC
surface and be present in the contact area of the CTL-TC conjugate;
ii) it should not interfere with conjugate formation between CTL
and TC; iii) the properties of a protein carrier should not be
altered after coupling to XL; iv) antibody to the protein carrier
should be available; and v) protein carrier tightly bound to TCs
should not be able to interact with radiolabeled CTLs on its own.

Concanavalin A was chosen as a protein carrier because it meets
these requirements and can serve as a vector for delivering XL to
the contact area of the CTL-TC conjugate. The reasons which justify
the use of XL·Con A are as follows: 1) Con A is firmly bound to
structures which are diffusely distributed on the TC surface and
which also appear to be present in the contact areas of CTL-TC conjugates (observed by immunofluorescence microscopy); 2) XL·Con A
binding to the TC does not impair the ability of TCs to be recognized
and lysed by antigen-specific CTLs in the ^{51}Cr-release assay and in
visible conjugate formation assay (9); 3) coupling of 4-6 XL molecules per tetramer of Con A does not detectably alter the binding
and biological properties of Con A (as tested in ^{125}I-labeled Con A
binding assay, [3]HTdR incorporation into Con A- and XL·Con A-treated
normal spleen cells, and its ability to mediate LDCC (data not
shown)); 4) once bound to the TC surface, Con A no longer functions
as a free lectin, i.e., these TC-bound molecules do not transfer to
CTLs or simultaneously bind to glycoproteins on the surface of the
contacting CTL and TC. If XL·Con A on the TC surface were still
able to interact with Con A-binding glycoproteins on CTLs, then
any crosslinked material on CTLs could obviously not be considered

as CTL "contact proteins". This important issue has been dealt with in a detailed study which is described below (Figs. 2 and 3).

Surface Radiolabeling of CTLs

According to the experimental design, the procedure for CTL radiolabeling should be efficient and at the same time mild, so as not to impair the ability of the CTLs to form conjugates and deliver the lethal hit. Several procedures for the cell surface ^{125}I- or ^{3}H-radiolabeling were tested and mock cell surface labeling experiments were performed to estimate the effect of the treatment on conjugate formation and on ^{51}Cr-release from the TCs. ^{125}I-cell surface labeling using lactoperoxidase, glucose oxidase, and glucose proved to be both efficient and mild in not affecting CTL functions. On the basis of these and other considerations, the following procedure was adopted for detection and isolation of cell-cell contact proteins from the CTLs.

Procedure for the Isolation of Cell-Cell "Contact Proteins" from the CTL Surface

Cloned CTLs were twice washed with α-MM in an attempt to remove residual Con A introduced into the culture medium by means of T cell growth factor (IL-2) containing Con A supernatant of rat spleen cells. Dead stimulator cells (BALB/c spleen cells) were removed by Ficoll-Hypaque centrifugation and purified CTLs were ^{125}I-radiolabeled using lactoperoxidase, glucose oxidase, and glucose. Radiolabeled CTLs ($2x10^6$ cells in 0.2 ml of CFM) were then mixed with XL·Con A-P815 ($2x10^6$ cells in 0.2 ml of CFM) in 15 ml conical tubes and centrifuged 3 minutes at 100 x g to facilitate conjugate formation (12,13) followed by incubation at 26° C. After 10 minutes incubation time the cells were resuspended in CFM (in some experiments N_2-saturated CFM was used to decrease UV light induced, oxygen mediated interactions between CTLs and Con A-treated TCs) and a standardized shearing force was applied using a Pipetman micropipette to disperse nonspecific conjugates. After UV light irradiation of the CTL-TC conjugates the cell mixtures were treated with α-MM to remove any traces of noncovalently bound Con A from the surface of radiolabeled CTLs as described in (9). Extraction with detergents and immunoprecipitation with Ab to Con A was then performed. It must be emphasized that the extraction buffer contained 10 mM iodoacetic acid (to prevent possible disulfide exchange between intracellular SH groups and disulfide groups of the XL molecules) and a high concenration of α-MM (200 mM) to preclude the possibility of sugar-specific noncovalent binding of Con A to the radiolabeled CTL proteins in the extraction buffer. Immunoprecipitated "contact proteins" were then treated with the sample buffer and analyzed by SDS PAGE under reducing conditions.

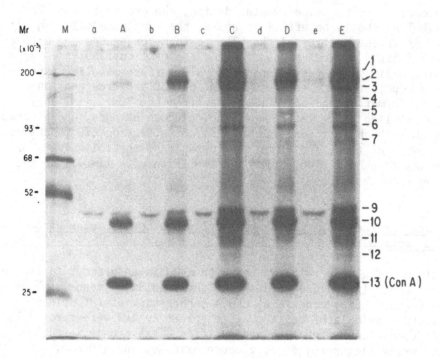

Figure 1. "Contact proteins" from ^{125}I-surface radiolabeled CTL clone 2C (anti-H-2^d) analyzed by SDS-10% PAGE.

Radiolabeled CTL surface proteins are immunoprecipitated according to the procedure for isolation of "contact proteins" after interaction with TCs in different conditions.

Lane A,a: Conjugates were formed between radiolabeled CTLs and Con A-P815 TCs (in absence of XL); B,b: Conjugates were formed between CTLs and XL·Con A-P815 TCs, but they were not UV light irradiated; C,c: Conjugates were formed between CTLs and XL·Con A-P815 TCs in the presence of 25 mM α-MM; after UV light irradiation "contact proteins" were isolated according to the standard procedure; D,d: "Contact proteins" involved in the interaction between CTLs and nonspecific TCs (XL·Con A-EL4); E,e: Radiolabeled CTL surface proteins which are immunoprecipitated with anti-Con A Abs after solubilization of UV irradiated conjugates between CTLs and XL·Con A-P815, according to the standard procedure; M: Radioactive markers. (See legends to Figure 2.)
Lanes a,b,c,d,e: control immunoprecipitates; cell extracts were immunoprecipitated with irrelevant Abs (anti-azobenzenearsonate). Lanes A,B,C,D,E: specific immunoprecipitates with anti-Con A Abs: immunoprecipitated samples were reduced with DTT.

Isolation of "Contact Proteins"

Using the above procedure, a set of radiolabeled CTL surface proteins was immunoprecipitated. The results of a characteristic experiment are shown in Figure 1, Lane E. Approximately 13 protein bands were revealed on the autoradiograph. The most prominent bands are 1 (210 Kd), 2 (190 Kd), 3 (180 Kd), 9 (47 Kd), 10 (43 Kd), 13 (27 Kd) and, in some cases, 11 (38 Kd) and 12 (33 Kd), which are not well seen on this autoradiograph. Which of these bands represent "contact proteins"? According to the experimental design and procedure, the following predictions can be made concerning the isolation of "contact proteins": 1) no "contact proteins" should be immunoprecipitated by anti-Con A Ab if Con A-P815 were used instead of XL·Con A-P815; 2) no "contact proteins" are expected to be immunoprecipitated by anti-Con A Ab when conjugates between CTL and XL· Con A-P815 are not UV light irradiated; and 3) addition of 25 mM of α-MM to the CFM should not affect the SDS PAGE pattern of isolated "contact proteins". Protein bands which correspond to these requirements can be considered as "contact proteins".

The following control experiments were performed to define "contact proteins" among the 13 immunoprecipitated bands (Fig. 1, Lane E). When Con A-P815 formed conjugates with radiolabeled CTLs (Fig. 1, Lane A) instead of XL·Con A-P815, only bands 10 and 13 could be seen in immunoprecipitates isolated according to the same procedure. A faint band with Mr of approximately 45 Kd was revealed in immunoprecipitates with control (irrelevant) Abs and is probably a result of nonspecific precipitation. Band 13 with Mr 27 Kd represents molecules of Con A which were nonspecifically absorbed by CTLs cultured in the presence of rat spleen cells Con A supernatant and subsequently ^{125}I-radiolabeled and immunoprecipitated with Abs to Con A. Band 10 (43 Kd) may represent radiolabeled actin. Other bands (1,2,3,4,5,6,7,8,9,11,12) may be considered as "contact proteins" on the basis of these criteria.

This set of "contact proteins" was missing in immunoprecipitates if conjugates of radiolabeled CTLs and XL·Con A-P815 were not UV light irradiated (Fig. 1, Lane B). Band 2 (in Lane B) was seen at a much lower intensity than after UV light irradiation (Fig. 1, Lane E). Immunoprecipitation of band 2 in Lane B may be the result of nonspecific (not photo-induced) reactions of the disulfide exchange.

When conjugate formation between radiolabeled CTLs and XL·Con A-P815 was performed in the presence of 25 mM α-MM, the same set of "contact proteins" was immunoprecipitated with anti-Con A Abs (Fig. 1, Lane C). We have shown that 25 mM of α-MM very effectively prevents binding of Con A to the cells but is able to release only about 40 % of tightly bound Con A from Con A-TCs.

In another control experiment, "contact proteins" were not

immunoprecipitated if specific conjugate formation was impaired by EDTA, 2-deoxyglucose, cytochalasin D or low temperature (data not shown). On the basis of these experiments, we believe that protein bands 1, 2, 3, 4, 5, 6, 7, 8, 9, 11, 12 correspond to "contact proteins" which are located in the contact area of CTL-TC conjugates.

According to the definition, "contact proteins" must include recognizing structures (T cell receptor) and structures that reinforce and stabilize CTL-TC conjugates (13). Also, cell surface "bystanders", which are irrelevant for CTL effector functions, may be isolated as "contact proteins" from the contact area of the CTL-TC conjugate.

Analysis of the "contact proteins" with mAbs to known CTL surface antigens is in progress, but on the basis of Mr estimation it is possible to suggest that band 2 (190 Kd) probably represents T200, bands 3 (180 Kd) and 6 (105 Kd) probably represent α- and β-chains of LFA-1 (6). It is tantalizing to note that T200 and LFA-1 antigens are the sites of action of N^{α}-tosyl-L-lysyl chloromethyl-ketone (TLCK) on the surface of cloned CTLs (14). TLCK inhibits serine proteases by covalent modification of the active site. Also, T200 and LFA-1 are part of the set of high affinity Con A receptors which we implicated in CTL functions in another study (10). Band 9 (47 Kd) may be a part of a T cell receptor (15,16). The faint band 12 (33 Kd) may represent Lyt-2 antigen (4,5).

It should be noted, however, that the exact chemical mechanism of the interactions between the photosensitive groups of the XL used in these studies and proteins is still not completely clear. Because of this we consider that the set of eleven "contact proteins" may be underestimated; using different crosslinking reagents (carbene-based, for example) and other procedures of radiolabeling, we expect to detect more "contact proteins".

The set of "contact proteins" we isolated using a crosslinking reagent may also include structures which are involved in the assembly of tubular complexes ("ring-like structures") on target membranes (17,18) after interactions with CTL or NK cells.

The approach described here may provide a new way to isolate "contact proteins" not only from the surface of effector cells, but also from the surface of target cells (e.g., NK-sensitive tumor cells) provided that a suitable carrier is available.

It is of great interest to note that the same set of "contact proteins" is involved in the interaction of CTLs with Ag-specific TCs (XL·Con A-P815) (Fig. 1, Lane E) and with nonspecific TCs (XL·Con A-EL4) (Fig. 1, Lane D). It can be argued, however, that Con A-treated, Ag-specific TCs (P815) behave and interact with CTLs as Con A-treated, nonspecific TCs (EL4). Results of two independent experiments support the notion that Con A-P815 are interacting with CTLs in the same way as untreated Ag-specific TCs (P815). First, the same dependence of ^{51}Cr-release on the effector/target cell ratio was reported for P815 and Con A-P815 (10; unpublished results with CTL clones) while up to a ten time greater E/T ratio was necessary to achieve comparable ^{51}Cr-release from Con A-EL4 after interaction with our clones 1D or 2C. Second, Ab to Con A dramatically inhibited CTL-mediated ^{51}Cr-release from Con A-EL4 but did not affect ^{51}Cr-release from Con A-P815.

Despite these significant differences in efficiency of killing and in effect of Ab to Con A, the similarity between the pattern of the "contact proteins" involved in the Ag-specific and nonspecific cytotoxicity (Fig. 1, Lanes D and E) suggests a common mechanism for Ag-specific and lectin-dependent cytotoxicity (LDCC), in agreement with (29). The evaluation of the exact role of the lectin is crucial for understanding the mechanisms of LDCC and Ag-specific cytotoxicity. We therefore used a biochemical approach to address this issue.

Cell Surface Biochemical Approach to Studying the Role of Lectin in LDCC

It is well known that Ag-specific CTLs kill nonspecific TCs, including syngeneic cells, in the presence of lectins (19,20) such as Con A. The exact role of the lectin in this phenomenon (generally refered to as LDCC) is not understood.

Three possible mechanisms have been proposed:

1. Initially, it was suggested that the lectin merely brings effector and target cells into close contact by agglutination (the "Agglutination Model") (19,20). Other studies, however, have indicated that while agglutination may be necessary it is not sufficient because some agglutinating agents are unable to mediate cytotoxicity (21-23).

2. It has also been proposed that only lectins that are both agglutinating and mitogenic for T-cells (i.e., are able to "activate" or "trigger" T cells) will support LDCC (22). However, LDCC can be caused by non-mitogenic lectins, such as wheat germ agglutinin (23; Sitkovsky, unpublished observations). Moreover, the concentration of Con A routinely used for LDCC (10 μg/ml) is hardly mitogenic for murine T-lymphocytes.

3. A third mechanism, the "Recognition Model" (24,25), proposes that CTL can recognize lectin-modified Ags on TCs. This suggestion was based on the observation that LDCC can occur when target cells alone are pretreated with lectin (21,22).

Thus the "recognition" model of LDCC assumes that TC-bound Con A does not bridge CTL to Con A-TC, whereas the "activation" and "agglutination" models require bridging of CTL to TC by Con A. To distinguish between these contradictory requirements we have undertaken a systematic study of the properties and fate of TC-bound Con A.

Binding and Dissociation of Con A from the Cell Surface

Using ^{125}I-Con A we were able to show that one of the interesting features of the process of binding of Con A to cell surface receptors is that an haptenic sugar (α-MM) is much more efficient in preventing the binding of Con A to cells than in displacing cell-bound Con A (data not shown). Similarly, unlabeled ("cold") Con A competes effectively with ^{125}I-Con A (*Con A) for binding to TCs, while the same high concentrations of "cold" Con A are unable to displace cell-bound *Con A (data not shown). Although cell-bound *Con A cannot be displaced by high concentrations of free Con A, 70% of the cell-bound Con A could be eluted from the cell surface by α-MM at very high concentration (200 mM). These results probably reflect the multivalency of Con A and the low probability of spontaneous dissociation of Con A molecules from the cell surface (see below).

To estimate the amount of Con A which can be released from Con A-TCs during incubation with CTLs, radiolabeled Con A was used. *Con A-TCs (1×10^6/ml) were incubated at 37° C and after 3.5 hours the cells were separated from the supernatant and the amount of *Con A on the cells and in the supernatant was determined. In a representative experiment it was found that after incubating EL4 cells with *Con A at 10 µg/ml (37° C, 45 minutes) approximately 1.0 µg of *Con A per 10^6 cells was strongly bound (i.e., remained on the TC surface after six consecutive washes). After 3.5 hours at 37° C approximately 16% of the TC-bound *Con A was released into the culture medium (approximately 0.16 µg of *Con A per 10^6 cells) in immunoreactive form, i.e. all of the *Con A in the supernatant could be immunoprecipitated with anti-Con A Ab and seemed structurally intact (by SDS PAGE analysis).

To determine whether the immunoreactive *Con A released into the supernatant from Con A-EL4 could bind to CTL, the following experiment was carried out. *Con A released from *Con A-EL4 (5×10^6 cells) was added to 5×10^6 pelleted, cloned CTLs. The volume was adjusted to 1 ml with culture medium, the cells were resuspended, and after 1 hour at 37° C the binding of *Con A to CTLs was estimated in the presence or absence of α-MM. Only a negligible amount of *Con A was found to bind to the CTLs (equivalent to 2 ng of Con A); in contrast, after addition of the same amount of "fresh" *Con A to the same number of CTLs a fourfold greater amount of the control *Con A was bound to the CTLs (but still only approximately 9 ng of *Con A). Evidently the amount of Con A released from the TC surface

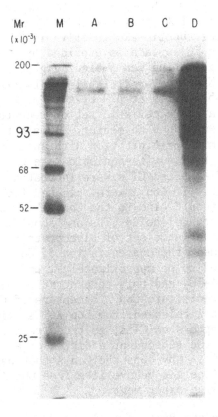

Figure 2. The Con A released from the surface of Con A-TC during incubation at 37°C does not interact with ^{125}I-labeled CTL surface glycoproteins.

[125]I-labeled CTLs (5x10[6] cells) were incubated with either Con A-TC (5x10[6] cells), or free Con A, or alone in 500 µl of culture K medium. After 35 hours at 37°C the cells were pelleted, solubilized in NP-40, and complexes of Con A with radiolabeled CTL surface glycoproteins were immunoprecipitated using antibody to Con A. Samples were reduced with 2-mercaptoethanol and subjected to SDS-10% PAGE and autoradiography. Radioactive standard proteins of known molecular weight (myosin, 200,000 Mr; phosphorylase B, 92,500 Mr; albumin, 68,000 Mr; IgG heavy chain, 52,000 Mr; IgG light chain, 25,000 Mr) (lane M).
Lane A, immunoprecipitates of ^{125}I-labeled CTLs incubated alone; Lane B, immunoprecipitates of ^{125}I-labeled CTLs incubated with Con A-P815; Lane C, immunoprecipitates of ^{125}I-labeled CTLs incubated with Con A-EL4; Lane D, immunoprecipitates of ^{125}I-labeled CTLs incubated with free Con A (1 µg/ml); M, radioactive markers.

is very small and its ability to bind to cells was impaired.

In parallel experiments we examined supernatants of unlabeled Con A-TCs (incubated for 3.5 hours at 37° C) and found that they did not agglutinate CTLs and EL4 (tested with cloned 2C cells). Additional evidence for the functional "inactivation" of Con A that had been released from the TC surface is provided by experiments based on the procedure for isolating Con A-binding glycoproteins, using anti-Con A Ab (10). When ^{125}I-radiolabeled CTLs are incubated with Con A (1 μg/ml) for 45 minutes at 37° C, some of the Con A molecules are tightly bound to a characteristic set of receptors and cannot be removed by extensive washing with medium. This set of receptors can then be isolated by immunoprecipitation with anti-Con A Ab after solubilization of Con A-CTLs with nonionic detergents (Fig. 2, Lane D). Accordingly, ^{125}I-labeled CTLs were incubated with Con A-TCs for 3.5 hours at 37° C. If Con A were released from the Con A-TCs in reactive form, it should bind to the Con A-binding glycoproteins on the surface of the radiolabeled CTLs and should be immunoprecipitated with this characteristic set of glycoproteins (Fig. 2, Lane D). In the present experiment the concentration of Con A released from Con A-TCs was estimated to be approximately 1 μg/ml (based on a parallel assay with *Con A-TC) and this concentration of free Con A is sufficient to immunoprecipitate Con A receptors of CTLs (Fig. 2, Lane D). However, Con A released from Con A-TCs evidently failed to bind to the Con A-receptors on CTLs, as these receptors were not immunoprecipitated by the subsequent addition of anti-Con A Abs (Fig. 2, Lanes B and C). Why does the Con A that has been released from the Con A-TC surface not behave like free Con A? The answer is provided by the following experiment.

Con A is Released from the Surface of Con A-TCs as a Complex with the Target Cells' Con A Binding Glycoproteins

As was shown, *Con A bound to TCs cannot be displaced with "cold" Con A, indicating that spontaneous dissociation of tetravalent Con A from Con A receptors on the cells is a very slow process. Nevertheless, we were able to detect *Con A released from the TC surface medium. It seemed possible, therefore, that the released Con A is not free Con A, but rather that it is associated with the target cells" Con A binding glycoproteins in soluble ligand-receptor complexes. To test this possibility ^{125}I-labeled TCs were coated with Con A, washed, incubated for 4 hours at 37° C and the culture medium (containing released Con A) was immunoprecipitated with anti-Con A Abs. We expected that, if Con A released into the medium from Con A-TCs were complexed with the radiolabeled glycoproteins of the TC surface, then Abs to Con A would immunoprecipitate a specific set of Con A receptors. If, however, Con A is released into the medium as a free molecule then no radioactivity would be immunoprecipitated from the culture medium with Abs to Con A.

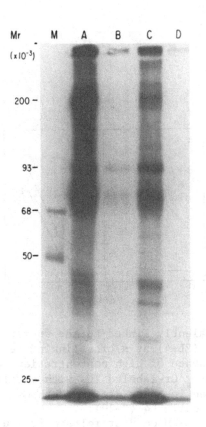

Figure 3

Con A is released from the surface of Con A-TC as a complex with TC Con A-binding proteins.

EL4 cells were ^{125}I-labeled (*EL-4) and Con A-*EL4 were prepared as described for Con A-TC in Materials and Methods. Con A-*EL4 (5x10[6] cells) were incubated at 37°C in 1 ml of RPMI 1640-0.2% BSA and after 3.5 hours the cells were pelleted. Cell pellets were solubilized with extraction buffer and immunoprecipitated with anti-Con A Ab (lane A) or as a control, with anti-DNP Ab (lane B). Cell culture supernatants, containing Con A released from Con A-TCs, were immunoprecipitated with anti-Con A Ab (lane C) or with control, anti-DNP Ab (lane D). Lane M: radioactive markers (see Figure 2).

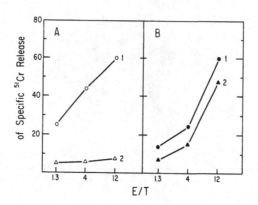

Figure 4. Con A covalently linked to the surface of an Ag-non-specific target cell (EL-4) by a crosslinking reagent can mediate LDCC even in the presence of high concentrations of α-MM. Details of the preparation of ^{51}Cr-labeled TCs with covalently attached XL·Con A are described in Materials and Methods. CTL: clone 1D (anti-H-2D^d); Target cell EL4 (H-2^b).

Panel A: Effect of α-MM on ^{51}Cr release from untreated EL-4 in the presence of XL·Con A and CTLs (absence of light).

1 – Untreated EL4 cells (wrong target) were mixed with CTLs and XL·Con A (final concentration 10 μg/ml); reaction in the dark avoided crosslinking of XL·Con A to the target cells.

2 – The same as in (1); α-MM (0.2M) was also included.

Panel B: Effect of α-MM on ^{51}Cr release from TCs with covalently linked XL·Con A in the presence of CTLs.

(1) XL Con·A was covalently linked to the TC surface by UV light irradiation of XL·Con A-TC (^{51}Cr-labeled) and mixed with CTLs. (2) The same as in (1); α-MM (0.2M final concentration) was also included.

As can be seen in Figure 3, anti-Con A Abs immunoprecipitated the same set of radiolabeled Con A receptors from the culture supernatant containing released Con A as it did from Con A-TC. These results strongly suggest that Con A-receptor complexes, not free Con A, are "shed" from Con A-TC. Thus, it is understandable that the released Con A cannot react as a lectin which agglutiantes CTLs and TCs and causes LDCC.

The possibility still existed, however, that molecules of Con A, tightly bound to TCs, could use one or two of their four binding sites to bridge neighboring CTLs to Con A-TCs. To exclude this possibility, we carried out a cytotoxicity assay in the presence of α-MM, which completely prevents the binding of Con A to CTLs.

Con A Covalently Linked to the TC Surface Can Mediate LDCC Even in the Presence of α-MM

To perform the cytotoxicity assay in the presence of α-MM some measures had to be taken to prevent elution of TC-bound Con A from the cell surface. To "fix" Con A on the TC surface we used a bifunctional, non-cleavable crosslinking reagent (N-succinimidyl-6(4'-azido-2'-nitrophenylamino) hexanoate (Lomant reagent II)) which was coupled to Con A in the dark (XL·Con A) (see Materials and Methods). After binding the XL·Con A to ^{51}Cr-labeled TCs and washing the cells extensively to remove unbound (or weakly bound) XL·Con A, the cells were irradiated with UV light to initiate the photoinduced crosslinking of Con A to the cell surface of glycoproteins. In a parallel experiment with unlabeled TCs we found that multiple washings with α-MM removed 30% of the photoactivated XL·Con A from the cells, leaving 70% irreversibly bound.

In the experiment outlined in Figure 4, UV light irradiated, ^{51}Cr-labeled XL·Con A-TCs were used as targets in a ^{51}Cr-release assay in the presence of α-MM. As can be seen from these results, α-MM completely inhibited LDCC when ^{51}Cr-labeled TCs were mixed with CTLs and soluble XL·Con A at 10 µg/ml (reaction in the dark) (Fig. 4, Panel A). In contrast, α-MM at 200 mM had little effect on ^{51}Cr-release from XL·Con A-TCs in which the XL·Con A was covalently linked to the TCs (Fig. 4, Panel B). This concentration of α-MM virtually excludes specific interactions between CTLs and Con A, including the Con A covalently bound to the TC surface; nevertheless, LDCC was observed (Fig. 4, Panel B). Pretreatment of TCs with XL-modified soybean lectin did not result in LDCC (data not shown); this excludes the possibility of a nonspecific effect of XL molecules as the cause of ^{51}Cr-release. The results of the experiments presented here demonstrate clearly that Ag-specific killing of Con A-TCs by CTLs is not due to bridging of CTLs to Con A-TCs.

The most compatible with our results is the "recognition" model of LDCC (24,25) which was based on observations (21,22) that Con A-

TCs are susceptible to lysis by CTLs. The main assumptions of this model are:

1. Con A on the surface of Con A-TCs does not link these cells to CTLs.

2. The TC-bound lectin acts by modifying the MHC antigens on the TC surface so that these antigens can then interact with the antigen-recognizing receptors of the CTLs.

In arguing for the first assumption it was shown (24,25) that Con A-pretreatment of CTLs does not lead to effective LDCC. Interpretation of these results was based on the additional assumption, now known to be incorrect, that Con A-CTLs express the same level of cytotoxicity as untreated CTLs. In fact, Con A-CTLs have greatly reduced cytotoxic activity (9,26) probably because Con A binds tightly on these cells to LFA-1 (10), which is evidently necessary for cytotoxicity (27,28).

For these reasons it was important to explore more thoroughly the possibility that Con A which has been shed from the surface of Con A-TCs, or even Con A that is still attached to the TCs, might still be able to link the Con A-TCs to neighboring CTLs.

Our results show that the Con A released from Con A-TCs could not bind to (Fig. 2) or agglutinate CTLs and TCs because the Con A released into the medium was in the form of lectin-high affinity receptor complexes (Fig. 3). Moreover, even if it were functionally active the amount and concentration of the released Con A (calculated for the conditions of the usual ^{51}Cr-release assay) would be too low to mediate LDCC. Finally, the most convincing evidence against the possibility that LDCC requires bridging of CTL to TC by a lectin was shown by the failure of α-MM to block Ag-specific lysis by CTLs of TCs to which Con A was covalently attached by a crosslinking reagent (Fig. 4).

Taken together, these data point to lectin-induced changes on the TC surface as the basis for TC-lysis by CTLs in LDCC. The identitiy of the TC surface structures that bind Con A with relatively high affinity (Con A-receptors on Con A-TCs) and the ability of monoclonal antibodies to these receptors to substitute for Con A in LDCC (a new phenomenon of Ab-dependent CTL-mediated cytotoxicity) will be described elsewhere.

REFERENCES

1. Berke, G. Cytotoxic T-lymphcytes: How do they function? Immunol. Rev. 72:5 (1983).
2. Martz, M., W. Heagy, and S.H. Gromkowski. The mechanism of

CTL—mediated killing: monoclonal antibody analysis of the roles of killer and target cell membrane proteins. Immunol. Rev. 72: 73 (1983).

3. Bonavida, B., T. Bradley, J. Fan, J. Hiserodt, R. Effros, and H. Wexler. Molecular interactions in T-cell mediated cytotoxicity. Immunol. Rev. 72:119 (1983).

4. Shinohara, N. and D.H. Sachs. Mouse alloantibodies capable of blocking cytotoxic T-cell function. I. Relationship between the antigen reactive with blocking antibodies and the Lyt-2 locus. J. Exp. Med. 150:432 (1979).

5. Nakayama, E., H. Shiku, E. Stockert, H.F. Oettgen, and L.J. Old. Cytotoxic T cells: Lyt phenotype and blocking activity by Lyt antisera. Proc. Natl. Acad. Sci. 76:1977 (1979).

6. Davignon, D., E. Martz, T. Reynolds, K. Kurzinger, and T.A. Springer. Lymphocyte function-associated antigen 1 (LFA-1): a surface antigen distinct from Lyt-2,3 that participates in T lymphocyte-mediated killing. Proc. Natl. Acad. Sci. 78:4535 (1981).

7. Krensky, A.M., F. Sanchez-Madrid, E. Robbins, J.A. Nagy, T.A. Springer, and S.J. Burakoff. The functional significance, distribution, and structure of LFA-1, LFA-2, and LFA-3: cell surface antigens associated with CTL-target interactions. J. Immunol. 131:611 (1983).

8. Cantor, H., M. Kasai, F.W. Shen, J.C. Leclerc, and L. Glimcher. Immunogenetic analysis of "natural killer" activity in the mouse. Immunol. Rev. 44:3 (1979).

9. Sitkovsky, M.V., M.S. Pasternack, and H.N. Eisen. Inhibition of cytotoxic T lymphocyte activity by Concanavalin A. J. Immunol. 129:1372 (1982).

10. Sitkovsky, M.V., M.S. Pasternack, J.P. Lugo, J.P. Klein, and H.N. Eisen. Isolation and partial characterization of Concanavalin A receptors on cloned cytotoxic T lymphocytes. Proc. Natl. Acad. Sci. 81:1519 (1984).

11. Schwarz, M.A., O.P. Das, and R.O. Hynes. A new radioactive crosslinking reagent for studying the interactions of proteins. J. Biol. Chem. 257:2343 (1982).

12. Schick, B. and G. Berke. Competitive inhibition of cytotoxic T lymphocyte-target cell conjugation. A direct evaluation of membrane antigens involved in cell-mediated immunity. Transplantation 27:365 (1979).

13. Shortman, K. and P. Goldstein. Target cell recognition by cytolytic T cells: different requirements for the formation of strong conjugates or for proceeding to lysis. J. Immunol. 123:833 (1979).

14. Pasternack, M.S., M.V. Sitkovsky, and H.N. Eisen. The site of action of N^{α}-Tosyl-L-Lysyl Chloromethylketone (TLCK) on cloned cytotoxic T lymphocytes. J. Immunol. 131:2477 (1983).

15. Haskins, K., R. Kubo, J. White, M. Pigeon, J. Kappler, and P. Marrack. The major histocompatibility complex restricted antigen receptor on T cells. I. Isolation with a monoclonal

antibody. J. Exp. Med. 157:1149 (1983).

16. Acuto, O., R.E. Hussey, K.A. Fitzgerald, J.P. Protentis, S.C. Heuer, S.F. Schlossman, and E.L. Reinherz. The human T cell receptor: appearance in ontogeny and biochemical relationship of and subunits on IL-2 dependent clones and T cell tumors. Cell 34:717 (1983).

17. Henkart, M.P. and P.A. Henkart. Lymphocyte-mediated cytolysis as a secretory phenomenon. In "Mechanisms of Cell-Mediated Cytotoxicity." W.R. Clark and P. Goldstein, eds. Plenum Press, New York, p. 243 (1982).

18. Dennert, G. and E.R. Podack. Cytolysis by H-2 specific T killer cells: assembly of tubular complexes on target membranes. J. Exp. Med. 157:1483 (1983).

19. Forman, J. and G. Moller. Generation of cytotoxic lymphocytes in mixed lymphocyte reactions. J. Exp. Med. 138:672 (1973).

20. Bevan, M.J. and M. Cohn. Cytotoxic effects of antigen- and mitogen-induced T-cells on various targets. J. Immunol. 114: 559 (1975).

21. Bonavida, B. and T. Bradley. Studies on the induction and expression of T cell-mediated immunity. V. Lectin-induced nonspecific cell-mediated cytotoxicity by alloimmune lymphocytes. Transplantation 21:54 (1976).

22. Green, W.R., Z.K. Ballas, and C.S. Henney. Studies on the mechanism of lymphocyte-mediated cytolysis. XI. The role of lectin in lectin-dependent cell-mediated cytotoxicity. J. Immunol. 121:1566 (1978).

23. Parker, W.L. and E. Martz. Lectin-induced nonlethal adhesions between cytolytic T-lymphocytes and antigenically unrecognizable tumor cells and nonspecific "triggering" of cytolysis. J. Immunol. 124:25 (1980).

24. Berke, G., V. Hu, E. Mcvey, and W.R. Clark. T lymphocyte-mediated cytolysis. I. A common mechanism for target recognition in specific and lectin-dependent cytolysis. J. Immunol. 127:776 (1981).

25. Berke, G., E. McVey, V. Hu, and W.R. Clark. T lymphocyte-mediated cytolysis. II. Role of target cell histocompatibility antigens in recognition and lysis. J. Immunol. 127:782 (1981).

26. Beretta, A., N. Persson, T. Ramos, and G. Moller. Con A inhibits the effector phase of specific cytotoxicity. Scand. J. Immunol. 16:181 (1982).

27. Davignon, D., E. Martz, T. Reynolds, K. Kurzinger, and T.A. Springer. Lymphocyte function-associated antigen one (LFA-1): a surface antigen distinct from Lyt-2/3 that participates in T lymphocyte-mediated killing. Proc. Natl. Acad. Sci. 78:4535 (1981).

ACKNOWLEDGEMENTS

This work was supported in part by research grants (CA-15472 and CA-28900), a Center Grant (CA-14051), and a Training Grant (CA-09255) from the National Cancer Institute. M.V. Sitkovsky is a recipient of a New Investigator Research Award (NIH Grant 1-R23 CA/AI 37439-01).

DISCUSSION

V. Hu: A point of clarification: were you suggesting that the unreactivity of the Con A treated CTLs was because Con A was inhibiting CTL activity?

M. Sitkovsky: Yes, Con A inhibits all CTL clones that I have tried, as well as CTL from MLC.

V. Hu: I think we did an experiment with Berke and Clark which showed that Con A-treated CTLs can kill Con A-treated targets.

M. Sitkovsky: Yes, but the effect is two-times less.

G. Berke: I think this point needs to be clarified (it has been reviewed extensively in the last Immunol. Rev. volume 72). Con A-pretreated effector cells can undergo two processes. One, they can self-annihilate due to lectin-pretreated killer cells interacting with either lectin-pretreated or non-pretreated killer cells. So there is a lymphocyte-lymphocyte interaction that on the average would render the population annihilated. What you present is a different explanation for that annihilation, namely, that Con A interacting with a CTL annihilates it as such. What we would argue is that this annihilation (Ben [Bonavida] has shown that it does occur) is not due to the Con A effect on the killer, but is because Con A affects some killer cells and renders them as target cells to other killer cells in the population. As a matter of fact, I think a direct study, which I refer to in my review, actually showed this. Besides that, I absolutely agree with you in the thesis that Clark and myself have been thinking about, namely, that killer cells utilizing their specific antigen receptors can recognize target cell entities that are modified by either lectin, or, as you showed, perhaps by antibodies.

M. Sitkovsky: This possibility, that is self-kill, was addressed in my first publication. We labelled the CTL clone, then added the same CTL cells unlabelled, Con A was added, and there was only 15% chromium release. This showed two things. CTL themselves are very poor targets. Second, that in our hands, inhibition cannot be explained by self-kill.

E. Martz: I would like to caution against the interpretation that because anti-clonotype blocks these kinds of non-specific killing (Con A induced or anti-target antibody induced killing) we can conclude that the clonotypic receptor on the killer is a direct participant in those nonspecific kinds of killing. Logically, its the same problem we have with anti-LFA-1-mediated inhibition. The fact that the antibody inhibits does not prove that the antigen, in this case the clonotype, is a direct participant in the process. It may simply be called in by the antibody to deliver a negative signal.

M. <u>Sitkovsky</u>: Of course, I agree.

SECTION 5. POST-BINDING EVENTS IN THE CYTOTOXIC PROCESS

INTRODUCTION

The nature of the biochemical events in the killer cell after binding of the target cell has been the subject of numerous
investigations, largely through the effect of drugs on the post
binding events as defined by the approaches worked out in the
1970s by several groups. This approach is exemplified in this
section by the chapter by Redelman and Hudig, using new agents to
further define both the binding and post binding processes. The
initial chapter by Russell and Howe discusses several new
approaches to delineate post-binding events. These involve
manipulation of cloned CTL to give cells which can bind targets
but do not go on to kill.

Studies on the events in the dying target cell have been
stimulated by Russell's description of a rapid DNA breakdown
induced by CTL but not by agents causing colloid osmotic lysis.
In this section both Tirosh and Berke, and Cohen et al., discuss
their rather different theories of target cell damage, and Sears
and Christiaansen show that the rapid target cell DNA breakdown
is observed with ADCC as well as CTL killing.

The final two chapters in this section are concerned with
rather different subjects. In Mechanisms of Cell-Mediated
Cytotoxicity, Yael Kaufmann described CTL hybridomas whose growth
is not dependent on exogenous IL-2. In this section she
describes experiments which suggest that these cells are actually
closer to CTL memory cells, in that a post-binding element in
their cytotoxic pathway is inoperative until antigen stmulation
occurs. The final chapter is a quantitative analysis of single
CTL cytotoxicity experiments by Perelson, et al., which
eliminates some models of post-binding CTL-target interactions.

EVIDENCE FOR THE MOLECULAR DISSOCIATION OF BINDING AND POST-BINDING FUNCTIONS IN CYTOTOXIC T LYMPHOCYTES

John H. Russell and Rawleigh C. Howe

Department of Pharmacology
Washington University Medical School
660 South Euclid Ave., St. Louis, Mo 63110

INTRODUCTION

The interaction between the cytotoxic T lymphocyte (CTL) and its target cell has been a model of immune cellular interaction for several years because of the relatively short time course between the actual receptor-ligand interaction and its functional expression in target cell lysis. The nature of the lethal event within the target remains unclear but recent experiments from our laboratory and others have suggested that CTL mediated lysis involves not only the production of an osmotic lesion in the plasma membrane but also rapid changes in nuclear and chromatin structure (see ref. #1 for review). This nuclear lesion distinguishes CTL mediated lysis from cell death mediated by Ab+C[1] or hypotonic shock.

It has previously been demonstrated that both the cytoplasmic (2,3) and nuclear (4) lesions can be functionally divided into binding and post-binding events. The binding event involves a recognition step between the CTL and target followed by a stable adhesion between the two cells. This step requires Mg^{+2} but not Ca^{+2}, and occurs equally well at 20° and 37° but not at 0°. This binding step is reversible in that targets can be rescued after incubation of effector target conjugates under conditions that are permissive for binding but non permissive for post-binding effects to occur.

The post-binding stage of the lytic sequence under normal conditions occurs only in the presence of Ca^{+2} and at tempera tures > 30°. It is during this period of time that irreversible damage is initiated in the target. In order to better understand the link between these functional processes, it is important to know if this separation of functional activity represents separate functions of a single molecule or multiple molecules with specific functions.

Over the past several years it has become apparent that antibodies to a variety of molecules on both the effector (5,6) and the target (6) can interfere with CTL mediated lysis. Most of these molecules appear to interfere with the binding step of the lytic process either directly through their interaction with the receptor or indirectly through their interaction with accessory molecules involved in stabilizing the adhesion between the CTL and its target. It has been reported that the molecule recognized by OKT 3 blocks a post-binding event (7) but this interpretation has been disputed by other laboratories (5).

The recent experiments of Harris et al. on the transfer of specific lytic activity from the CTL to lymphocytes (including B cell tumors) with no demonstrable lytic activity of their own (8) suggest a simple relationship between the receptor and the lytic apparatus. Because this transfer is accomplished by means of a simple membrane fusion between the acceptor cell and liposomes prepared from cell extracts of CTL clones, these authors have suggested that lysis is mediated either by the receptor itself or a relatively simple molecular complex from the CTL. The latter observation would appear to be inconsistant with the involvement of intracellular components described by others (9).

In this report we have addressed the issue of single or multiple molecules being involved in the binding and post-binding events by asking whether the two functions are coordinately regulated during the immune induction cycle. These results suggest that binding and post-binding are not coordinately expressed and therefore may be functions of independent molecular species. In addition we have found pretreatment of CTL clones with phorbol esters produces a cell that has apparently normal total binding capacity but reduced or no post-binding capacity. Recovery from PMA treatment does not require immune signals but does require protein synthesis which suggests that PMA can selectively deplete molecules involved in post-binding processes without affecting those molecules affecting binding.

MATERIALS AND METHODS

Media. The base medium for maintenance of cells and production of conditioned medium was RPM1-1640 supplemented with heat inactivated (56°, 45') fetal calf serum, glutamine, mercaptoethanol, non-essential amino acids, sodium pyruvate, penicillin-streptomycin and HEPES buffer as described previously. Cytotoxicity assays were performed in RPM1-1640 without bicarbonate but supplemented with 15 mM HEPES and 3-5% heat inactivated bovine calf serum. Sera were purchased from K.C. Biological (Lenexa KS) HEPES and mercaptoethanol from Sigma (St. Louis, Mo.). All other media components were from GIBCO (Grand Island, NB).

Reagents. 4β-phorbol and its esters were purchased from Sigma, dissolved (10^{-2} or 10^{-3}M) in dimethyl sulfoxide (DMSO, Sigma), aliquoted and stored at -70° until use. Cycloheximide (Sigma) was stored as 1 M aliquots in DMSO until use.

Animals: C57BL/6J ($H-2^b$), CBA/J ($H-2^k$), and DBA/2J ($H-2^d$) mice were purchased from The Jackson Laboratory (Bar Harbor, ME).

CTL clones. C57BL/6 anti DBA/2 clones were derived from secondary mixed lymphocyte cultures by a modification of the method of Glasebrook and Fitch (10) as described previously (11). CTL 3 is a heteroclitic clone that is strongly lytic against D^k (12). CTL 7 recogonizes a determinant shared by K^d and D^d (unpublished). Both clones are strongly Thy 1.2^+ and Lyt 2.2^+ with little or no reactivity to Lyt 1.2. Clones were maintained by weekly stimulation with irradiated DBA/2 spleen cells and conditioned medium from 30-36 h secondary mixed lymphocyte cultures as previously described (11). CTL 3 and 7 are constituitively lytic. That is their lytic activity on a per cell basis is constant throughout the weekly stimulation cycle.

The cloned continuous cell line CTL-108 was propogated as described (11). Briefly, $5X10^4$ CTL were stimulated every 7-8 days with $3X10^6$ irradiated DBA/2 spleen cells and 12-30% secondary MLC SN in 1.5 ml RPM1 media in 16 mm diameter Linbro plates. The line was recloned every 6-12 wk at limiting dilution in Falcon Microtest II plates in the presence of 10^6 irradiated DBA/2 spleen cells plus 25-33% MLC SN in a volume of 300 μl. Proliferating subclones were maintained for 2-3 weekly stimulations with above supplement in microwells prior to expansion in larger (16 mm) wells.

Targets. The murine tumors P815 ($H-2^d$) and EL-4 ($H-2^b$) were maintained and labeled with ^{125}iodo-5'-deoxyuridine (^{125}IUdR Amersham, Arlington Hgts, IL) as previously described (4). Lymphoblast targets were prepared by harvesting spleen cells, lysing red blood cells and incubating for two days at $2x10^6$/ml in medium containing 2 μg/ml concanavalin A (Con A). Lymphoblasts were labelled with ^{125}IUdR as described (4).

<u>Cytotoxicity assays.</u> A 1 hr. detergent soluble ^{125}IUdR release
assay was used with tumor targets and a similar 1.5 hr assay for
lymphoblast targets (4). Briefly, 5×10^3 target cells in 100 µl
cytotoxicity medium were mixed with 100 µl of medium containing
$0-1 \times 10^5$ effector cells in 12x75 mm polystyrene tubes. The mixture was centrifuged 200 x g, 2' and incubated for the appropriate time (37°) in a water bath. The assay was terminated by
adding 1 ml of buffered saline containing 0.2% Triton X-100
(Sigma) centrifuging 700 x g, 5' and separating one-half (0.6
ml) of the supernatant from the remainder of the supernatant
plus the pellet. % specific release (%S.R.) was calculated as
described (4).

In general, spontaneous release was < 10% for tumor targets and
< 20% for lymphoblast targets.

<u>Inhibition of Lytic activity</u> CTL harvested 4-6 days after the
previous stimulation were washed and plated at $4-10 \times 10^5$/ml in
6 or 16 mm wells (Linbro, Flow Laboratories, McLean, VA) in 0.2
or 1 ml of medium containing 10% MLC conditioned medium respectively. To each well was added either nothing or DMSO with or
without phorbol compounds. The highest concentration of DMSO
was .01% which has no effect on lytic activity or clonal proliferation (unpublished). At the appropriate time, cultures were
harvested, centrifuged, resuspended in cytotoxicity medium,
diluted and assayed for lytic activity. Aliquots were counted
and cell recoveries were within 10% of control.

In some experiments (Figs. 5,7), the inhibition of lytic
potential was determined by comparing the % specific release of
experimental/control X100 at E:T resulting in 15-50% specific
release by the control cultures (see Fig. 5). The results are
expressed as mean ± S.E.M. of 3-5 points on the E:T curve. This
method rather than the more traditional lytic units method was
adopted for two reasons. First, in situations where inhibition
is significant, it becomes very expensive in terms of cells to
observe an arbitrary 20-40% specific release value. Second,
because the lytic unit method compares activity at a single,
arbitiary % lysis, it does not provide information about changes
in the slope of the E:T curve. By comparing lysis at a number
of E:T ratios along what is the linear portion of the E:T curve
in the control, changes in slope are also incorporated in our
method. The weakness in the method used here is that, because
of the error in accurately assessing low levels of lysis, 5-10
fold changes (80-90% inhibition) in lytic efficiency cannot be
reliably distinguished from > 10 fold changes. Thus the % inhibition method described above allows a relative comparison of
the 10-80% reduction in lytic activity in the situations for
which it is used here, but can underestimate the overall change
in lytic activity.

Recovery from PMA. CTL clones were cultured with or without PMA as described above. After 15-16 hrs, cultures were harvested, centrifuged and washed four times in ice cold medium. Cells were counted and one aliquot removed for assessment of lytic activity. The remainder of cells were cultured (1×10^5/ml) for 3 hrs. at 37° in medium (1 ml) alone or medium containing 20% MLR conditioned medium. Cultures were harvested and lytic activity determined as described above.

Determination of protein synthesis. Cells were cultured as for determination of recovery from PMA inhibition. ^{35}S-methionine (New England Nuclear, Boston, MA) was added to some cultures (final concentration = 100 µCi/ml). After a seven hour incubation in ^{35}S- methionine, cultures were harvested, washed once and the pellets dissolved in 0.2 ml 0.1 N NaOH containing 1 mg/ml BSA (siliconized 12x75 mm glass tube). Tubes were incubated 37°, 30 min before adding 0.2 ml ice cold 20% TCA and incubated overnight at 4°. Pellets were centrifuged (2000 x g, 10 min) and washed four times with 1 ml ice cold 10% TCA. The final pellet was dissolved in 0.2 ml NCS (Amersham, Arlington Hgts. IL) by incubation at 37° for one hour. The solution was neutralized with glacial acetic acid and an aliquot counted in 4 ml PCS II (Amersham) by liquid scintillation spectrometry (Beckman, Palo Alto CA).

Binding and post binding assays. Binding was determined by mixing 50 µl of effectors ($0.1-2 \times 10^6$/ml) with 50 µl of targets ($2-4 \times 10^6$/ml) in 12x75 mm polystyrene tubes and centrifuging (200 x g, 2 min). Tubes were incubated 20 min, 20° before mixing by vigorous agitation followed by 6 up and down strokes of an adjustable pipettor. Aliquots were taken for determination of conjugates by counting (400Xphase contrast microscope). Effectors were distinguished from tumor targets by the difference in cell size. To determine the rate of post-binding events, cultures were diluted (5 ml) with warm (37°) cytotoxicity medium after dispersing conjugates as described above. At the indicated times after dilution, cultures were mixed by agitation and triplicate 100 µl aliquots were added to 1 ml PBS containing 0.02% Triton X-100 for determination of soluble ^{125}IUdR. To control for initiation of new conjugates during the post binding assays, a separate, parallel culture consisted of 50 µl of effectors and targets being added to the 5 ml of cytotoxicity medium without a prior centrifugation and binding incubation.

Single-cell assay in Agarose. The single cell assay was performed essentially as described (13). Conjugates were diluted to ~ 5×10^5 targets/ml, and added to an equal volume of 0.5% agarose (Type I, Sigma) which had been boiled and cooled to 39°C immediately before use. 100 µl of the cell suspension was spread in a thin layer over glass slides previously coated with

0.1% agarose. The slides were immersed in Coplan glass jars containing warm media, and incubated for various lengths of time at 37°C. Lysis was terminated by dipping the slides in 0.1% trypan blue for 5 minutes followed by a quick rinse in PBS. Slides were immediately examined under a phase contrast microscope or following fixation in 0.3% formalin. Results are expressed as % of conjugated targets lysed, corrected for background lysis of targets alone.

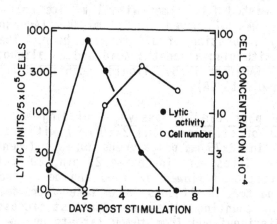

Figure 1

Time course of CTL-108 proliferation and lytic activity. Cells were assayed on day 0 and at the indicated times after stimulation of 2×10^5 CTL with 10^7 irradiated DBA/2 spleen cells plus 25% MLC SN in 4.5 ml Falcon T25 flasks placed in the upright position. Varying numbers of CTL were mixed with 5×10^3 ^{125}IUdR labelled targets and % specific release determined after 5 h at 37°C. One lytic unit is defined arbitrarily as the absolute number of CTL required to lyse 30% of P815 targets, extrapolated from the linear portion of E:T curves. Spontaneous isotope release ranged from 2.4±1 to 5.6±0.5%.

RESULTS

We have isolated a cloned CTL that has the characteristic increase in lytic activity after stimulation with antigen and conditioned medium (Fig. 1) that had been observed earlier for a secondary response of CTL in culture (11). The increase in lytic activity is subsequently lost so that with each weekly stimulation the cells rapidly change from a weakly or non lytic state to a highly lytic state and slowly return to the weakly lytic state. We have previously demonstrated that the increase in lytic activity is antigen specific, is on a per cell basis and is the result of a single clone (11).

Thus this clone allows us to investigate the changes in the lytic properties of the cell at various states of activation. We considered two possible explanations at the level of the lytic mechanism to explain these changes in functional activity. The first was that there would be no changes in the lytic properties of individual cells but simply alterations in the relative frequencies in the population of cells with or without lytic activity. The second possibility was that the lytic efficiency of the individual cells would change as a result of immune induction.

Others have shown that, from the standpoint of the CTL, the lytic process can be dividied into two stages. Initially the CTL binds to the target cell in a process that occurs equally well at temperatures from 20°-37° but not at 0° and requires Mg^{+2} but not Ca^{+2} (2,3). The second or post-binding stage is that part of the process where irreversible damage is done to the target and requires temperatures >30° and under normal situations extracellular Ca^{+2} but not Mg^{+2} (2,3).

The capacity of the cells to carry out the binding process can be approximated by allowing the cells to bind under permissive conditions for binding but not post binding, dispersing the conjugates and enumerating the fraction of effector cells binding to specific or non specific targets. Changes in the post-binding process can be determined again by allowing effectors and targets to bind under conditions permissive for binding but not post-binding, dispersing the conjugates and changing the conditions to those that are permissive for post binding events. Measuring the subsequent rate of target cell destruction allows an estimation of the post-binding efficiency.

We tested the binding capacity of optimally induced and non induced cells against specific $H-2^d$ (P815) and non specific (K562 or EL-4) targets. The results (Fig. 2) demonstrated that a large fraction of both effector populations could form antigen specific conjugates but higher cell densities in the pellet were

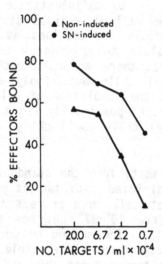

Figure 2. Effect of cell concentration on conjugate formation. CTL-108 were harvested 6d following stimulation with allogeneic cells plus MLC SN (open figures), or following 2 days SN induction (closed figures). Cells were washed and mixed on ice with P815 tumor targets at an E:T of 0.3:1, and the resulting mixture was serially diluted into several tubes. Following centrifugation, tubes were placed in a 20°C water bath for 30 minutes, and shear force resistant conjugates enumerated under a phase contrast microscope. The data shown represent the average of duplicate samples. Greater than 200 cells were counted in each of the samples.

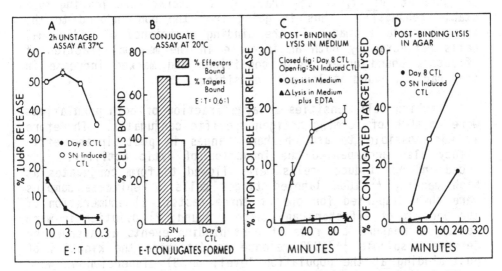

Figure 3   Induction of binding and programming capacity of CTL-
108.   CTL-108 cells were harvested from day 8 cultures following
stimulation with allogeneic cells plus MLC SN or following MLC
SN alone.   Panel A: Varying numbers of effector cells were
added to 5×10^3 P815 targets and cytolysis monitored in a 2h
Triton-developed ^{125}IUdR assay.   Panel B: 6×10^4 CTL (induced or
non-induced) were added to 10^5 targets and conjugate formation
(shear force resistant) determined after 20 minutes at 20°C.
Total effector cell counts were 138 (non-induced CTL-target
mixtures) and 60 (induced CTL-target mixtures).   Total target
cell counts were 552 (non-induced CTL target mixtures) and 138
(induced CTL-target mixtures).   Panel C: Conjugates were
diluted to 10^3 targets /ml for the indicated lengths of time.
EDTA was added to 1.0 mM, the tubes vortexed vigorously and
incubated an additional 60 minutes, and cytolysis assessed by
the addition of Triton X - 100 to 0.2% (circles).   The
additional   incubation   was   included   to   allow   additional
expression of killer-cell independent lysis (KCIL).   Treatment
of conjugates with 10 mM EDTA following the 20 minute binding
incubation at 20°C resulted in less than 1% specific release
when assayed after dispersion for 100 minutes at 37°C.   This
indicates that no programming for lysis occured during the
binding incubation.   Spontaneous release and recycling control
values were $\leq$ 2% for all time points tested.   Panel D:
Conjugates were diluted to 2.5×10^5 targets/ml and added to an
equal volume of molten agar and incubated at 37° for various
times as described in materials and methods.

required for the non induced cells to achieve similar fractional binding. Since the E:T ratio was constant over the entire binding, curve the differences in binding probably reflect changes in apparent avidity or the fraction of interactions leading to a stable conjugate. Thus in going from the non induced to the induced state a change in the binding efficiency of individual cells reflected by both an increase in the maximal fraction of effectors bound under these conditions and marked increase in the fraction bound at low cell densities.

At high cell densities a large fraction of both populations were capable of forming antigen specific conjugates. Therefore it was possible to ask whether changes in post-binding efficiency also accompanied the induction of lytic activity. Induced and non induced cells were allowed to form conjugates at high density ^{125}IUdR labeled target cells. Replicate samples were then dispersed for one of three tests: 1) enumeration of the percent of effectors and targets bound; 2) dilution in warm medium to measure the rate of post-binding events as assayed by detergent soluble ^{125}IUdR release to determine the kinetics of post-binding at the population level; or 3) dispersion in warm agarose (13) to determine post-binding at the level of individual cells (trypan blue uptake of bound targets). These results (Fig. 3) demonstrate that marked changes in the efficiency (rate) of lysis of bound targets accompanies induction of lytic activity with T cell conditioned medium. This is reflected both in the isotope release assay and in the single cell assay in agarose. Since the induced cells bound ~ 40% of the targets (Panel B) the 20% specific release in 100 minutes (Panel C) would represent 50% lysis of bound targets. This is approximately equivalent to the lysis in the single cell assay after 4 hrs (Panel D). Lysis by non induced cells was much slower such that < 10% of the attached targets were lysed in 100 minutes in the isotope assay (Panel C) and less than 20% by 4 hrs in the single cell assay (Panel D). Thus by either assay, marked changes in post-binding efficiency are observed between optimally induced and non induced cells.

Based on these experiments it was of interest to evaluate the lytic mechanism of cells with intermediate overall activity. This was accomplished by comparing the binding and post-binding capacities of cells taken 4 days after stimulation with antigen and conditioned medium (intermediate activity) with those taken 6 days after stimulation (low activity) or similar cells after a 24 hour induction with conditioned medium (high activity). The results (Fig. 4) demonstrated that cells with intermediate overall activity have the binding properties of high activity CTL but the post-binding efficiency of low activity CTL. This suggests that these two functional activities can be separated in individual cells.

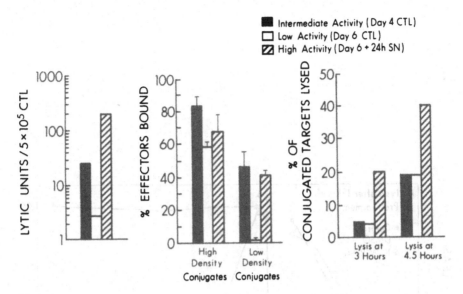

Figure 4

Binding and post-binding capacities of CTL with intermediate, low, and high lytic activity.

CTL-108 cells were harvested after 4 or 6 days of culture with DBA/2 spleen cells plus MLC SN. CTL were seeded at $3x10^4$/ml. Cell concentration at day 4 and day 6 was $4.2x10^5$/ml, and $5.4x10^5$/ml, respectively. A separate aliquot of day 6 cells was washed and recultured at $3x10^4$/ml in the presence of MLC SN alone. Recovery after 24h was 68% of input. Left panel: CTL were assayed in the continuous 2h Triton soluble ^{125}IUdR assay targets against P815. Middle panel: Conjugates were formed at high cell density ($5x10^4$ CTL + $2x10^5$ targets) or low cell density ($1.8x10^3$ CTL + $7x10^3$ targets) for 30 minutes at 20°C. Results are expressed as total effector cells bound to P815 tumor cells. Greater than 100 total effector cells were counted in each sample. Non-specific conjugates formed with K562 targets at high and low density, respectively: Day 4 cells (15%, 15%), Day 6 cells (11%, 10%) and SN induced cells (34%, 21%). Right panel: conjugates were diluted in agar and target lysis determined as in Figure 3. The data shown are representative of 3 experiments with similar results.

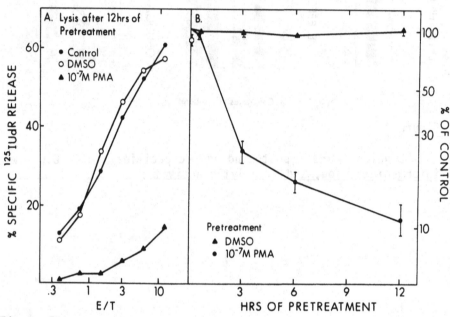

Figure 5

Time course of PMA inactivation of lytic activity, A) Cloned CTL (CTL 3) were plated at 1×10^6/ml in 10% conditioned medium alone (•), .01% DMSO (o) or 10^{-7} M PMA (▲). After 12 hrs of treatment the cells were washed and assayed for lytic activity (1.5 hr) against ^{125}IUdR labeled con A blasts (CBA). B) Similar cultures were harvested at the indicated times and assayed as in $\underline{A}$. The open symbol (o) in panel B represents an assay in which untreated CTL were assayed for lytic activity in the presence of 10^{-7} M PMA.

The results of the examination of lytic process as a function of activation state suggested that binding and post-binding events could be uncoupled within the same cell. A similar interpretation (14) could be given to CTL pretreated with 4β phorbol myristate acetate (PMA). The clones tested here do not vary in their lytic activity capacity with time after stimulation. Figure 5 is a time course of the loss of lytic activity in a CTL clone pretreated with 10^{-7} M PMA. It is characterized by a brief (30-60 min) lag and a rapid decrease such that by 6 hrs CTL have ~ 20% of the overall lytic capacity of control (untreated) cells. Preliminary experiments indicated that PMA treated cells retained similar, total binding capacity (high density conjugates). Comparison of the change in post-binding efficiency (rate of lysis) with the overall lytic activity (Fig. 6) suggested that the change in post-binding efficiency was quantitatively similar to the alteration in the overall change in lytic efficiency of the population. Thus PMA appears to be relatively selective in its effects on post-binding process (14).

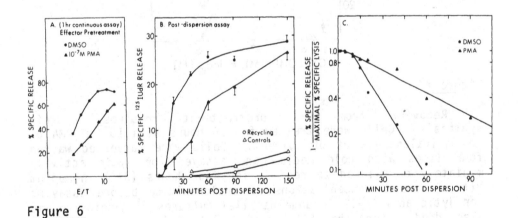

Figure 6

Effect of PMA on post binding events. CTL treated for six hours were assessed for overall lytic activity (A) or the capacity induce lysis in preformed conjugates (B). In this assay the control (DMSO treated) cells bound 38% of the targets and the PMA treated cells bound 36% of the targets. Panel C is a replot of the data from panel B to allow a more accurate assessment of the difference in post-binding rates of the two populations.

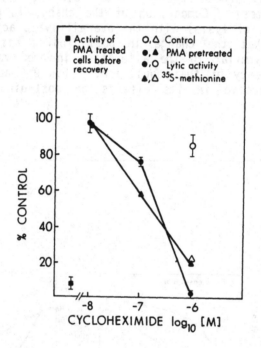

■ Activity of PMA treated cells before recovery	O,△ Control
	●,▲ PMA pretreated
	●,O Lytic activity
	▲,△ ^{35}S-methionine

Figure 7

Recovery from PMA pretreatment requires protein synthesis. Cells were treated for 16 hours with 10^{-7} M PMA or an equivalent amount of solvent. Cells were harvested washed four times with cold medium and assayed for lytic activity mediately or allowed to recover for four hours (37°) in medium with different concentrations of cycloheximide before assaying for lytic activity. In some parallel cultures ^{35} methionine was also added to test the efficacy of cycloheximide treatment.

The recovery of lytic activity after removal of PMA was very rapid (within 4 hrs) and did not require exposure to T cell conditioned medium (14). This was true even after prolonged (16 hrs) PMA pretreatment. Similarly the total binding activity of the clones was not affected by a 16 hr PMA pretreatment (Russell, unpublished). However Figure 7 demonstrates that recovery of lytic activity after PMA pretreatment is blocked by an inhibitor of protein synthesis, cycloheximide. The degree of inhibition of recovery at different doses correllates well with the degree of inhibition of protein synthesis as measured by the incorporation of ^{35}S methionine into a TCA precipitable form. Since the binding ability of PMA treated cells appears intact, the observation that recovery of post-binding activity requires the synthesis of new protein(s) strongly suggests that binding and post-binding activities are carried out by independent molecules.

DISCUSSION

Two major points are addressed in the experiments reported here. The first is that the functional binding and post-binding processes can be uncoupled within the same cells. This was observed by examination of a cloned CTL line at different times in its activation cycle. As it went from low activity to high activity, both binding and post-binding activities changed. However, as the overall lytic activity declined with time after stimulation, the post-binding efficiency appeared to be lost at a faster rate than the binding activity. This was reflected in the observation that cells with intermediate activity possessed the high binding phenotype of induced cells but the slow post-binding phenotype of non induced cells. Similarly PMA pretreatment of cells markedly reduced post-binding activity but had little effect on the CTL's binding capacity. Thus two independent systems demonstrated discordant expression of binding and post-binding function suggesting the possibility of independence of the molecular basis of these functional activities.

Cells (CTL) that had been treated with PMA recovered their lytic activity within hours after removal of PMA. However PMA treated cells failed to recover lytic activity when inhibitors of protein synthesis were included in the medium. Since the binding capacity of the cells appeared intact, the requirement for protein synthesis for the restoration of post-binding activity strongly suggests that post-binding is effected by an independent molecule.

While the evidence above is consistant with an independent molecular basis for binding and post-binding functions, several qualifying points must be made. The principal difficulty in interpreting this data is that it is difficult to measure the binding capacity of the cells in a way that can be kinetically related to the binding function in the normal continuous assay. Thus while the PMA and control cells have indistinguishable "total" binding capacity it is possible that PMA changes binding in a subtle fashion not detected in this assay. Similarly it is possible that PMA or changes in the cell's activation state do not directly affect a component of the lytic apparatus but rather have their affect on accessory components that merely establish the permissive state for post-binding events (e.g. a metabolic function).

Experiments are currently underway to more precisely define the molecules altered during the activation cycle of our CTL clone and those affected by PMA treatment. When such molecules have been identified and their functions understood it will be possible to more definitively address the issue of molecular independence of binding and post-binding functions within the CTL.

REFERENCES

1. Russell, J.H. 1983. Internal disintegration model of cyto-toxic lymphocyte-induced target damage. Immunol. Rev. 72:97.

2. Golstein, P. and E.T. Smith. 1977. Mechanisms of T-cell mediated cytolysis: the lethal hit stage. Contemp. Top. Immunol. 4:273.

3. Martz, E. 1977. Mechanism of specific tumor cell lysis by alloimmune T lymphocytes: resolution and characterization of discrete steps in the cellular interaction. Contemp. Top. Immunol. 4:301.

4. Russell, J.H. and C.B. Dobos. 1980. Mechanisms of immune lysis. II. CTL-induced nuclear disintegration of the target begins within minutes of cell contact. J. Immunol. 125:1256.

5. Reinherz, E.L., S.C., Meuer and S.F. Schlossman. 1983. The human T cell receptor: analysis with cytotoxic T cell clones. Immunol. Rev. 74:83.

6. Martz, E., W. Heagy and S.H. Gromkowski. 1983. The mech-anism of CTL-mediated killing: monoclonal antibody analysis of the roles of killer and target-cell membrane proteins. Immunol. Rev. 72:73.

7. Tsoukas, C.D., P.A. Carson, S. Fong and J.H. Vaughan. 1982. Molecular interactions in human T cell-mediated cyto-

toxicity to EBV. II. Monoclonal antibody OKT3 inhibits a post-killer-target recognition/adhesion step. J. Immunol. 129:1421.

8. Harris, D.T., H.R., MacDonald and J.-C., Cerottin. 1984. Direct transfer of antigen specific cytolytic activity to noncytolytic cells upon fusion with liposomes derived from cytolytic T cell clones. J. Exp. Med. 159:261.

9. Dennert, G. and E. Podack. 1983. Cytolysis by H-2 specific T killer cells: Assembly of tubular complexes or target membranes. J. Exp. Med. 157:1483.

10. Glasebrook, A.L., M. Sarmiento, M.R. Loken, et al., 1980. Murine T lymphocyte clones with distinct immunological functions. Immunol. Rev. 51:93.

11. Howe, R.C. and J.H. Russell. 1983. Isolation of alloreactive CTL clones with cyclical changes in lytic activity. J. Immunol. 131:2141.

12. Russell, J.H. and C.B. Dobos. 1983. Characterization of a "heteroclitic" cytotoxic lymphocyte clone: heterogeneity of receptors or signals? J. Immunol. 130:538.

13. Bonavida, B., T.P. Bradley and E.A. Grimon. 1983. Frequency determination of killer cells by a single-cell cytotoxic assay. Meth. in Enzymology. 93:270.

14. Russell, J.H. 1984. Phorbol esters inactivate the lytic apparatus of cytotoxic T lymphocytes. J. Immunol. (in press).

DISCUSSION

[Editors Note: Although omitted from the preceding paper, the talk given by Dr. Russell at the Workshop included a review of his work on nuclear disintegration induced in target cells during CTL-mediated killing. The following Discussion largely concerns this phenomenon, as do the subsequent papers by Cohen and Sears. Since there is no overview of this phenomenon in the present Volume, the reader is directed to a recent review by Dr. Russell, Immunol. Rev. 72:97, 1983.]

S. Bhakdi: The major argument is that you can pretreat your targets with antibody and complement, and post-treat with CTL, and you won't get the release of DNA fragments. Are you quite sure that the CTL reacted towards the antibody and complement-treated target cells in the same manner as towards the living target cells?

J. Russell: No, we obviously can't address that issue. What that experiment says is that the nuclear damage, the nuclear lesion, is an integral part of the lytic process of the cells and not a nonspecific result of secretion of enzymes by the CTL.

S. Bhakdi: [But the CTL] ... may be introducing nuclease or protease into the target.

J. Russell: That's completely open. I don't know where the nucleases or proteases are coming from. I don't think anybody has satisfactorily addressed the issue of whether the nucleases that are involved are coming from the CTL or the target.

S. Bhakdi: But you can say there are nucleases, so it could be a secondary nonspecific process.

J. Russell: I think that the nuclear damage is not primary to the lytic process.

Y. Kaufmann: Concerning the role of the nucleus in CTL-mediated killing, I'd like to say that we studied binding and lysis of cytoplasts, or enucleated cells, by killer cells. Although they could be specifically bound by the CTL, almost no lysis could be detected (Berke & Fishelson, Transplant. Proc. 9:671, 1977). [Editor's Note: see also Siliciano & Henney, J. Immunol. 121:186, 1978; Sanderson & Thomas, Immunol. 37:373, 1979.]

J. Russell: I would not say that the nucleus is required for lysis. My own experiments do not address that issue: the fact that you can get lysis of cytoplasts, the fact that if you separate the point of attack you can get the destruction of membrane material without the nuclear attack. I think that both events are secondary to some primary lesion.

P. Henkart: I'd like to clear up what may be a wrong impression that I may have given in discussing our work with the cytolysin. We regard the granules as being a possible differentiated organelle for cytotoxic cells. There is obviously a cytolysin in there which is capable of making these membrane lesions, which we've demonstrated. But I think it is quite possible that there are other potent enzymes which can contribute the sort of events which John [Russell] so nicely documented. We are actively looking at these granules for other components which may be responsible for such things.

J. Ding-E Young: One has a pore of the diameter that we are seeing under the electron microscope. It would be perfectly possible for a second lytic molecule to go through the channel. It would be large enough for that possibility.

J. Russell: I think these nuclear changes occur very early, before any evidence of an osmotic lesion, and I don't have any trouble seeing pores as part of the lytic machinery. I have a problem seeing them as functionally the same as in antibody and complement. They may very well be injection sites of things from the CTL to the target.

W. Clark: What do you see in the case of ADCC where antibody is part of the mediating process? Have you looked at ADCC?

J. Russell: I have -- we did these experiments a number of years ago -- and we didn't see nuclear changes early on.

W. Clark: So its a CTL-specific phenomenon.

J. Russell: Well, I won't say that because with NK's, we see a very heterogeneous kind of something in between. Its not clear when you use NK's. You do see some, but not as much.

G. Berke: If I understood, the crux was that you could detect nuclear damage prior to membrane damage. If a pore were created in the membrane, and if that pore were solely responsible for killing the cells ... then one could have great difficulties in proposing a mechanism where the nucleus disintegrates before chromium effluxes.

P. Henkart: I would challenge the statement that you can show that the DNA breaks down before any membrane damage, because it seems to me that the thing you're really measuring is chromium release. Is that really the measurment that you want for "membrane damage".

J. Russell: (Pointing to an electron micrograph) Its things like this, the fact that you're getting these really drastic changes in the chromatin at a time when there's no evidence of osmotic damage in the cytoplasm that says to me that if those pores are serving a purpose in the lytic process, they're functionally different from the pores that result from antibody and complement.

S. Bhakdi: There might be some analogy to the action of complement and lysozyme on bacteria, where complement is making a hole, and lysozyme can come in and destroy the peptidoglycan.

IMMUNE CYTOLYSIS VIEWED AS A STIMULATORY PROCESS OF THE TARGET

Reuven Tirosh and Gideon Berke

Department of Cell Biology
The Weizmann Institute of Science
Rehovot 76100, Israel

ABSTRACT

Humoral and cellular mechanisms of immune cytolysis, as effected by antibody and complement (Ab+C') or by cytolytic T lymphocytes (CTL), have traditionally been considered the end result of early but terminal membrane damage, in turn causing colloid-osmotic lysis of the target cell. A comprehensive theory explaining and relating known <u>prelytic cellular events</u> to subsequent membrane damage is lacking, nor is there a specific picture as to the role and mode of action of Ca^{2+}, which appears to be involved in both complement- and cell-mediated cytolysis (C'MC and CMC, respectively). Recent studies are in support of the view that both Ab+C' and CTL induce a comparable series of prelytic events, in the TC, initiated by membrane depolarization, which in turn bring about voltage-dependent Ca^{2+} influx or its intracellular release. Persistent elevation of cytosolic Ca^{2+} can induce massive stimulation of cellular ATPases (actomyosin, Ca^{2+}) and cause exhaustive depletion of ATP. Consequently, Na^+-pumping is slowed down and colloid-osmotic lysis ensues. Hence, in our view, membrane damage in immune cytolysis is the result rather than the cause of intracellular events culminating in lysis.

INTRODUCTION

While substantial strides have been made towards defining the cells involved and characterizing individual steps of the lytic process, the mechanism whereby cytolytic T lymphocytes (CTL) kill their target cells (TC) has remained an enigma (for review see Clark and Golstein, eds., 1982; Immunol. Rev. 72, 1983; Contemp.

Topics Immunobiol. Vol. 7, 1977). A number of early events
(Ca^{2+}-dependent; Martz, 1977; Golstein and Smith, 1977), beyond
initial CTL-TC conjugation (Mg^{2+}-dependent; Stulting and Berke,
1972) have been demonstrated (Berke and Amos, 1973; Martz, 1977;
Henney, 1977; Golstein and Smith, 1977; Berke, 1980; Sanderson,
1981; Russell, 1983). These include: Rb^+ efflux, prelytic nuclear
disintegration, cytoplasmic streaming and membrane blebbing
('zeiosis'), Ca^{2+} involvement, low temperature and osmotic protection of the terminal phase (post-lethal hit), to mention just a
few. The nature of these pre-lytic events may be a key to understanding the mechanism of lysis. Let us consider the early and
substantial increased efflux of $K^+(Rb^+)$, observed before or concomitantly with delivery of the lethal hit (Martz, 1976; Sanderson,
1981). Traditionally, Rb^+ efflux has been taken as an indication
for early membrane damage giving rise to a leaky, expandable
'hole' (Ferluga and Allison, 1974; Henney, 1974; Martz et al.,
1974). However, this possibility has been questioned (Sanderson,
1976, 1981). We would like to suggest that early efflux of Rb^+
from affected cells may be considered as an indication of (physiological) depolarization of the target cell membrane rather than
'hole' formation. Indeed, a comparable (and reversible) pre-lytic
depolarization of target cell membrane has been observed in Ab+C'
mediated lysis (Stephens and Henkart, 1979; Jackson et al., 1981).
What is important to stress is that early membrane depolarization
(K^+-efflux) must not be simply equated with terminal membrane
damage (although this is also possible), as persistent membrane
depolarization, by and of itself, may stimulate a lethal process,
e.g., by exciting exhaustive activation of ATP-consuming processes. In this context, (membrane depolarization) $^{86}Rb^+$ efflux may
be considered an important link between CMC and C'MC, rather than
as evidence for a common primary membrane lesion (Mayer, 1977,
1982).

The plasmalema is undoubtedly the primary site of C' attack
(Müller-Eberhard, 1975; Mayer et al., 1981; Esser, 1982; Lachmann,
1979). Evidence has been presented that membrane-bound C' components (C5b-C9) form (trans)membrane 'channels' (the 'doughnut'
model) and/or 'leaky patches,' which perturb permeability barriers
of the cell membrane. Such perturbation is assumed sufficient to
impair the active state of osmotic balance, allowing net influx of
water and membrane rupture as a result of 'colloid-osmotic' burst.
Indeed, distinct 'ring-like' structures imbedded in the membrane
have been observed by electron microscopy following C' attack;
what is not at all clear is whether formation of these membrane-
bound structures alone is sufficient for the onset of lysis
(Ohanian et al., 1978).

Under low levels of Ab+C' attack of nucleated cells, evidence
has been accumulated suggesting functional involvement of intracellular activities similar to those observed in CMC. That is,

early Rb^+ efflux, Ca^{2+} dependency, osmotic and low temperature
protection of affected target cells and variation in susceptibility during the various stages of cell cycle (Burakoff et al., 1975;
Ohanian et al., 1978; Mayer et al., 1981; Boyle et al., 1976a, b;
Ramm et al., 1983; Taylor et al., 1982). The possibility that TC
actively participate in their own lysis is further indicated by
the demonstration of threshold doses of Ab+C' (like ConA and
A23187) below which cellular activities (motility, secretion,
proliferation) are stimulated, while slightly higer doses are
lethal (Shearer et al., 1976). However, involvement of cellular
metabolism in the lytic process has been questioned in view of
lytic effects by purified terminal C' components against synthetic
liposomes (see Lachmann, 1983). But in liposomes, viruses,
bacterial outer membranes and red blood cell ghosts, a detergent-
like ('non-colloid osmotic') effect, in Ab+C' excess, must be
considered (Mayer et al., 1981; Esser, 1982).

Four similar pre-lytic events in C'MC and CMC suggesting a physio-
logical process during immune cytolysis

Several common prelytic events have been demonstrated in target
cells under low level of Ab+C' attack and during CTL-TC interaction. These include: (a) Initial efflux of $^{86}Rb^+$ (Burakoff et
al., 1975; Martz, 1976; Sanderson, 1976; Ferluga and Allison,
1974; Mayer 1977); (b) temperature and Ca^{2+} dependency of progressive events of the lethal phase (Berke et al., 1972; Berke and
Sullivan, 1973; Henney and Bubbers, 1973; Berke and Gabison, 1975;
Martz and Benacerraf, 1975; Golstein and Smith, 1976; Martz,
1982); (c) enhanced terminal phase of cellular activity, reflected
in cytoplasmic streaming, blebbing and membrane extrusions
(zeiosis), followed by quiescent swelling (Ginsburg et al., 1969;
Sanderson, 1981); (d) osmotic and low temperature protection
preventing leakage of cellular content during advanced phase of
lysis (Berke et al., 1972; Burakoff et al., 1975; Martz, 1977;
Mayer, 1977).

Lysis is usually deduced from the release of intracellular
content (^{51}Cr-labeled) or entry of impermeable dyes (e.g., trypan
blue), both indicative of membrane damage; but the phase of the
lytic process at which the membrane is damaged is unknown.
Prevailing notions of immune cytolysis view it as the result of a
primary and terminal membrane assault. No matter how reasonable
this conclusion is, it has led to models that do not consider
known prelytic events as integral parts of the lytic mechanism.
If, however, prelytic events are significant for the lytic
process, then the lytic pathway exhibits characteristic features
in common with physiological phenomena of cellular stimulation,
like axonal conduction and synaptic transmission of nerve impulse,

muscle contraction, cellular motility and secretion. Of course, these cellular processes are triggered by transmembrane stimulation effected by external agents, without injuring the membranes. In immune cytolysis, we propose the following 4-step stimulative mechanism in the TC, ultimately leading to target cell dissolution:

(1) Transmembrane stimulation of depolarization effected by Ab+C' fixation or CTL-TC interaction under permissive temperature and ionic conditions;

(2) temperature-dependent Ca^{2+} influx, probably through voltage-sensitive channels in the TC;

(3) exhaustive activation of ATP hydrolysis by the Ca^{2+} regulated ATPases like actomyosin or the Ca^{2+} pump.

(4) colloid-osmotic swelling of the intact, semipermeable plasma membrane of the ATP-deprived cell.

Let us analyze available facts relevant to these effects.

1. Depolarization and initial efflux of K^+ and its analog $^{86}Rb^+$

Electrical measurements performed on cultured nerve and muscle cells have revealed complement-mediated membrane depolarization, reversible upon dilution (Stephens and Henkart, 1979; Jackson et al., 1981). These electrical changes appear comparable to early prelytic efflux of $^{42}K^+$ and its analog $^{86}Rb^+$ (Ferluga and Allison, 1974; Sanderson, 1976). Since $^{86}Rb^+$ efflux precedes the (lethal) insertion of the terminal complement component C-9 (Boyle et al., 1976a), there is no longer consensus that it must indicate an early and expandable lesion (Sanderson, 1981). Alternatively, these K^+ and Rb^+ fluxes can be generated in response to electrical depolarization of the plasma membrane, since distribution of these cations (unlike H_2O^+, Na^+ and Ca^{2+}) across the plasma membrane is governed by the electric potential difference according to the Nernst equation. We can therefore employ efflux of $^{86}Rb^+$ as a probe for (intact) membrane depolarization.

How is depolarization triggered and what may be its direct effect(s)? These are two central and general issues in the physiology of cellular stimulation that go beyond immune cytolysis. Current approaches to immune cytolysis do not consider membrane depolarization as an important step of the process. Of course membrane depolarization will be irrelevant in treating a lytic lesion ('holes' or 'leaky patches'), causing short-circuiting of the membrane to electrolytes. Under physiological conditions however, immune cytolysis can be induced by a single (molecular) hit of the complement transmembrane-complex, proposed to be effective in breaking permeability barriers of the cell membrane (Mayer, 1981). In terms of efficiency, however, the amount of cationic flux sufficient to induce depolarization is negligible compared to that needed for substantial osmotic effect. Consequently, energetic demands for triggering lysis are minimized in the case of a stimulative effect of depolarization, especially if enhanced by influx of cations down their concentration gradient.

In CMC current notions of a membrane lesion were adopted from putative 'holes' proposed in the complement system (see Henkart and Henkart, 1982). There is, however, no convincing evidence for such early and lethal holes in CMC (Berke, 1980; Kalina and Berke, 1976; Sanderson, 1977; Biberfeld and Johansson, 1975; Liepins et al., 1977). The initial efflux of the potassium analog $^{86}Rb^+$ from the target cell before or concomitantly with the lethal hit (Martz, 1976) may indicate membrane depolarization, as has been observed under Ab+C' attack. This functional similarity is further supported by electrical measurements of ion flow across Ab-coated, antigenic lipid bilayers attacked by lymphocytes (ADCC) or complement (Henkart and Blumenthal, 1975; Michaels et al., 1976). It is also of interest that the change in conductance produced by lymphocytes or complement can be observed only when a positive potential is applied on the side of the (effector) attack. Most interesting is the demonstration that similar voltage-sensitive gating of conductive channels can be generated in pure phospholipid membranes due to hydrolysis of acetylcholine by acetylcholinesterase inserted in black lipid membranes (Silman and Karlin, 1967; Kaufmann and Silman, 1980). Thus, a proton flux may be considered as a primary inducer of ionic gating, an idea that is developed below.

2. Micromolar elevation of Ca^{2+} levels in the cytosol of the TC due to influx and/or internal release

Involvement of external Ca^{2+} ($[Ca^{2+}]_{ext}$) in the mM range, in inflicting the lethal hit is well documented in both Ab+C' (Shearer et al., 1976) and CTL attack (Martz, 1982), but its role is poorly understood. Ca^{2+} is known to be involved in the fixation and activation of the C' system. Evidence has been presented for $[Ca^{2+}]_{ext}$ requirement at a post-fixation stage (Boyle et al., 1976b), and for cytosolic elevation of Ca^{2+}, in the micromolar range, necessary for the lethal hit (Campbell et al., 1981). In CMC, neither the site (effector or target) nor the mode of action of Ca^{2+} are known. It may act inside the target, inside the effector and/or at external membranes (Martz, 1982). Recently we have obtained evidence that Ca^{2+} may exert its (lethal) effect at the target cell and not the CTL (Tirosh and Berke, 1984). We have found that for a given CTL population, the lytic requirement for $[Ca^{2+}]_{ext}$ varies, depending on the TC: some TC (type II), like L1210, are strictly dependent on $[Ca^{2+}]_{ext}$ while others (type I), like EL4 or P815 cells (MacLennan, Gotch and Golstein, 1980) are not (Fig. 1).

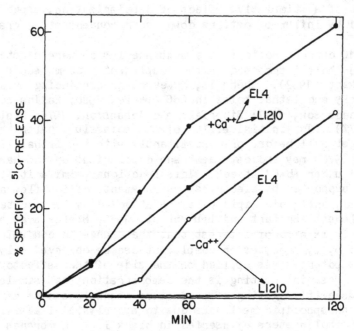

FIGURE 1. Influence of $[Ca^{2+}]_{ext}$ on lymphocyte-mediated cytolysis of L1210 and EL4 cells.
Effectors were BALB/c anti-EL4 peritoneal exudate (PEL) CTL.
Lysis of L1210 was performed against ConA (10 ug/ml) treated cells (LDCC).
+ $[Ca^{2+}]_{ext}$ = Assay performed in PBS+FCS 10%. - $[Ca^{2+}]_{ext}$ = As above in addition of 2 mM Mg_2 EGTA.

The Ca^{2+} channel blocker verapamil, inhibiting lysis of type II but not of type I TC exposed to the same effectors, support the above conclusion. Further, effector cells that lyse EL4 cells (type I) in the absence of $[Ca^{2+}]_{ext}$ require it when used themselves as TC, showing that the effector cells do not require $[Ca^{2+}]_{ext}$ for killing. The results suggest effector-cell induced cytosolic mobilization of Ca^{2+} in the TC, either by influx through voltage-sensitive channels and/or by release from internal stores (Tirosh and Berke, 1984; see also Fig. 2B).

Ca^{2+} influx to the TC could be induced by membrane depolarization, as discussed above. Na^+ influx may enhance this phase of electric depolarization (like that of the nerve action potential). Such a modulatory role of Na^+ has been verified by a delay of ^{51}Cr released from EL4 by replacing external Na^+ by choline$^+$ ions (Tirosh and Berke, 1984). Ca^{2+} release from internal stores is possible due to Ca^{2+}/H^+ exchange (Lehninger et al., 1978), but this effect in the lysis of type I cells remains to be shown. It is, however, interesting to note that a proton influx into the target cell (as mentioned above) could induce both membrane depolarization and cytosolic acidification and thus trigger the two potential pathways of Ca^{2+} mobilization. Fast depolarization may be induced by a regenerative influx of Na^+ as mentioned. Acidification, however, would be hampered by the buffering of the TC cytosol. Thus, the delay of cytolytic response in EL4 cells, in the absence of $[Ca^{2+}]_{ext}$ (Fig. 1), could be explained.

It has recently been proposed that in CTL-TC conjugates, an electrochemical gradient of protons is generated by ATPase activity of the actomyosin system, polarized on both sides of the CTL-TC contact zone (cited in Berke, 1983). The CTL-receptor TC-MHC complex has been proposed to facilitate conductance of protons from the effector into the TC. It has been suggested that the primary effect of proton influx could induce gating of Na^+ and Ca^{2+} channels. In recent studies (Tirosh and Berke, 1984), Na^+ has been found not to be involved in electrolytic effects of lysis but only play a modulatory role in conjunction with Ca^{2+} influx into the target cell, as mentioned above.

A CTL-induced Ca^{2+}-mediated (lethal) effect in the TC has been considered and tested before by using mast cells as TC of C'MC and CMC (Martz et al., 1982). Antigen-triggered secretion from mast cells is known to be induced via Ca^{2+} influx; this response has therefore been employed to probe prelytic influx of Ca^{2+} into the TC. Sequential release of ^{14}C-serotonin secretion followed by ^{51}Cr release has been observed under Ab+C' but not CTL attack. Moreover, in the latter system, a prelytic <u>inhibition</u> of secretory activity of mast cells has been observed. The authors suggested that "the inhibitory effect does not exclude the possibility that the CTL produces early calcium influx into the target cell simultaneously with other effects (such as depletion of ATP) which block secretion" (Martz et al., 1982). Surprisingly, this interesting possibility was not followed up. Martz et al. also argued against extracellular Ca^{2+} as a mediator in the anti-target action of diverse cytolysins (see Schane, Kane and Farber, 1979), by demonstrating $[Ca^{2+}]_{ext}$-independent toxic effects on certain cells, e.g., P815. However, their own results do not exclude mobilization of intracellular Ca^{2+} in the target cell tested. Interestingly, P815 cells have previously been shown to be independent of $[Ca]_{ext}$ under CTL attack (MacLennan et al., 1980). Therefore, two pathways of Ca^{2+} mobilization (influx and internal release), widely recognized in physiological responses, may be considered in cytolytic processes.

What may be the role of intracellular Ca^{2+} in the cytolytic mechanism?

3. Exhaustive activation of ATP hydrolysis by Ca^{2+}-regulated ATPases

Ca^{2+} plays a pivotal role in the activation of a wide range of cellular processes. A major energy-consuming process is likely to be the Ca^{2+}-regulated actomyosin system, involved in cytoplasmic streaming, endo- or exocytosis and intercellular interactions. Other ATPases (e.g., Na^+/K^+, Ca^{2+}, H^+ pumps) may also be involved. We have recently demonstrated by ^{31}P-NMR spectroscopy selective depletion of high energy phosphates, induced in nucleated cells by antibody and complement (Tirosh et al., 1984). Within 10 min of Ab+C' attack, before onset of overt lysis, we observed a marked, selective reduction in the intracellular content of phosphocreatine (PCr) and ATP. A longer attack was accompanied by a total depletion of either PCr or ATP in residual cells, which preserved other phosphate compounds, such as sugar phosphates. These results indicated that in nucleated cells formation of C'-dependent membrane channels stimulates exhaustive hydrolysis of ATP. ATP deprivation could in turn lead to colloid osmotic swelling, membrane rupture and cell lysis. In CMC, prelytic depletion of ATP has also been demonstrated (Fishelson and Berke, 1983; Fig. 2A). Using intracellularly trapped fluorescent probes, preliminary results in CMC also indicate prelytic mobilization of Ca^{2+} in TC, and prelytic effects of transient fluctuations in pH inside a single target cell undergoing a CTL attack (Fig. 3B, C).

At low MgATP levels, the actomyosin system may exhibit a well-recognized effect of superprecipitation, during which time the rate of ATP hydrolysis increases. The whole effect may be due to an apparent increase in the enzymatic concentration, leading to a catalytic surge of ATP hydrolysis coupled to enhanced mechanochemical effects of cytoplasmic streaming. This may explain the process of 'zeiosis' during CTL-mediated lysis (Sanderson, 1981).

A similar sequence of terminal events, namely cytoplasmic activity followed by swelling and lysis, is observed microscopically in cells undergoing Ab+C' attack, with one distinct difference, the lack of 'zeiosis' (Sanderson, 1981). This difference, however, may reflect various levels of otherwise similar enhancement of terminal cytoplasmic streaming. This variance in the final surge of cytoplasmic streaming in the TC may explain also early nuclear disruption under CTL but not under Ab+C' attack (Russell and Dobos, 1982; Russell, 1983).

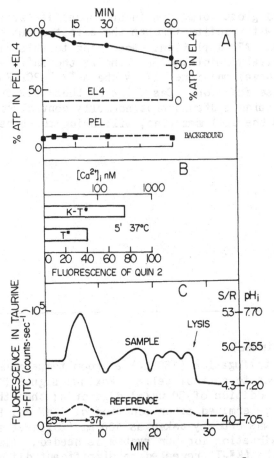

FIGURE 2. Fluctuation in intracellular ATP, Ca^{2+} and pH during
CTL-TC interaction. Preliminary results.
Specific cytolysis of EL4 cells was effected by BALB/c anti-EL4
CTL at $37^{\circ}C$ after forming conjugates by a 10 min centrifugation
(150 xg) at room temperature (with similar treatment to control
target cells).
(A) Intracellular content of ATP in PEL, EL4 and in conjugated
PEL+EL4 incubated at 37°. ATP in cell lysates (obtained by NRS)
was determined by the luciferin/luciferase enzymatic test.
Measurements were performed by a LUMAC Biocounter M2010, LUMAC BV,
Holland. Reagents (NRS, enzymes, buffers) were from LUMAC; a few
assays were performed with firefly lantern extracts obtained from
Sigma.
(B) $[Ca^{2+}]_i$ was measured using the fluorescent indicator 'quin 2'
which shows a fivefold fluorescence enhancement on binding Ca^{2+}
(Tsien et al., 1982). Quin 2 was trapped inside EL4 cells (T*) by
incubation with its membrane-permeant intracellularly hydrolysable
acetoxymethyl ester (Amersham; ($4x10^6$ cells/ml, 20 uM ester, 0.5%
DMSO, 60 min, $37^{\circ}C$). Fluorescence at 480 nm excited at 340 nm was
measured on a Perkin Elmer fluorescence spectrophotometer at $37^{\circ}C$.
Effector/target ratio (K/T) was 2. Conjugates K-T* were induced
(continued)

481

Swelling and ghost formation in our model is explained as the result of net water influx through the affected but intact plasmalema, upon ATP depletion. According to this view, osmotic balance is actively maintained as long as the Na^+/K^+-ATPase (Ouabain sensitive) and more likely the Na^+/K^+-2Cl-Furosemide sensitive ATPase function. Cessation of these ATP-fueled ions (and water) pumping systems, that normally control colloid-osmotic balance across the cell membrane, will bring about net water

---

(FIGURE 2, continued)

by a 10 min centrifugation (150 xg) at room temperature with similar treatment to control cells. Maximum signal (100) was obtained after addition of 50 ug/ml digitonin; then the lowest signal (0) was determined after addition of 5 mM Mg_2 EGTA. Half ways intensity was crudely taken as 100 nm (Tsien et al., 1982) but careful calibration for our system is needed. Similar probing of effector cells (K*-T) revealed no significant difference from that of control (K*).

(C) pH_i of a single, conjugated EL4 cell was measured using fluorescent indicator composed of two FITC molecules covalently attached to taurine (an ester of this probe was kindly obtained from Prof. C. Gitler). The ester diffuses into the cytosol where the probe is released by hydrolysis and trapped in its highly charged, hydrophilic form. Loading conditions of EL4 in PBS: $5x10^6$ cells/ml, 1 ug/ml ester, 0.5% DMSO, 15 min, $37^{\circ}C$. To monitor a signal from single cells, epifluorescence microscopy was used (Zeiss system). The fluorescence radiation (excitation 450-490 nm, FT 510 nm, LP 520 nm) was collected by the objective lens (oil immersion x63, 1.4 NM) through a field diaphragm onto a sensitive photomultiplier tube connected to photon counting electronics (Schlessinger and Elson, 1982). Intermittently, another filter (LP 570 nm) was inserted on the way of the fluorescence signal (sample in the figure) to give a reference signal. The ratio of the fluorescent intensities: sample/reference was calibrated as a pH indicator. A drop of the conjugates sample was enclosed between microscope slide and coverslip spaced by a siliconized parafilm ring. Heating to $37^{\circ}C$ was performed by thermostated ventilation. (Experiments were carried out in the laboratory of Dr. J. Schlessinger.)

482

influx, and cell burst. It is of interest to note that a parallel
sequence of blebbing, swelling and finally lysis is also observed
during the terminal pathway of cell death due to senescence
(Bessis, 1973).

4. Osmotic and low temperature protection and recovery

An intermediate step of CTL-affected target cells has been
identified (Berke et al., 1972). The fate of the target at that
stage is highly temperature-dependent (Q_{10} 25°-35° = 3-4; Berke
and Amos, 1973). Similarly, the lysis of affected target cells
can be prevented by increasing the osmotic pressure outside, e.g.
by Dextran (Martz, 1977). These two effects, found similarly in
C'MC and CMC, are difficult to reconcile with accepted views of
early membrane damage (see discussion in Burakoff et al., 1975).
If, as a result of C'MC and CMC, rupture of the membrane (formation of holes) in the target is the exclusive cause of cell death,
how could dextran when placed outside prevent net influx of water
through a strained membrane? Likewise, how would lowering the
temperature stop lysis, effectively drastically and reversibly?
However, in the model presented herein (summarized in Fig. 3)
membrane damage is the result of an otherwise 'vital' temperature
dependent process. Thus, osmotic and low temperature protection,
and possible recovery of the TC, are predicted and explained.

Naturally, if lysis is believed to be initiated and completed
solely from without and the target is considered merely as an
osmotic bag (Bubbers and Henney, 1975), membrane damaging mechanism must and have repeatedly been proposed. These include:
cytolytic function of the plasma membrane (Ferluga and Allison,
1975; see however Kahn-Perles and Golstein, 1978); CTL-associated
complement-like components transferred from the CTL to bound TC
(Mayer, 1977); localized extracellular secretion of nonspecific or
specific toxins (Gately et al., 1976; Hiserodt et al., 1979);
tangential shearing and tearing of the TC membrane as a result of
movement of the TC-bound CTL (Seeman, 1974; Grimm et al., 1979);
alteration of ion permeability as a direct result of CTL-receptor
TC-MHC antigen interaction (Berke and Clark, 1982); and secretion
of degradative enzymes at the CTL-TC contact zone (Bykovskaya et
al., 1978; Zagury, 1982). The recent studies on NK (natural
killer) like tumor cells and some CTL lines, but not on in vivo
generated CTL, have resulted in the isolation of granules capable
of inserting into membrane and lysing a wide range of target
cells, including NK-resistant cells, RBC and liposomes (Henkart
and Henkart, 1982; Millard et al., 1984). While most investigators today favor the theory that lysis occurs solely from without,
that is, initiated and completed via drastic and lethal damage to
the targets' membrane, a detailed explanation of how lysis occurs

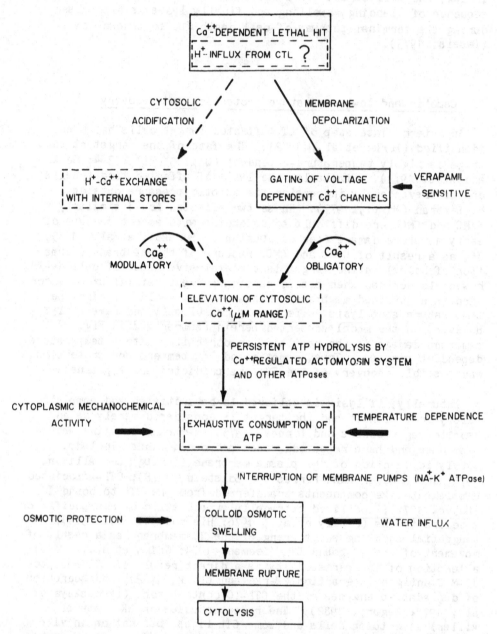

FIGURE 3. Working hypothesis of stimulation of exhaustive activation of the target cell during immune cytolysis.
Continuous line, frames and arrows refer to known effects. Broken line, frames and arrows refer to predicted effects.

is lacking. We emphasize the importance of prelytic intracellular events common to C'MC and CMC). The mechanism proposed herein (see scheme, Fig. 3) suggests that lymphocytotoxicity is not initiated and completed solely at the target cell membrane, as intracellular events occurring in the target (and possibly in the CTL) precede cytolysis. In other words, membrane damage is viewed as the result rather than the cause of lymphocytotoxicity. Pertinent to the above mechanism is the observation that target cells must preserve certain metabolic activities so as to be affected by CTL (see Berke, 1980). Another observation suggesting active participation of the target in the process is the variable susceptibility of target cells at different stages of the cell cycle (Sanderson and Thomas, 1976), as well as the observation that nuclear disintegration occurs before membrane damage (Russell, 1983). Evidence has been accumulating recently that the mere expression of appropriate MHC-Ag on TC, although necessary, is by itself not sufficient for specific CTL-TC interaction which may explain the failure to observe consistently, specific interactions of isolated MHC-Ag with CTL (Mescher, 1982). The importance of not only the membrane milieu but of also a viable target for functional presentation of MHC-Ag has been stressed recently by demonstrating that isolated TC membrane components that contain MHC-Ag, but which do not specifically bind to CTL or inhibit CTL-TC interaction, exhibit these activities upon insertion into membranes of antigenically irrelevant TC (Schick et al., 1983). The foregoing arguments for a viable involvement of the TC in CMC have been raised also with respect to C'MC (Mayer et al., 1981).

Finally, we would like to draw an analogy between the prelytic response of cells to CTL or AB+C' and a wide range of stimulators, including growth and chemotactic factors. This analogy is promoted by common effects of Ca^{2+} mobilization and metabolic stimulation. Persistent transmembrane stimulation during CTL-TC interaction or sustained fixation of the complement complex (Shearer et al., 1979; Ramm et al., 1983), unlike transient interactions with hormones or growth factors which undergo rapid clustering, endo- or exocytosis (Schlessinger, 1980) may be a major factor determining the lethal sequence of prelytic events in the TC during CMC and C'MC.

REFERENCES

Berke, G. (1980) Interaction of cytotoxic T lymphocytes and target cells. Prog. Allergy 27:69.
Berke, G. (1983) Cytotoxic T lymphocytes. How do they function? Immunol. Rev. 72:5.
Berke, G. (1984) The function and mode of action of the cytolytic T lymphocyte. In: "Micobiological Sciences," Oxford: Blackwell, in press.
Berke, G., and Amos, D.B. (1973) Mechanism of lymphocyte-mediated cytolysis. The LMC cycle and its role in transplantation immunity. Transplant. Rev. 17:71.

Berke, G., and Clark, W.R. (1982) T lymphocyte-mediated cytolysis
  - A comprehensive theory (I, II). In: "Mechanisms of Cell-
  Mediated Cytotoxicity," eds. W.R. Clark and P. Golstein, New
  York: Plenum Press, p. 57.
Berke, G., and Gabison, D. (1975) Energy requirements for the
  binding and lytic steps of T lymphocyte-mediated cytolysis of
  leukemic cells in vitro. Eur. J. Immunol. 5:671.
Berke, G., and Sullivan, K.A. (1973) Temperature control of
  lymphocyte-mediated cytotoxicity in vitro. Transpl. Proc.
  5:421.
Berke, G., Sullivan, K.A., and Amos, D.B. (1972) Rejection of
  ascites tumor allograft. II. A pathway for cell-mediated
  tumor destruction in vitro by peritoneal exudate lymphoid
  cells. J. Exp. Med. 136:1594.
Bessis, M. (1973) Living Blood Cells and Their Ultrastructure.
  Translated by R.I. Weed, Berlin-New York: Springer Verlag.
Biberfeld, P., and Johansson, A. (1975) Contact areas of cytotoxic
  lymphocytes and target cells: An electron microscopic study.
  Exp. Cell Res. 94:79.
Boyle, M.D.P., Ohanian, S.H., and Borsos, T.Y. (1976a). Lysis of
  tumor cells by antibody and complement, VII. Complement-dependent ^{86}Rb release: A nonlethal event? J. Immunol.
  117:1346.
Boyle, M.P.D., Ohanian, S.H., and Borsos, T. (1976b) Studies on
  the terminal stages of antibody-complement mediated killing
  of a tumor cell, III. Effect of membrane active agents. J.
  Immunol. 117:106.
Bubbers, J.E., and Henney, C.F. (1975) Studies on the synthetic
  capacity and antigenic expression of glutaraldehyde-fixed
  target cells. J. Immunol. 114:1126.
Burakoff, S.J., Martz, E., and Benacerraf, B. (1975) Is the primary complement lesion insufficient for lysis? Failure of cells
  damaged under osmotic protection to lyse in EDTA or at low
  temperature after removal of osmotic protection. Clin.
  Immunol. Immunopathol. 4:108.
Bykovskaya, S.N., Rylenko, A.N., Rauschenbach, M.O. and Bykovsky,
  A.F. (1978) Ultrastructural alteration of cytolytic T
  lymphocytes following their interaction with target cells.
  I. Hypertrophy and change of orientation of the Golgi appara-
  tus. Cell. Immunol. 40:164.
Campbell, A.K., Daw, R.A., Hallet, M.B., and Luzio, J.P. (1981)
  Direct measurement of the increase in intracellular free
  calcium ion concentration in response to the action of
  complement. Biochem. J. 194:551.
Clark, W.R., and Golstein, P., eds. "Mechanisms of Cell-Mediated
  Cytotoxicity." New York: Plenum.
Contemporary Topics in Immunobiology, Vol. 7, eds. O. Stutman, New
  York: Plenum.
Esser, A.F. (1982) Interactions between complement proteins and
  biological and model membranes. In: "Biological Membranes,"
  Vol. 4, ed. D. Chapman, New York: Academic Press, p. 277.

Ferluga, J. and Allison, A.C. (1974) Observations on the mechanism by which T-lymphocytes exert cytotoxic effects. Nature (London) 250:673.

Ferluga, J., and ALlison, A.C. (1975) Cytotoxicity of isolated plasma membranes from lymph node cells. Nature (London) 255:708.

Fishelson, Z., and Berke, G. (1983) CTL devoid of lytic activity can lower ATP levels of target cells. In: "Communication and Leucocyte Function," eds. J.W. Parker and R.L. O'Brien, New York: John Wiley and Sons, p. 601..

Gately, M.K., Mayer, M.M., and Henney, C.S. (1976) Effect of anti-lymphotoxin on cell-mediated cytotoxicity. Evidence for two pathways, one involving lymphotoxin and the other requiring intimate contact between the plasma membranes of killer and target cells. Cell. Immunol. 27:82.

Ginsburg, h., Ax, W., and Berke, G. (1969) Functional implications of cellular immunity. An analysis of graft reaction in cell culture. In: "Pharmacological Treatment in Organ and Tissue Transplantation, Excerpta Medica Inter. Congr. Serie 196, p. 85.

Golstein, P. (1982) Sequential analysis of T cell mediated cytolysis: A brief reminder of some possibly informative markers at the recognition and lethal hit stages. In: "Mechanisms of Cell-Mediated Cytotoxicity," W.R. Clark and P. Golstein, eds., New York: Plenum Press, p. 111.

Golstein, P., and Smith, E.T. (1976) The lethal hit stage of mouse T and non-T cell-mediated cytolysis: Differences in cation requirements and characterization of an analytical "cation pulse" method. Eur. J. Immunol. 6:31.

Golstein, P., and Smith, E.T. (1977) Mechanism of T-cell mediated cytolysis: The lethal hit stage. In: "Contemporary Topics in Immunobiology," Vol. 7, ed. O. Stutman, New York: Plenum Press, p. 273.

Grimm, E., Price, Z., and Bonavida, B. (1979) Effector-target junction and target cell membrane disruption during cytolysis. Cell. Immunol. 46:77.

Henkart, P., and Blumenthal, R. (1975) Interaction of lymphocytes with lipid bilayer membranes: A model for lymphocyte-mediated lysis of target cells. Proc. Natl. Acad. Sci. 72:2789.

Henkart, M.P., and Henkart, P.A. (1982) Lymphocyte mediated cytolysis as a secretory phenomenon. In: "Mechanisms of Cell-Mediated Cytotoxicity," eds. W.R. Clark and P. Golstein, New York: Plenum Press, p. 227.

Henney, C.S. (1974) Estimation of the size of a T-cell induced lytic lesion. Nature (London) 249:456.

Henney, C.S. (1977) T-cell mediated cytolysis: An overview of some current issues. In: "Contemporary Topics in Immunobiology," Vol. 7, ed. O. Stutman, New York: Plenum Press, p. 245.

Henney, C.S., and Bubbers, J.E. (1973) Studies on the mechanism of
    lymphocyte-mediated cytolysis. I. The role of divalent
    cations in cytolysis by T lymphocytes. J. Immunol. 110:63.
Hiserodt, J.C., Tiangco, G.J., and Granger, G.A. (1979) The LT
    system in experimental animals. IV. Rapid specific lysis of
    ^{51}Cr-labeled allogeneic target cells by highly unstable high
    mw lymphotoxic receptor complex(ex) released in vitro by
    activated alloimmune murine T lymphocytes. J. Immunol.
    123:332.
Jackson, M.B., Stephens, C.L., and Lecar, H. (1981) Single channel
    currents induced by C' in antibody-coated cell membranes.
    Proc. Natl. Acad. Sci. 78:6421.
Kahn-Perles, B., and Golstein, P. (1978) Cell membrane-mediated
    cytolysis by membranes from noncytolytic cells. Eur.
    J. Immunol. 8:71.
Kalina, M., and Berke, G. (1976) Contact regions of cytotoxic T
    lymphocyte-target cell conjugates. Cell. Immunol. 25:41.
Kaufmann, K., and Silman, I. (1980) The induction of ion channels
    through excitable membranes by acetylcholinesterase. Natur-
    wissenschaften 67:608.
Lachmann, P.J. (1979) Complement. In: "The Antigens," Vol. V, ed.
    M. Sela, New York: Academic Press, p. 277.
Lachmann, P.J. (1983) Are complement lysis and lymphocytotoxicity
    analogous? Nature 305:473.
Lehninger, A.L., Reynafarje, B., Vercesi, A. and Tew, W.P. (1978)
    Transport and accumulation of calcium in mitochondria. In:
    "Calcium Transport and Cell Function," eds A. Scarpa and E.
    Carafoli, Ann. N.Y. Acad. Sci. 307:160.
Liepins, A., Faanes, R.B., Lifter, J., Choi, Y.S., and de Harren,
    E. (1977) Ultrastructural changes during T lymphocyte-medi-
    ated cytolysis. Cell. Immunol. 28:109.
MacLennan, I.C.M., Gotch, F.M., and Golstein, P. (1980) Limited
    specific T-cell mediated cytolysis in the absence of extra-
    cellular Ca^{2+} Immunology 39:109.
Martz, E. (1976) Early steps in specific tumor cell lysis by
    sensitized mouse T lymphocytes. II. Electrolyte permeability
    in the target membrane concomitant with programming for
    lysis. J. Immunol. 117:1023.
Martz, E. (1977) Mechanism of specific tumor-cell lysis by alloim-
    mune T lymphocytes: Resolution and characterization of
    discrete steps in the cellular interaction. In: "Contempo-
    rary Topics in Immunobiology," Vol. 7, ed. O. Stutman, New
    York: Plenum Press, p. 301.
Martz, E., and Benacerraf, B. (1975) T lymphocyte-mediated cytoly-
    sis: Temperature dependence of killer cell dependent and
    independent phases and lack of recovery from the lethal hit
    at low temperatures. Cell. Immunol. 20:81.
Martz, E., Burakoff, B., and Benacerraf, B. (1974) Interpretation
    of the sequential release of small and large molecules from
    tumor cells by low temperature during cytolysis mediated by

immune T cells or complement. Proc. Natl. Acad. Sci. USA
71:177.

Martz, E., Parker, W.L., Gately, M.K., and Tsoukas, C.D. (1982)
The role of calcium in the lethal hit of T lymphocyte-mediated cytolysis. In: "Mechanisms of Cell-Mediated Cytotoxicity," eds. W.R. Clark and P. Golstein, New York: Plenum
Press, p. 121.

Mayer, M.M. (1977) Mechanism of cytolysis by lymphocytes: A
comparison with complement. J. Immunol. 119:1195.

Mayer, M.M. (1982) Membrane attack by C' (with comments on cell-
mediated lysis). In: "Mechanisms in Cell-Mediated Cytotoxicity, eds. W.R. Clark and P. Golstein, New York: Plenum
Press, p. 193.

Mayer, M.M., Michaels, D.W., Ramm, L.E., Whitlow, M.B., Whillough-
by, J.B., and Shin, M.L. (1981) Membrane damage by complement. Crit. Rev. Immunol. 2:133.

Mescher, M.F. (1982) The interaction of MHC antigens with the
plasma membrane and the other cellular components. In:
"Histocompatibility Antigens: Structure and Function (Receptors and Recognition, Series B, Vol. 14), eds. P. Parham and
J. Strominger, New York: Chapmann and Hall, p. 55.

Michaels, D.W., Abramovitz, A.S., Hammer, C.H., and Mayer, M.M.
(1976) Increased ionic permeability of planar lipid bilayer
membranes after treatment with C5b-9 cytolytic attack mechanism of complement. Proc. Natl. Acad. Sci. US 73:2852.

Millard, P.J., Henkart, M.P., Reynolds, C.W., and Henkart, P.A.
(1984) Purification and properties of cytoplasmic granules
from cytotoxic rat LGL tumors. J. Immunol. 132:1.

Müller-Eberhard, H.J. (1975) Complement. Ann. Rev. Biochem.
44:697.

Ohanian, S.H., Schlager, S.I., and Borsos, T. (1978) Molecular
interactions of cells with antibody and complement: Influence of metabolic and physical properties of the target on
the outcome of humoral immune attack. Contemp. Top. Mol.
Immunol. 7:153.

Ramm, L.E., Whitlow, M.B., Koski, C.L., Shin, M.L., and Mayer,
M.M. (1983) Elimination of complement channels from the
plasma membranes of U937, a nucleated mammalian cell line:
Temperature dependence of the elimination rate. J. Immunol.
131:1411.

Russell, J.H. (1983) Internal disintegration model of cytotoxic
lymphocyte-induced target damage. Immunol. Rev. 72:97.

Russell, J.H., and Dobos, C.B. (1980) Mechanisms of immune lysis,
II. CTL-induced nuclear disintegration of the target begins
within minutes of cell contact. J. Immunol. 125:1256.

Sanderson, C.J. (1977) The mechanism of T cell mediated cytotox-
ity. V. Morphological studies by electron microscopy. Proc.
R. Soc. Lond. B. 198:315.

Sanderson, C.J. (1976) The mechanism of T cell mediated cytotox-
ity. I. The release of different cell components. Proc.
R. Soc. Lond. B. 192:221.

Sanderson, C.J. (1981) The mechanism of lymphocyte-mediated cytotoxicity. Biol. Rev. 56:153.

Sanderson, C.J. (1982) Morphological aspects of lymphocyte-mediated cytolysis. In: "Mechanisms of Cell-Mediated Cytotoxicity," eds. W.R. Clark and P. Golstein New York: Plenum Press, p. 1.

Sanderson, C.J. and Glauert, A.M. (1979) The mechanism of T cell mediated cytotoxicity. VI. T cell projections and their role in target cell killing. Immunology 36:119.

Sanderson, C.J., and Thomas, J.A. (1976) The mechanism of T cell mediated cytotoxicity, III. Changes in target cell susceptibility during the cell cycle. Proc. R. Soc. Lond. B. 194:417.

Schanne, F.A.X., Kane, A.B., Young, E.E., and Farber, J.L. (1979) Calcium dependence of toxic cell death: A final common pathway. Science 206:700.

Seeman, P. (1974) Ultrastructure of membrane lesions in immune lysis, osmotic lysis and drug induced lysis. Fed. Proc. 33:2116.

Shearer, W.T., Atkinson, J.P., and Parker, C.W. (1976) Humoral immunostimulation, VI. Increased calcium uptake by cells treated with antibody and complement. J. Immunol. 117:973.

Silman, I., and Karlin, A. (1967) Effect of local pH changes caused by substrate hydrolysis on the activity of membrane-bound acetylcholinesterase. Proc. Natl. Acad. Sci. US 58:1664.

Stephens, C.L., and Henkart, P.A. (1979) Electrical measurements of complement-mediated membrane damage in cultured nerve and muscle cells. J. Immunol. 122:455.

Stulting, R.D., and Berke, G. (1973) Nature of lymphocyte-tumor interaction. A general method for cellular immunoabsorption. J. Exp. Med. 137:932.

Schick, B., and Berke, G. (1978) Is the presence of serologically-defined alloantigens sufficient for binding of cytotoxic T lymphocytes? Transplantation 26:14.

Schick, B., Jakobovits, A., Sharon, N., and Berke, G. (1983) Cytotoxic T lymphocytes specifically lyse antigenically irrelevant cells upon insertion of appropriate target cell antigens into their plasma membranes. Transplantation 36:84.

Schlessinger, J. (1980) The mechanism and role of hormone-induced clustering of membrane receptors. Trends in Biochem. Sci. 5:210.

Schlessinger, J., and Elson, E.L. (1982) Fluorescence methods for studying membrane dynamics. In: "Methods of Experimental Physics," Col. 20, eds. G. Ehrenstein and H. Lecar, New York: Academic Press, p. 197.

Taylor, B.W., Knoll, H.P. and Bhakdi, S. (1983) Killing of Escherichia coli LP1092 by human serum. Immunobiology 164:304.

Tirosh, R., and Berke, G. (1984) T lymphocyte-mediated cytolysis as a stimulatory process of the target, I. Evidence that the target is the site of Ca^{2+} action. Submitted for publication.

Tirosh, R., Degani, H., and Berke, G. (1984) Prelytic depletion of high energy phosphates induced by antibody and complement in nucleated cells. ^{31}P-NMR study. Submitted for publication.

Tsien, R.Y., Pozzan, T., and Rink, T.J. (1982) T cell mitogens cause early changes in cytoplasmic free Ca^{2+} and membrane potential in lymphocytes. Nature 295:68.

Zagury, D. (1982) Direct analysis of individual killer T cells: Susceptibility of target cells to lysis and secretion of hydrolytic enzymes by CTL. In: "Mechanisms of Cell-Mediated Cytotoxicity," eds. W.R. Clark and P. Golstein, New York: Plenum Press, p. 149.

DISCUSSION

J. Ding-E Young: I love this idea of a stimulatory process.
Actually, we spent several years working on the mouse macrophage Fc
receptor, as you know. We showed there (inaudible) that we can
induce pore formation, stimulatory processes, and they are
coupled. However every single piece of data you mentioned, as far
as I can see, is totally consistent with the pore formation model.
The (complement?)-mediated efflux. That's perfect. I'll challenge
anyone in the audience who can show a pore over 20 nm of size and
not show rubidium efflux or calcium influx. You mentioned ATP
depletion. I would like to say, if you perturb the cell with that
gigantic hole, I'll again challenge anyone in the audience who will
tell me that the cell, in order to try to recover the ionic
equilibrium will not deplete its ATP resources trying to pump out
(inaudible) . . . its still consistent. You talk of an osmotically
protected step. That's well known for any type of (inaudible)
where you have a molecular sieving effect. You should expect
osmotic protection. Temperature: that's consistent with ionic
perturbation and the fact that you have to have a polymerized
species which occurs only at 37 degrees -- this is well
characterized. Endocytosis: we believe, as many people believe,
that endocytosis is a protective mechanism by the simple fact that
you can deplete a piece of membrane containing a pore and
internalize it and eliminate the effect. Also, the final point you
made, that the result of all these effects can cause zeiosis, you
mentioned that the pore formation is a consequence of a sum of all
these effects. I'd like to point out that we can really pin down
at this point the pore formation to a structural protein. Maybe
Pierre [Henkart] has the purified species -- we still don't have
the purified species -- but as far as we can see you can really
correlate functional activity with a structural entity. This is not
to refute a stimulatory process, which may occur simultaneously
with the pore formation. You should expect stimulatory signals.
So I'm not really refuting anything you've said, except that I
think that what you've said is completely consistent with the pore
formation model.

G. Berke: I think it boils down to answering the question: if a
pore is being created, is the pore required and sufficient for a
cell to undergo lysis? Because we cannot define, if that pore is
small, as we think, namely becoming a conducting channel or a
stimulatory channel, or as you think, its a big hole which is
required and sufficient for lysis. That's actually the crux of my
presentation.

DNA FRAGMENTATION IN TARGETS OF CTL: AN EXAMPLE OF PROGRAMMED CELL DEATH IN THE IMMUNE SYSTEM

J. John Cohen, Richard C. Duke, Robert
Chervenak, Karen S. Sellins and
Lori K. Olson.

Department of Microbiology and Immunology
University of Colorado Medical School
Denver, Colorado 80262

INTRODUCTION: PROGRAMMED CELL DEATH

Our studies of T cell-mediated cytotoxicity grew out of an interest in the mechanism of programmed cell death. The death of cells in the metazoan body can be categorized functionally, morphologically and biochemically. On the functional level, cell death is often acceptable or desirable for the system; it is part of the design. Examples of this programmed cell death include morphogenetic death, which occurs during early development and helps shape organs and limbs; death in systems with a normal cell turnover, for example epithelia or polymorphonuclear neutrophils; and the involution of hormone-dependent tissues. Opposed to this functionally acceptable cell death is accidental death, such as might follow physical, chemical or anoxic injury, and certain bacterial and viral infections.

Morphologically, cell death has been classified as either necrotic or apoptotic (1). Necrosis is in general the morphological correlate of accidental cell death, and is characterized by early cytoplasmic changes, especially mitochondrial swelling. In apoptosis, which is usually observed when cell death can be considered to be programmed, the earliest changes are a condensation of nuclear chromatin and blebbing of nuclear and plasma membranes (zeiosis); pathologic changes in cytoplasmic organelles occur later.

Less is known about the biochemical processes which distinguish the two forms of cell death. In necrosis the mitochondrial swelling is accompanied by a loss of energy production, followed shortly by the cell's inability to osmoregulate; the nuclear chromatin is spared during this process. In contrast, Wyllie observed that apoptosis in rat thymocytes is characterized by the reduction of chromatin to nucleosome-sized fragments (2). This correlated with the observed early condensation of chromatin, and suggested that this was the event that led eventually to the cell's death and lysis. It was obvious that the chromatin was being cleaved by an enzyme, and Wyllie suggested that the enzyme involved might be Hewish and Burgoyne's endogenous endonuclease (3,4,5).

THE ENDOGENOUS ENDONUCLEASE

This enzyme was first described in the 1970's in isolated liver and lymphocyte nuclei. If calcium and magnesium were added to the buffer in which these nuclei were incubated, the chromatin was rapidly fragmented to small multiples of an approximately 200 base-pair unit. We have repeated this observation with mouse thymocyte nuclei. Figure 1 shows the characteristic ladder of bands that are obtained on agarose gel electrophoresis of DNA from nuclei incubated with calcium and magnesium. Not all nuclei contain this enzyme activity, however (Table 1); by far the richest cells are lymphocytes, both immature (thymus) and mature (spleen and lymph node). Bone marrow cell nuclei do not contain detectable enzyme activity; neither do the nuclei of mitogen-activated T cells or any of the tumor lines we have examined. The enzyme is easily eluted from nuclei that contain it by incubation in buffered saline. The preparation of enzyme so obtained can be assayed on tumor cell nuclei; it requires calcium and magnesium and produces the fragments seen in Fig. 1. It apparently cuts DNA in the relatively exposed linker region between nucleosomes, which are regularly spaced on chromatin about 200 bases apart. It will also cleave the SV40 minichromosome, which has nucleosomes, but it is much less active on naked DNA. We have not found another cation which can substitute for calcium for activation. The enzyme is very strongly inhibited by zinc (6).

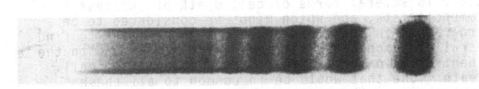

Fig. 1. DNA fragments obtained following activation
of the endogenous endonuclease in isolated
mouse spleen cell nuclei. Nuclei obtained
from Balb/c spleen cells by Dounce
homogenization were incubated with 10 mM
$MgCl_2$ and 5 mM $CaCl_2$ for 90 min at 37°C.
DNA was extracted and subjected to
electrophoresis in 0.8% agarose for 2 hr at
90 V. DNA was visualized with ethidium
bromide.

Table I. Tissue Distribution of Calcium- and Mag-
nesium-Dependent Endonuclease Activity

Nuclei	% fragmented DNA[*]	
	Mg^{2+}	$Mg^{2+} + Ca^{2+}$
Spleen	7	70
Thymus	2	47
Lymph node	6	44
Liver	1	17
Human PBL	3	36
P815 mastocytoma	3	4
PSW lymphoma	1	3
Bone marrow	1	3
Con A blasts	9	10
HT-2 T cell line	1	1
CTLL-20 T cell line	2	3
MLR blasts	2	2

[*]Nuclei were isolated from the cells shown and
incubated for 90 min at 37°C in tris-buffered saline
containing 10 mM $MgCl_2$ with or without 5 mM $CaCl_2$
added. Nuclei were then washed and lysed and
centrifuged at 13,000 x g for 10 min. DNA was measured
in the pellet (intact DNA) and in the supernatant
(fragmented DNA); further details are in reference 6.

We decided to determine whether changes in DNA occur in several forms of cell death of interest to immunologists, and which might be considered to be programmed in the broad sense. We hoped thus to find parallels among these systems which might lead to the identification of a "final common pathway" of cell death: one that would be in common to all these systems, even though the means by which they were initiated differed. If this were so, we might then be able to infer mechanisms in one system from studies in another; this is a great advantage, since some systems are better characterized or easier to study than others. What follows is a summary of where we are after about two years.

GLUCOCORTICOID-INDUCED THYMOCYTE DEATH

When mouse thymocytes are exposed in vitro to glucocorticoids at levels within the physiological range (0.1 to 1 uM) they are killed within 8 to 20 hours, as assessed by exclusion of a dye such as eosin Y. About four hours before the cells die their chromatin begins to break up into fragments; on an agarose gel these show a regular pattern, and are approximately 200, 400, 600 and so on bases long, similar to those shown in Figure 1. DNA cleavage is prevented, and cell death very much delayed, if protein or RNA synthesis is inhibited during the exposure to glucocorticoid. Since we already knew that the thymocyte nucleus contains the endonuclease, but like all nuclei is essentially devoid of the calcium which the enzyme requires, we concluded that the necessary proteins could include a calcium transporter (6). Thus the glucocorticoid might induce the synthesis of this transport protein, which would become loaded with calcium in the cytoplasm and then move into the nucleus, where its calcium would activate the endogenous endonuclease. This still seems to be a reasonable explanation, although we have not yet been able to isolate a calcium transport protein in glucocorticoid-treated thymocytes.

We cannot at this stage prove that the activation of the endonuclease, and the fragmentation of DNA that results, directly leads to cell death, although of course any nucleated cell in which the majority of the DNA is reduced to nucleosome-sized pieces is certainly doomed. We have observed that cell death is prevented when DNA fragmentation is prevented, for example by inhibiting protein synthesis or in the presence of zinc. To establish the connection rigorously we need a thymocyte line that lacks functional structural genes for the endonuclease; would such a cell be unkillable by glucocorticoids?

It must be stressed at this point that the fragmentation of DNA is not merely a concommitant of cell death, regardless of cause. If cells are killed by heat, or freezing, or sodium azide, or by antibody and complement, no DNA fragmentation is observed even after the cells are dead by dye uptake.

The killing of thymocytes by glucocorticoids is not, in our view, solely a pharmacological or pathophysiological event. The ease of activation of the endonuclease at low steroid concentrations, well within the range that is achieved at the peak of the circadian cycle, suggests that such activation is part of a normal physiological process. We propose that lymphocytes which arrive at or develop within the thymus have a day or so to be selected for further maturation and export, on the basis of displaying an appropriate MHC-restricted receptor. One of the maturational changes in such selected cells is the acquisition of the resistance to glucocorticoids which is characteristic of peripheral T cells (7). The vast majority (greater than 99%) are not selected to mature and may be induced to die as the blood glucocorticoid level reaches its peak. This effect of glucocorticoids would be moderated by adequate tissue zinc concentrations, since zinc inhibits the endonuclease. Although this view of one aspect of the regulation of lymphopoiesis in the thymus may seem a bit ad hoc, its logical predictions are supported by experimental observations. When mice are adrenalectomized, the thymus becomes enlarged, up to three times normal (8, and our own unpublished observations). Conversely, mice on a low zinc diet have atrophic thymuses, which are restored to normal when zinc is added back to the diet (9). Furthermore, the thymuses of zinc-deficient mice do not involute if the animals are also adrenalectomized (10).

In conclusion, if the notion that thymocyte number is regulated by normal glucocorticoid levels is correct, then the mechanisms of this example of programmed cell death can serve as useful models to compare to other systems.

"INTERPHASE DEATH" OF IRRADIATED LYMPHOCYTES

Lymphocytes are the most sensitive cells in the body to ionizing radiation and are unusual in that they are killed in interphase, whereas most other cells are much more sensitive when actively dividing (11). The dose of radiation which can kill a lymphocyte is as low as 5 R (12). Skalka and coworkers (13) showed that this death is accompanied by extensive DNA breakage, which is surprising because at these low doses double-stranded breaks in chromosomes are rare. We found (14) that low-dose irradiation of thymocytes or spleen cells in vivo or in vitro produced DNA fragmentation identical to that seen with glucocorticoid-treated thymocytes. Again, the DNA cleavage was prevented with cycloheximide or zinc. Thus ionizing radiation also induces the activation of the endogenous endonuclease in lymphocytes (at these low doses the DNA remains intact in other organs).

Why are lymphocytes so easily killed by ionizing radiation? We do not know, but we suggest that it is because a damaged lymphocyte is so potentially dangerous to the body. Lymphocytes are the only cells in the body which are normally permitted to undergo clonal expansion. If a lymphocyte were to sustain damage of a type that could lead to mutation, that mutation might be in the genes for its receptor. Should the new receptor be autoreactive, the risk to the organism would not be just from that lymphocyte, but also from the clone to which it would rapidly give rise. This is so dangerous from the organism's point of view that we believe that evolution has built a "better dead than wrong" mechanism into lymphocytes. Our preliminary results suggest that hydroxyl radicals are involved in the process which leads to activation of the endogenous endonuclease.

DEATH DUE TO LACK OF INTERLEUKIN-2

Hematopoietic hormones have a number of properties in common: they stimulate proliferation in their target cell, they may also stimulate differentiation, and they keep their target cell alive; this has been demonstrated for erythropoietin-sensitive red cell precursors (15) and myeloid (16) and T cell precursors (17). Certain subpopulations of T cells, notably cytotoxic cells, require a hormone or growth factor, interleukin 2 (IL-2), for proliferation after initial antigen stimulation, and these IL-2 dependent cells will die if the factor is removed. This observation forms the basis for the common bioassay of IL-2 preparations. To examine the mechanisms of this form of death, we used two cell lines which are extremely IL-2 dependent and are used to assay IL-2: CTLL-20 and HT-2. We also used spleen cells which had been stimulated with concanavalin A and maintained for 10 doublings on IL-2. All cells were grown in tissue culture medium containing IL-2 and then split and recultured with or without added IL-2. Cells remained viable in the presence of the growth factor, but began to die, as measured by eosin Y uptake, about 12 hr after its removal. Several hours before the cells died, their DNA had begun to fragment in the now-familiar nucleosomal pattern (Table II). This DNA fragmentation could be prevented and the cells kept alive for at least 24 hr, if protein synthesis were inhibited by a low concentration (5 ug/ml) of cycloheximide. We were less successful in preventing cell death with zinc, because the particular cells used seem to effectively exclude this cation.

Is IL-2 deprivation an example of programmed cell death? We believe that this may represent one of the ways in which the immune system is controlled. Upon

Table II. DNA Fragmentation and Cell Death Following IL-2 Removal from CTLL-20 Cells

Condition	Time (hr)	% fragmented DNA	% dead
+ IL-2	6	8	1
	10	5	1
	14	6	3
NO IL-2	6	8	0
	8	35	2
	10	62	10
	12	81	38
	14	87	55
NO IL-2 + cyclohex	6	16	1
	10	10	5
	14	10	15

proper presentation of antigen, helper or inducer cells are activated and begin to secrete IL-2. Effector cell precursors, seeing antigen, become responsive to IL-2; they proliferate and differentiate into active effectors (for example, killers) which assist in the removal of antigen or the destruction of infected cells. When antigen has been eliminated, the helpers, no longer stimulated, stop their production of IL-2; the IL-2 dependent cells, no longer necessary, then die. This view is consistent with the evidence that most immunological memory seems to inhere in helper rather than effector populations.

DEATH BY CYTOTOXIC T CELL

When we began to study the effects of cytotoxic T cells (CTL) on their targets, we quickly confirmed Russell and Dobos's finding (18) that DNA fragmentation is an early event; in our hands it precedes chromium release by about 90 minutes (the exact time seems to depend on the activity of the CTL population; when effective killing occurs at low killer:target ratios, chromium release occurs more rapidly). The fragments are a regular array of nucleosome multiplets as seen in the other systems (19). We observe this fragmentation within five minutes of adding CTL to their targets, and it is immunologically specific and CTL-dose related.

The nuclear envelope is normally resistant to solubilization by detergents. Russell and Dobos (18) noted that a "nuclear lesion" develops in the targets of CTL, such that DNA can be released from the cell by Triton X-100. They suggested that this lesion may be an earlier event than DNA fragmentation. In our hands DNA fragmentation and the nuclear lesion develop pari passu, since the total fragmented DNA in the cell (measured after complete lysis of the cell and its nucleus with hypotonic detergent-containing buffer) is always equal to the fragmented DNA released from the cell by detergent alone (Table III); we do not see intact DNA released from CTL targets by detergent, as would be expected if the nuclear lesion preceded DNA fragmentation.

The cleavage of DNA by the endogenous endonuclease does not in itself produce a nuclear lesion. If thymocyte nuclei are incubated with calcium,, up to 80% of the DNA will be fragmented within 90 minutes, but

Table III. Appearance of Total Fragmented DNA, Triton-Soluble DNA, and Chromium Release During T Cell-Mediated Cytolysis

Time (min)	% specific fragmented DNA	% specific triton-soluble DNA	% specific chromium release
5	21	20	1
20	45	41	5
40	55	49	8
60	60	54	28
120	69	61	62
180	81	76	82

CBA spleen cells were stimulated with irradiated BALB/c spleen for 5 days, and maintained on IL-2 for an additional 5 days. They were assayed on P815 target cells which had been labelled with either ^{125}IUdR or ^{51}Cr. Effector:target ratio was 1:1. For complete experimental details see reference 19.

none of the fragments leak out into the medium, and Triton does not release them; hypotonic lysis is required. Nicholson and Young (20) have described increased nuclear fragility in thymocytes and sensitive tumor cell lines exposed to glucocorticoids, but we have not found that the DNA of such cells becomes Triton-soluble. Thus, we do not think that the nuclear lesion is secondary to DNA fragmentation, nor that there is much evidence that the reverse is true. It seems most likely that these are separate events, perhaps brought about by separate enzymes.

If we isolate nuclei from either CTL or any of the usual target cells, including tumors and lymphoblasts, we find no endogenous endonuclease that we can activate with calcium. Nonetheless, mixing the two cell types results in cleavage of target cell chromatin within minutes. Where did the enzyme come from? We do not know yet, but one intriguing possibility is that it is injected by the CTL, perhaps via the same granules that insert ring structures (21,22). If the enzyme were confined in cytoplasmic vesicles in the CTL, it could do no harm (and in fact, CTL chromatin remains quite intact during the killing process), but upon injection as free enzyme into the target's cytoplasm it might rapidly bind calcium and be transported into the cell's nucleus. It is known that lymphocytes can transfer certain enzymes to other cells (23).

Alternatively, the enzyme may be within the target cell in an inactive form. In that case, changes in the cell's cytoplasmic composition, such as might follow opening of ion channels, might activate the enzyme; or the killer cell might activate it by injecting a cofactor. We are working on making an antibody to the enzyme so that we can trace its movements.

In considering mechanisms by which CTL destroy their targets, a vital question is whether DNA fragmentation is the direct cause of cytolysis, especially since zinc blocks both phenomena (Table 4). We see no evidence that this is so, because cytolysis follows too quickly upon DNA cleavage (30 to 90 minutes) to result from interruption of macromolecular synthesis. Furthermore, we have preliminary evidence that the two processes can be separated. When CTL are mixed with their targets in the presence of manganese, DNA fragmentation takes place normally, but chromium release, our measure of cytolysis, is inhibited (Table IV). Thus, fragmentation does not inevitably lead to lysis within the time frame studied. We favor the view that DNA cleavage and cell lysis are separately signalled to the target cell.

Table IV. Inhibition of DNA Fragmentation and Chromium Release by Zinc and Magnanese

Expt	Ions added	% specific fragmented DNA	% inhib	% specific chromium release	% inhib
1	-	95		89	
	1 mM Zn^{2+}	0	100	8	91
	1 mM Mn^{2+}	79	17	19	79
2	-	83		97	
	1 mM Mn^{2+}	69	17	24	75

CONCLUSIONS

We have described four immune system-related types of cell death, which have in common the fragmentation of DNA into oligonucleosome units as an early event which precedes cell lysis. In each case, calcium and magnesium are required for, and zinc inhibits, both DNA fragmentation and cytolysis. In each case, as discussed above, we believe that these are examples of programmed cell death, in that their outcome is good for the organism as a whole.

We have included the killing of target cells by CTL in this group, because we think that such death can be considered programmed. The question is basically philosophical. It is accepted that the immune system has the role of surveillance of cell surfaces for the detection of altered self. A cell which displays such alterations may be harmful, and the good of the organism is served by its destruction. It would be simple enough to lyse the offending cell, but it seems that we have evolved other protective modalities in addition to lysis; one of these is induced DNA fragmentation.

In the four systems described above, the common feature is DNA fragmentation, but an important difference is that CTL killing does not require protein synthesis by the target cell. This is a good design feature, since a major role of CTL is to kill virus-infected cells before the virus have had a chance to replicate within them; and many viruses shut off host cell protein synthesis early after infection. If the expression of endonuclease activity in the target cell were to require new protein synthesis, the virus, by preventing it, could escape destruction. Thus, the CTL may have two effective and complementary viricidal strategies: it rapidly destroys DNA (and possibly RNA), impairing the replication of most viruses, and then it lyses the target.

ACKNOWLEDGEMENT

The work discussed in this review was supported by NIH Grant AI-11661.

REFERENCES

1. Wyllie, A.H. Cell death: a new classification separating apoptosis from necrosis, in "Cell Death in Biology and Pathology", I.D. Bowen and R.A. Lockshin, eds. Chapman and Hall, London (1981).

2. Wyllie, A.H. Glucocorticoid-induced thymocyte apoptosis is associated with endogenous endonuclease activation. Nature 284:555 (1980).

3. Hewish, D.R. and L.A. Burgoyne. The calcium-dependent endonuclease activity in isolated nuclear preparations. Relationships between its occurrence and the occurrence of other classes of enzymes found in nuclear preparations. Biochem. Biophys. Res. Comm. 52:475 (1973).

4. Hewish, D.R. and L.A. Burgoyne. Chromatin sub-structure. The digestion of chromatin DNA at regularly spaced sites by a nuclear deoxyribonuclease. Biochem. Biophys. Res. Comm. 52:504 (1973).

5. Burgoyne, L.A., D.R. Hewish and J. Mobbs. Mammalian chromatin substructure studies with the calcium/magnesium endonuclease and 2D polyacrylamide gel electrophoresis. Biochem. J. 143:67 (1974).

6. Cohen, J.J. and R.C. Duke. Glucocorticoid activation of a calcium-dependent endonuclease in thymocyte nuclei leads to cell death. J. Immunol. 132:38 (1984).

7. Cohen, J.J. and H.N. Claman. Thymus-marrow immunocompetence. V. Hydrocortisone-resistant cells and processes in the hemolytic antibody response of mice. J. Exp. Med. 133:1026 (1971).

8. Shortman, K. and H. Jackson. The differentiation of T lymphocytes. I. Proliferation kinetics and interrelationships of subpopulations of mouse thymus cells. Cell. Immunol. 12:230 (1974).

9. Fraker, P.J., P. DePasquale-Jardieu, C.M Zwicki, and R.W. Leuke. Regeneration of T-cell helper function in zinc-deficient adult mice. Proc. Natl. Acad. Sci. USA 75:5660 (1978).

10. DePasquale-Jardieu, P. and P.J. Fraker. Further characterization of the role of corticosterone in the loss of humoral immunity in zinc-deficient A/J mice as determined by adrenalectomy. J. Immunol. 124:2650 (1980).

11. Trowell, O.A. The sensitivity of lymphocytes to ionizing radiation. J. Path. Bact. 64:687 (1952).

12. Anderson, R.E., G.B. Olson, J.R. Autry, J.L. Howarth, G.M. Troup and P.H. Bartels. Radiosensitivity of T and B lymphocytes. IV. Effect of whole body irradiation upon various lymphoid tissues and numbers of recirculating lymphocytes. J. Immunol. 118:1191 (1977).

13. Skalka, M., J. Matyasova and M. Cejkova. DNA in chromatin of irradiated lymphoid tissues degrades in vivo into regular fragments. FEBS Letters 72:271 (1976).

14. Sellins, K.S. and J.J. Cohen. Protein synthesis-dependent induction of endogenous endonuclease in irradiated thymocytes. Fed. Procs. 43:1640 (Abs.) (1984).

15. Cantor, L.N., A.J. Morris, P.A. Marks and R.A. Rifkind. Purification of erythropoietin-responsive cells by immune hemolysis. Proc. Natl. Acad. Sci. USA 69:1337 (1972).

16. Metcalf, D. Studies on colony formation in vitro by mouse bone marrow cells. II. Action of colony stimulating factor. J. Cell Physiol. 76:89 (1976).

17. Cohen, J.J. and S.S. Fairchild. Thymic control of proliferation of T cell precursors in bone marrow. Proc. Natl. Acad. Sci. USA 76:6587 (1979).

18. Russell, J.H. and C.B. Dobos. Mechanisms of immune lysis. II. CTL-induced nuclear disintegration of the target begins within minutes of cell contact. J. Immunol. 125:1256 (1980).

19. Duke, R.C., R. Chervenak and J.J. Cohen. Endogenous endonuclease-induced DNA fragmentation: An early event in cell-mediated cytolysis. Proc. Natl. Acad. Sci. USA 80:6361 (1983).

20. Nicholson, M.L. and D.A. Young. Effect of glucocorticoid hormones in vitro on the structural integrity of nuclei in corticosteroid-sensitive and -resistant lines of lymphosarcoma P1798. Cancer Res. 38:3673 (1978).

21. Dennert, B. and E.R. Podack. Cytolysis by H-2 specific T killer cells. Assembly of tubular complexes on target membranes. J. Exp. Med. 157:1483 (1983).

22. Milliard, P.J., M.P. Henkart, C.W. Reynolds and P.A. Henkart. Purification and properties of cytoplasmic granules from cytotoxic rat LGL tumors. J. Immunol. 132:3197 (1984).

23. Olsen, I., H. Muir, R. Smith, A. Fensom and D.J. Watt. Direct enzyme transfer from lymphocytes is specific. Nature 306:75 (1983).

DISCUSSION

W. Clark: Does manganese cause conjugates to fall apart?

E. Martz: Manganese not only does not inhibit conjugate formation, but it is able to replace magnesium [otherwise required for conjugate formation], as Maury Gately showed a while back (Cellular Immunol. 61:78, 1981). Also it blocks programming for lysis. I think John [Cohen] has made an extremely interesting observation.

E. Podack: Is this nuclear disintegration inhibited by protein synthesis inhibitors in the CTL system?

J. Cohen: No, it is not.

E. Podack: The comment that I have is the observation that I mentioned in my talk, that zinc is strongly inhibitory of granule-mediated lysis. The suggestion that I made was that while it may be involved in polymerization, it may also be involved in protein synthesis.

J. Cohen: Yes, its important to point that out. I think we all tend to make our system sound most important. There are at least 130 enzymes that have been described that use zinc as a cofactor, regardless of how many are inhibited by it.

S. Bhakdi: Where does the chromium come out? We have the kiss of death --wouldn't you expect the chromium to be released there? Or would you think that would be a secondary phenomenon.

P. Henkart (?): I think John Russell has got probably the best system going for looking at that. If you kill a neurite up here, you could actually see whether chromium is released from the cell even though its a mile away.

J. Russell: We've tried to label the neurons with chromium and they leak like a sieve.

G. Berke: Regarding the question just posed as to whether the chromium is coming out at the site of certain cell contacts, I don't think anybody has a straightforward answer to that question. But, one can ask the quesion if you were to label the cells with a fluorescent dye, say, fluorescein diacetate (FDA), with cinematography under ultraviolet light. We addressed the question whether the fluorescent tag would come out at the site of the CTL-target contact region. We were surprised to see that the dye would come out as a big aura surrounding the cell, and not at the site of cell-to-cell contact.

<u>S. Bhakdi</u>: What were the kinetics?

<u>G. Berke</u>: The kinetics of FDA release were as quick as those of chromium release.

<u>S. Bhakdi</u>: Or as slow.

<u>G. Berke</u>: When you say slow, you have to define it. There is only one agent that effluxes [from] the target with [more] rapid kinetics than chromium, and this is rubidium [86]. This will be brought up in my discussion. Maybe there is in the audience somebody who has demonstrated a cellular constituent which effluxes with greater kinetics than that of chromium, which is not rubidium.

<u>E. Martz</u>: We showed many years ago that nicotinamide effluxes more rapidly than does chromium during CTL-mediated lysis [Proc. Nat. Acad. Sci. USA 71:177, 1974].

<u>T. Springer</u>: I have a comment on the idea of whether there are two separate signals, one forming a hole, and the other one causing nuclear damage. Or whether the findings which have been presented are still consistent with a single signal being just the damage of the cell membrane. Its been shown that a number of kinds of signals can cause this nuclear disintegration, irradiation of the cells, glucocorticoids, removal of IL2. It seems that this system is very sensitive to changes occurring in the intercellular environment. It still remains possible that because the hole is larger, at least the hole in ADCC, is larger than the hole that is caused by complement-mediated killing, that the intracellular environment may be different. There may be different molecules leaking out. Its possible that this could trigger this kind of nuclear disintegration.

<u>J. Hiserodt</u>: I was wondering if you would generalize this to other species, or whether its unique to rodents, or whether you see this kind of nuclear disintegration in human thymocytes, or human CTLs or rats...

(unknown): This is obviously a set-up ... Duane [Sears] is about to get up here and say no.

508

MECHANISM OF RAPID TUMOR LYSIS BY HUMAN ADCC: MEDIATION BY MONOCLONAL ANTIBODIES AND FRAGMENTATION OF TARGET CELL DNA

Duane W. Sears and Jeffrey E. Christiaansen

Department of Biological Sciences
University of California, Santa Barbara
Santa Barbara, CA 93106

INTRODUCTION

Immunologically programmed cell destruction is an important defense mechanism for limiting the spread of invasive intracellular parasites and malignant cells in the body (1,2). However, when such processes are misdirected, in autoimmune diseases for example, they can be very harmful to normal tissues and can interfere with vital tissue functions (2). Thus, it is of considerable value to understand the mechanisms of cytolytically induced cell destruction as mediated by the immune system. Several such mechanisms have evolved with the immune system of man, and each is characterized by distinct antigen recognition requirements and/or distinct lytic processes. Some cytolytic mechanisms require only the secreted products of cells and not the direct intervention of an effector cell for cytolysis to occur, as with complement plus antibody-mediated cytotoxicity (CAMC), for example. Other mechanisms, however, do require that intimate contact be made between an effector cell and its target cell. Various lymphocytes, such as cytotoxic T lymphocytes (CTL), natural killer (NK) cells, and killer (K) cells all appear to initiate the lytic process only after contact is made with the target cell (1-4).

K cell-mediated killing -- i.e., antibody-dependent cellular cytotoxicity (ADCC) -- is particularly intriguing when compared in potency and mechanism to the other cytolytic processes. In effect, K cells bridge humoral and cellular immunity in that both antibody and effector cells are required for the lytic process to occur. However, ADCC is considerably more potent than its humoral counterpart -- i.e., CAMC -- since the former mechanism

509

requires 10- to 100-fold lower concentrations of antibody than the latter mechanism in order to achieve efficient target cell lysis (5). Although K cells and CTL are comparable in their lytic potencies (i.e., equally efficient and equally rapid killing can be achieved with relatively low effector to target cells ratios with both effector types), K cells (as well as NK cells) are distinguished by the fact that they require no prior antigenic education. Thus, K cells are always in a ready state of action whenever appropriate antibody is present.

Because much is yet to be learned about the actual ADCC lytic mechanism mediated by K lymphocytes, a systematic study has been undertaken to find answers to two key questions concerning the process mediated by these cells. 1) What are the target cell recognition requirements for efficient ADCC by human nonadherent K lymphocytes? 2) How do the ADCC mechanism and K effector compare to other lytic processes and other effector lymphocytes?

MEDIATION OF ADCC BY MONOCLONAL ANTIBODIES

Most prior studies of ADCC have focused on target cell lytic events mediated by heteroantisera, although scattered reports are found in which monoclonal antibodies (MAbs) have been tested for their ability to mediate ADCC. Generally, these studies have found MAbs to be relatively inefficient mediators of ADCC. However, MAbs which are exceptions to these observations were described in a recent study from this laboratory (6) where a panel of IgG MAbs directed against a variety of murine cell surface antigens was examined in ADCC reactions with human effector cells. Although the majority of MAbs tested showed a profound lack of ability to mediate ADCC, even though they all bound target cells effectively, a few MAbs mediated ADCC extremely efficiently, in fact, nearly as efficiently as a hyperimmune rabbit heteroantiserum also tested. However, the most unexpected finding was that a clear relationship did not exist between the efficiency of a given MAb in the ADCC assay and its IgG subclass. The most effective MAbs were of the IgG2a and IgG3 subclasses, but, even so, not all IgG2a antibodies worked well and some did not work at all. These observations have been extended in the present study where another panel of MAbs, this time specific for a single cell surface antigen -- i.e. human β_2m (Hu β_2m) -- was tested in an ADCC assay with 8866 human tumor targets. As illustrated in Fig. 1, a wide variation is found in the ability of these MAbs to mediate ADCC, verifying our earlier findings. In this experiment, extremely low amounts (< 100 ng) of all IgG2a MAbs tested, except one (i.e., 26/114HLK), caused nearly complete target cell lysis within 4 hr and at low effector to target (E:T) ratios. The IgG3 MAb and one IgG2b MAb were moderately effective whereas the other IgG2bs and IgG1s tested were, at best, marginally active in the lytic process at

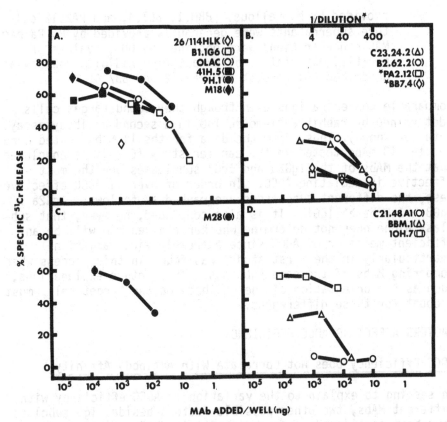

FIG. 1. MADCC activity OF γ2a (A), γ1 (B), γ3 (C), and γ2b (D).
anti-Hu β₂m MAbs with human leukocyte effectors. Duplicate samples of 1×10^4 ^{51}Cr-labeled human 8866 B
lymphoblastoid tumor cells (7) were incubated for 10 min
with log dilutions of MAb (except 26/114 HLK, tested at
a single dilution). 25×10^4 human effector cells were
then added to a final volume of 200 μl (E:T ratio =
25:1). After 4 hr, 100 μl of supernatant was removed
from each microtiter well including spontaneous-release
(SR) wells (no MAb and no effectors) and full-release
(FR) wells (NP40 lysed) to determine experimental
specific ^{51}Cr release. Human leukocyte effectors were
obtained from heparinized peripheral blood of healthy
donors followed by centrifugation over Ficoll-Hypaque
and removal of adherent cells by incubation in plastic
petri dishes for 1 hr at 37°C. Specific ^{51}Cr release
with MAb and no effectors or effectors and no MAb was
less than 5% in all cases. SR was always less than 10%
of FR. 26/114 HLK was purchased form Pel-Freez Bio-
logicals. OLAC (clone SRL-1) was purchased from OLAC,
Ltd. B1.1G6, B2.62.2, C21.48A1, and C23.24.2 purified
MAbs were generously provided by A. Liabeuf. 9H.1,
10H.7, and 41H.5 were generously provided by
M. Longnecker. M18 and M28 ascites were generously

provided by M. Fellous. BBM.1, BB7.4, and PA2.12 culture supernatants were generously provided by P. Parham.
MAb concentrations were obtained by OD_{280} values of
purified material or by competition radioimmunoassay as
described (6), except for PA2.12 and BB7.4.

comparable concentrations even though they bound target cells
(determined by rabbit anti-mouse IgG in a second-antibody assay;
data not shown). Thus, from the data for the 14 MAbs tested here
and the 13 MAbs tested in the earlier study (6), it is concluded
that the MAbs of the IgG2a and IgG3 subclasses are the most
effective in mediating ADCC. In order of overall ADCC effectiveness, the different subclasses are ranked as follows: IgG2a >
IgG3 > IgG2bs >> IgG1. It is also concluded, however, that subclass alone does not determine whether a given MAb will be an
efficient mediator of ADCC since extremely wide variation
(particularly in the first study) was found in this process when
comparing MAbs of the same subclass. Thus, other explanations,
such as the orientation of the antibody on the target cell, must
account for these differences.

FACTORS AFFECTING ADCC EFFICIENCY

ADCC Efficiency Does Not Correlate With Antibody Affinity

In seeking to explain to the variation in ADCC efficiency with
different MAbs, two other possible factors besides IgG subclass
have been considered -- antibody affinity and antibody orientation. In our earlier study (6), the importance of antibody
affinity was tested and it was discovered, somewhat surprisingly,
that one of the best MAbs in mediating ADCC (an IgG3) had the
lowest target cell affinity tested whereas a second MAb (an
IgG2a) did not initiate target cell lysis by ADCC even though it
bound exactly the same target cell antigen, but with very high
affinity. Thus, it was concluded that the ability of a MAb to
mediate ADCC was not critically dependent on antigen affinity, at
least in any obvious way.

Antibody Orientation is Critical for Efficient ADCC

In order to test the second possibility above - that ADCC efficiency depends in some way on the orientation of bound Ab relative to the target cell surface and the adjacent components of
the cell membrane - it was necessary to test target cells which
had the same antigen in different orientations. Thus, the ADCC
susceptibility of human tumor cells was compared to the ADCC susceptibility of murine cells with $Hu\beta_2m$ covalently attached
to them by a heterobifunctional cross-linking reaction recently
developed in this laboratory (8); this cross-linking method
randomly introduces about 10 million or more protein molecules

512

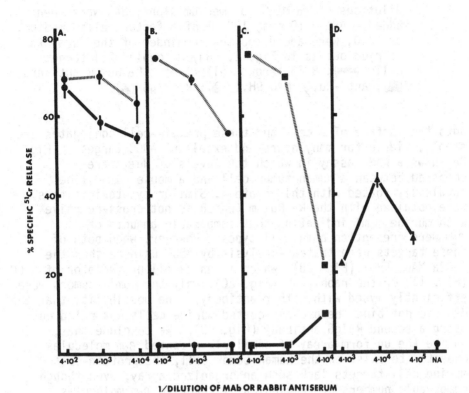

Fig. 2. Efficient ADCC requires a regular array of properly
oriented antibodies on the target cell surface. Purified Huβ_2m was covalently coupled to mouse C14 "null"
(Abelson virus-transformed) cells. 10 nmoles of Huβ_2m
in 35 μl of HBS (pH 8) was reacted with an equimolar
amount of SMCC for 10 min at r.t. This mixture was
added to 2 x 10^6 ^{51}Cr-labeled C14 cells in 100 μl which
had been reduced for 1 hr at 0°C with 10 mM DTT in 1 ml
PBS, and washed 3X. After a 10 min reaction at r.t.,
the Huβ_2m-coupled C14 cells were washed again 3X to
remove unreacted Huβ_2m. The presence of Huβ_2m on the
C14 cells was assayed by CAMC (A), and by ADCC (B-D),
and compared to human 8866 tumor targets. In (A), 2-
stage complement assays with log dilutions of 9H.1 were
performed identically on Huβ_2m-coupled C14 cells and
8866 cells in the same experiment. ADCC assays in (B)
and (C) were performed exactly as in Fig. 1 with 9H.1 or
Rα Huβ_2m, respectively. In (D), an indirect ADCC
reaction was employed using Rα MIgG to detect 9H.1 on
the surface of the Huβ_2m-coupled C14 cells. 1.5 x 10^5
Huβ_2m-coupled C14 cells were incubated with a 1/400
final dilution of 9H.1 for 20 min at r.t. and washed.
The cell pellet was resuspended in 750 μl, and 50 μl
aliquots were added to microtiter wells. 50 μl of log
(continued)

Fig. 2. (continued)

dilutions of Rα MIgG (or medium alone, NA) were then
added. After 10 min, 100 µl of effector cells, medium,
or NP40, were added and the remainder of the assay was
carried out as in Fig. 1. Huβ_2m-coupled C14 target
cells (▬); 8866 target cells (▭). Rα Huβ_2m antisera
(■); anti-Huβ_2m MAb 9H.1 (●); Rα MIgG (▲).

onto the surface of a cell and these protein-cell conjugates are
stable, viable for many hours and excellent ADCC targets. Fig.
2A shows a CAMC assay in which the levels of Huβ_2m are
compared between a human tumor cell and a mouse tumor line
covalently coated with this protein. Similar cytotoxic titers
were obtained with the Rα Huβ_2m (which is not cross-reactive
with murine β_2m) indicating that comparable amounts of
β_2m were present on both cell types. However, when both of
these targets were tested for lysis by ADCC using either the
IgG2a MAb, 9H.1 (Fig. 2B), which is an excellent mediator of ADCC
(Fig. 1), or the rabbit Ab (Fig. 2C), only the human tumors were
efficiently lysed with either antibody. The possibility that the
MAb did not bind the protein-coated murine cells was ruled out
using a second RaIgG antibody (Fig. 2D). We conclude that,
unlike the uniform array of similarly-oriented β_2m molecules
expected to exist on the human tumor cell, the protein-coated
murine cell targets lack such an organized array, even though
comparable numbers of serologically reactive β_2m molecules
are present. It could be argued that this reasoning may not
explain the differences in susceptibilities of the two targets
because the ADCC assay using the second antibody (Fig. 2D) should
not have worked. However, the outcome of this experiment many be
a result of the fact that many second antibodies can attach to
one mouse IgG MAb on the cell surface because of the large size
of immunoglobulins as compared to β_2m which may bind only a
few, at most, rabbit antibodies. Thus, local arrays of Abs may
be possible in the first but not the second case. The fact that
β_2m is the target antigen in these experiments may also
account for the fact that most of the IgG2a MAbs against this
molecule were efficient in ADCC (Fig. 1) whereas the majority of
IgG2a MAbs examined in our first study (6) where ineffective.
β_2m may exhibit only a limited region of antigenicity which
might cause most antibodies to bind in similar orientations. In
summary, it is concluded that a uniform array of properly
oriented antibodies on the target cell is necessary in order to
initiate interactions between the target and the effector cell Fc
receptors (FcR) leading to the initiation of the killing process.

INSENSITIVITY OF NORMAL LYMPHOCYTES TO ADCC

The question raised here is whether normal, nontransformed cells
are lysed as effectively as human and mouse tumor cells by ADCC.

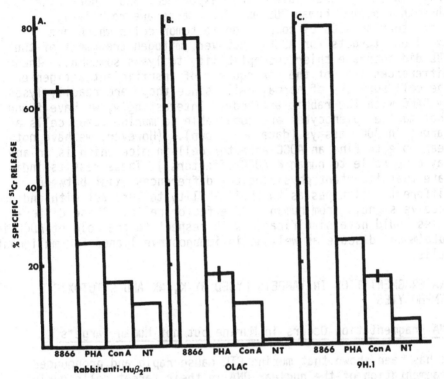

Fig. 3. Normal human peripheral blood leukocytes are less
susceptible to monoclonal ADCC than human tumor targets,
but increase in susceptibility after treatment with
mitogens. 1 x 10^7 Ficoll-Hypaque purified PBL were
cultured in 5 ml complete RPMI + 10% FCS for 3 d in the
presence of 10 µg/ml phytohemaglutinin (PHA), or 5 µg/ml
Concanavalin A (Con A). On day 3, fresh PBL were
obtained from the same donor - some of which were ^{51}Cr-
labeled and used for targets (NT) - while the remainder
were used as effectors after removal of adherent cells.
PHA, Con A, and NT PBL plus 8866 cells were used as
targets in ADCC assays over 4-log dilutions of Rα Huβ₂m
(A), OLAC (B), or 9H.1 (C). For brevity, the data shown
above represents the duplicate points of the particular
dilution resulting in the greatest lysis of the
untreated PBL targets; Rα Huβ₂m (1/40,000); OLAC
(1/400); 9H.1 (1/400). These dilutions of OLAC and 9H.1
also gave the greatest levels of lysis with the mitogen
treated PBL.

Thus, normal human PBL and PBL treated with mitogens were compared to 8866 human tumor cells in an ADCC assay as shown in Fig. 3. For this comparison Rα Huβ_2m (Fig. 3A) and two MAbs (Fig. 3B and C) where used. This experiment and others like it show that normal human PBL and PBL blasts are relatively refractory to ADCC by comparison to tumor cells which are excellent targets for ADCC. However, mitogen treatment of the PBL did increase thier susceptibility to lysis somewhat. These differences are not the consequence of insufficient antigen on the cell surfaces of normal cells since they were readily lysed by CAMC with the rabbit antibody. Interestingly, we have found that murine splenocytes are comparable to murine tumor cells as target in ADCC assays (data not shown). (However, we have not been able to find an ADCC effector cell in mice which is in any way comparable to human K ADCC effectors.) These results indicate that important physiological differences exist between different cell types as to their ability to interact with and/or receive signals from human ADCC effector cells. These differences could have significance with respect to the role of ADCC in autoimmune disease as well as in immunosurveillance for malignant cells.

DNA FRAGMENTATION IN TARGETS LYSED BY K, NK AND CYTOTOXIC T LYMPHOCYTES

DNA Fragmentation Occurs in Murine but not Human Targets

It has been shown that murine CTL cause rapid and pronounced fragmentation of the nuclear DNA in their target cells during cytolysis (9,10). In order to determine whether K and NK lymphocytes also induce fragmentation of the target cell DNA during lysis, various combinations of effector cells and targets were simultaneously assayed for both DNA fragmentation and lysis. To monitor fragmentation, target cells were labeled with ^{3}H-thymidine which was metabolically incorporated into newly synthesized DNA, and to monitor cytolysis target cells were labeled with ^{51}Cr. As shown in Fig. 4A, for all murine target cells tested (Pal3, a cloned T helper cell; YAC-1 murine T lymphoma cells; and B10.BR splenocyte Con A blasts), there was a rapid and complete (in 3 hr) degradation of target cell DNA which accompanied the lysis of the respective targets induced by human K, murine C3H normal splenocyte NK, and murine C57B1/6 anti-B10.BR CTL. The kinetics of fragmentation paralleled the release of ^{51}Cr from these cells into the surrounding medium. When the same target cells were also lysed by CAMC, or by heating for 10 min at 56°C, or by freeze-thawing, no DNA fragmentation occurred in the subsequent 2 hr following these treatments in agreement with previous findings (11). However, as shown in Fig. 4B, no DNA fragmentation accompanied the lysis of any human targets (8866 human B lymphoblastoid cells or K562 human myeloblastoma cells)

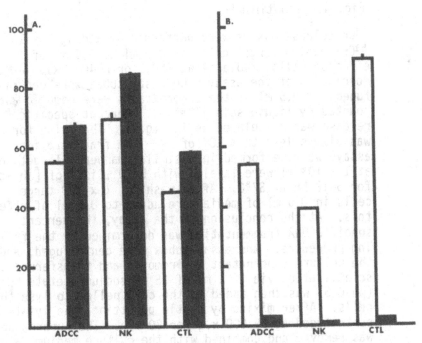

Fig. 4. Fragmentation of DNA occurs in mouse (A) but not human
(B) target cells regardless of lymphocyte effector type.
^{51}Cr release (open bars) and DNA fragmentation (solid
bars) assays were carried out in parallel on mouse and
human target cells lysed by K cells (ADCC), natural
killer cells (NK), or by cytotoxic T lymphocytes (CTL).
The data points shown were taken after 3 hr except for
the mouse NK assay in which the data points shown were
taken 14 hr after the beginning of the assay. The
effector (E) and target (T) cell combinations were the
following. For ADCC in (A), E = human nonadherent PBL
and T = mouse Pa13 cells preincubated with a 1/1000
final dilution of Rα MLS for 20 min at r.t.; E:T ratio =
25:1. For ADCC in (B), E = human nonadherent PBL and
T = 8866 cells preincubated with a 1/1000 dilution of Rα
Hu β₂m; E:T ratio = 25:1. For NK lysis in (A), E =
C3H/HeJ unimmunized nonadherent splenocytes and T = YAC-
1 cells; E:T ratio = 100:1. For NK lysis in (B), E =
human nonadherent PBL and K562 cells; E:T ratio = 25:1.
For CTL lysis in (A), E = C57/BL6 anti-B10.BR CTL
generated in a 5 d mixed lymphocyte culture and T =
48 hr Con A-blasted B10.BR splenocytes; E:T ratio =
25:1. For CTL lysis in (B), E = human anti-8866 CTL
generated in a 7 d mixed lymphocyte culture (1 x 10⁶ x-
irradiated 8866 cells as stimulators plus 20 x 10⁶ human
PBL) and T = 8866 cells; E:T ratio = 35:1.

(continued)

517

Fig. 4. (continued)

^{51}Cr release assays were performed by adding 1 x 10^5 ^{51}Cr-labeled target cells in 0.5 ml to 0.5 ml of effector cells, media alone (SR), or NP40 (FR). At the conclusion of the assay, the assay tubes were centrifuged and 0.5 ml of the supernatants were removed and counted by liquid scintillation. Percent specific ^{51}Cr release was calculated as in Fig. 1. The value for SR was always less than 10% of FR. DNA fragmentation assays were performed in a similar manner. Target cells at 1 x 10^6/ml were labeled with 5-20 μCi/ml of [^{3}H]-dThd for 6-12 hr at 37°C. After washing, 1 x 10^5 target cells in 0.5 ml of media were added to 0.5 ml of effectors. At the conclusion of the assay, the percent specific DNA fragmentation was determined by the following procedure: the assay tubes were centrifuged, and the culture supernatant was removed and transferred to a scintillation vial. 1 ml of 25 mM sodium acetate buffer (pH 6.5) was then added to the cell pellet to lyse the cells. After mixing by gentle pipetting, the lysate was centrifuged at 15,000 x g for 20 min. The supernatant was removed and combined with the culture medium, and counted by liquid scintillation. The percent specific DNA fragmentation is given by the formula:

$$\frac{CPM^{frags}_{exp} - CPM^{frags}_{spont}}{CPM^{frags}_{total} - CPM^{frags}_{spont}} \times 100$$

where CPM^{frags}_{exp} = CPM in the culture media and the 15,000 x g supernatant of the experimental samples.

CPM^{frags}_{spont} = CPM in the culture media and the 15,000 x g supernatant from target cells in the absence of antibody and effectors.

CPM^{frags}_{total} = total CPM in 1 x 10^5 target cells in 1 ml of media.

CPM^{frags}_{spont} was always less than 12% of CPM^{frags}_{total}.

Specific ^{51}Cr release or specific DNA fragmentation of ADCC target cells in the absence of antibody or in the absence of effector cells was always less than 1%.

lysed by human K, human NK, or human CTL. The uniform difference
between murine and human cells with respect to DNA fragmentation
is suggestive of three important aspects of the cytolytic mech-
anism(s) of lymphocytes: 1) DNA fragmentation per se is not an
inherent aspect of the lytic mechanism of lymphocyte effector
cells because human K cells lyse both human and murine targets by
ADCC but DNA fragmentation is observed only in the latter cell
type. 2) DNA fragmentation reflects a programmed physiological
difference between mouse and human cells and probably does not
reflect the delivery of a nuclease activity to the target cell by
a lymphocyte effector. 3) K cells, NK cells and CTL are likely
to have a common lytic mechanism.

Characterization of Fragmented DNA

In order to characterize the DNA fragmented in the murine target
cells lysed by human ADCC effectors, [125I]-deoxyuridine-labeled
target cell DNA was isolated at intervals during an ADCC assay
and fractionated by electrophoresis. The results of one such
experiment are shown in Fig. 5. Only DNA isolated from targets

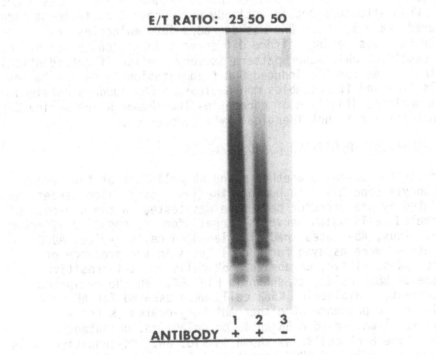

Fig. 5.   Agarose gel electrophoresis of human K cell induced
           fragmentation of target cell DNA. C14 cells (1 x
           10^6/ml) were labeled with 10 μCi/ml of [^{125}I]-dUrd,
           washed, and used as ADCC targets. 5 mls of ^{125}I-labeled
                                                        (continued)

Fig. 5. (continued)

C14 cells at 2 x 10^5/ml were incubated with a 1/1000 final dilution of rabbit anti-mouse lymphocyte (Rα MLS) antiserum for 20 min at r.t. 0.5 ml of these cells were added to 0.5 ml of human effectors. After 90 min at 37°C, the cells were centrifuged and the culture supernatant removed. 1 ml of 25 m$\underline{M}$ sodium acetate buffer (pH 6.5) was added to each cell pellet to lyse the cells. After mixing by gentle pipetting, the lysate was centrifuged at 15,000 x g for 20 min at 4°C. The supernatants were carefully removed then extracted 3 times with Tris-buffered phenol (pH 7.5) followed by 2 extractions with chloroform:isoamyl alcohol (24:1). The DNA was concentrated and run on a 0.75% agarose gel overnight at 20V. The gel was dried down onto filter paper and autoradiographed for 48 hrs at -80°C with a Dupont intensifying screen. Lanes 1 and 2 show target cell DNA fragments obtained at E:T ratios of 25:1 and 50:1, respectively. Lane 3 is a control performed exactly as in lane 2 except without the addition of antibody.

incubated with effectors and Ab showed fragmentation (Lanes 1 and 2). When effectors but no antibody were present no fragmentation occured (Lane 3). The DNA was degraded into molecules of discrete sizes having uniform differences in molecular weight. The resulting DNA ladder pattern is very similar if not identical to that found for CTL induced DNA fragmentation in murine target cells (10) and it resembles mononucleosome DNA ladders obtained from nuclease digestion of chromatin. Thus human K and murine CTL induce similar if not identical lytic processes.

THE RELATIONSHIP BETWEEN K AND NK CELLS

In order to determine whether K and NK cells are of the same lymphocyte population in humans, the lysis of labeled targets as mediated by one effector cell type was tested in the presence of unlabeled cells which serve as targets for the opposite effector type. Thus, Ab-coated, radiolabeled 8866 cells -- i.e. ADCC targets -- were assayed for K cell lysis in the presence of either NK-sensitive, unlabeled K562 cells or NK-insensitive, unlabeled 8866 cells, as shown in Fig. 6A. In the reciprocal experiment, radiolabeled K562 cells were assayed for NK cell lysis in the presence of either antibody-coated (K cell-sensitized) unlabeled 8866 cells or unlabeled, uncoated, NK-insensitive 8866 cells, as shown in Fig. 6B. NK-sensitive cells profoundly inhibited ADCC target cell lysis (Fig. 6A) whereas ADCC-sensitive targets profoundly inhibited the NK lysis of targets (Fig. 6B). These data agree with similar findings by others (12, 13). Although a possible explanation for the K562 inhibition of ADCC K cell effectors is that they may have Fc

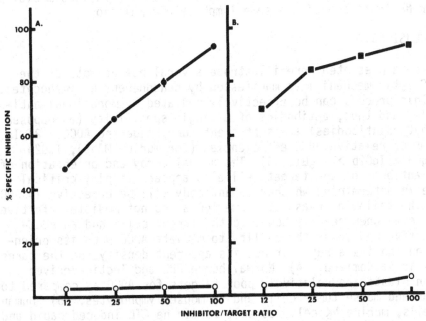

Fig. 6. Reciprocal inhibition of ADCC and NK. Unlabeled
         inhibitor cells were serially diluted in duplicate from
         100 x 10⁴ to 12 x 10⁴/well in 100 μl to give
         inhibitor:target ratios of 100:1 to 12:1. 1 x 10⁴ ⁵¹Cr-
         labeled target cells in 50 μl were added to each well
         containing inhibitor cells or just media. 20 x 10⁴
         human nonadherent PBL effectors were then added to each
         well (except SR and FR wells), resulting in an
         effector:target ratio of 20:1. In (A), targets for ADCC
         were 8866 cells precoated with Rα Hu β_2m (1/1000).
         Inhibitors were NK-sensitive K562 (●) cells, or NK-
         insensitive 8866 (○) cells. In (B), targets for NK were
         K562 cells. Inhibitors were Rα Hu β_2m-precoated 8866 (■)
         cells, or untreated 8866 (○) cells. Specific ⁵¹Cr
         release was determined after 4 hr. Percent specific
         inhibition was calculated from the decrease in percent
         specific ⁵¹Cr release observed in the absence of
         inhibitors (A, 45 ± 2%; B, 51 ± 1%), by the following
         formula:

$$\frac{\text{\% Specific }^{51}\text{Cr release with inhibitors}}{\text{\% Specific }^{51}\text{Cr release with no inhibitors}} \times 100.$$

receptors which compete for the binding of Ab-coated targets, K562 cells are unreactive with an anti-FcR MAb (B73.1) which does bind the ADCC effector and block its ability to lyse targets (14) (data not shown). Thus, it is concluded that effectors mediating K or NK lysis are of the same lymphocyte population.

CONCLUSIONS

The data presented here illustrate several new aspects of the ADCC lytic mechanism as manifested by nonadherent K lymphocytes. 1) This process can be effectively mediated by monoclonal antibodies and thus, antibodies of a single specificity (as opposed to heteroantibodies) are sufficient for triggering ADCC. 2) In terms of relative ADCC efficiencies (for murine MAbs), IgG2a > IgG3 > IgG2b >> IgG1. 3) The actual array and orientation of the antibody on the target cell also appears to play critical role in determining whether an antibody will be effective in ADCC for the following reasons: some IgG2as do not mediate effective ADCC even when readily bound to the target cell; and an ADCC-effective MAb loses the ability to mediate ADCC when its orientation and its array, but not its apparent density, on the target cell is randomized. 4) Normal human PBL and lectin-derived human blasts are relatively poor targets for ADCC as compared to human and mouse tumor cells and to mouse lymphocytes. 5) Human K cells, murine NK cells as well as murine CTL induced rapid and pronounced fragmentation of target cell DNA into discretely-sized pieces having MW differences approximating nucleosome-associated MW differences. 6) However, human K cells, human NK cells and human CTL did not induce DNA fragmentation in any human targets tested. 7) DNA fragmentation per se is not an inherent aspect of the lytic mechanism of lymphocyte effector cells because human K cells lyse both human and murine targets by ADCC but DNA fragmentation is observed only in the latter cell type. Therefore, DNA fragmentation reflects a programmed physiological difference between mouse and human cells and probably does not reflect the delivery of a nuclease activity to the target cell by a lymphocyte effector. 8) K/NK cells and CTL are likely to cause target cell lysis by very similar, if not identical, mechanisms. 9) In agreement with findings by others, we find that K and NK cells are of the same lymphocyte population in humans since targets of one effector function reciprocally block target lysis mediated by the other effector function.

ACKNOWLEDGEMENTS

We are grateful to Stephen Burnside for preparing Huβ_2m-coupled murine target cells and to Bryan Woods for purifying Huβ_2m. This work was supported by grant CA 24433 awarded by the NCI, DHHS. We also thank Dr. B. Bonavida for valuable discussion and for providing the K562 and YAC-1 cell lines.

REFERENCES

1. Perlman, P. and J.-C. Cerottini. 1979. Cytotoxic Lymphocytes. in The Antigens. M. Sela, editor. Academic Press, Inc. New York. 173-281.

2. Pearson, G.R. 1978. In vitro and in vivo investigations on antibody-dependent cellular cytotoxicity. Curr. Top. Microbiol. Immunol. 80:65.

3. Henney, C.S. 1977. T-cell-mediated cytolysis: an overview of some current issues. Contemp. Top. Immunobiol. 7:245.

4. Wright, S.C. and B. Bonavida. 1982. Studies on the mechanism of natural killer (NK) cell-mediated cytotoxicity (CMC). 1. Release of cytotoxic factors specific for NK sensitive target cells (NKCF) during coculture of NK effector cells with NK target cells. J. Immunol. 129:433.

5. Sissons, J.G.P. and M.A. Oldstone. 1980. Antibody-mediated destruction of virus-infected cells. Adv. Immunol. 29:209.

6. Christiaansen, J.E. and D.W. Sears. 1984. Unusually efficient tumor cell lysis by human effectors of ADCC mediated by monoclonal antibodies. Cancer Res. In press.

7. Pious, D., P. Hawley, and G. Forrest. 1973. Isolation and characterization of HLA-variants in cultured human lymphoid cells. Proc. Natl. Acad. Sci. 70:1397.

8. Christiaansen, J.E., D. Gallardo, S.S. Burnside, A.A. Nelson, and D.W. Sears. 1984. Rapid covalent coupling of proteins to cell surfaces: Immunological characterization of viable protein-cell conjugates. Submitted for publication.

9. Russell, J.H. and C.B. Dobos. 1980. Mechanism of immune lysis. II. CTL-induced nuclear disintegration of the target begins within minutes of cell contact. J. Immunol. 125:1256.

10. Duke, R.C., R. Chervenak, and J.J. Cohen. 1983. Endogenous endonuclease-induced DNA fragmentation: an early event in cell-mediated cytolysis. Proc. Natl. Acad. Sci. 80:6361.

11. Russell, J.H., V.R. Masakowski, and C.B. Dobos. 1980. Mechanism of immune lysis. 1. Physiological distinction between target cell death-mediated by cytotoxic T lymphocytes and antibody plus complement. J. Immunol. 124:1100.

12. Karen, H.S. and P.J. Jensen. 1980. Natural killing and antibody-dependent cellular cytotoxicity: independent mechanisms mediated by overlapping cell populations. in Natural Cell-Mediated Immunity Against Tumors. R.B. Herberman, editor. Academic Pres, Inc. New York. 347-363.

13. de Landazuri, M.O., A. Silva, J. Alvarez, and R.B. Herberman. 1979. Evidence that natural cytotoxicity and antibody-dependent cellular cytotoxicity are mediated in humans by the same effector cell populations. J. Immunol. 123:252.

14. Perussia, B., S. Starr, S. Abraham, V. Fanning, and G. Trinchieri. 1983. Human natural killer cells analyzed by B73.1, a monoclonal antibody blocking Fc receptor functions. II. Studies of B73.1 antibody-antigen interaction on the lymphocyte membrane. J. Immunol. 130:2142.

DISCUSSION

Weiss: Is it worth considering the possibility that the distinction, both in terms of species differences and also effector cell differences that you sometimes see, might be related to different routes of uptake of lytic vectors?

D. Sears: I have no information on that; it would be a formal possibility.

P. Henkart: How would you go about testing that idea?

Weiss: For example, if one needed some intracellular delivery mechanism by the usual routes that one trys to block, endocytic uptake, mechanisms by which viruses get taken up into the nucleus versus those that penetrate across the plasma membrane.

D. Sears: Your comment is hard to reconcile with our K cell lysis, or ADCC, where we have one effector cell population, the human K cell, lysing human and mouse targets and giving different results. You'd have to postulate that the human antibody-coated target somehow got the lytic factors differently than the mouse target. I find that hard to accept, but I can't rule it out.

W. Clark: John Russell, have you seen any difference morphologically in cell death beyond the nuclear stage in human versus mouse targets?

J. Russell: We haven't looked at that. We had looked at the human NK system, and the human ADCC system. We see similar results, except we do see a little more evidence of nuclear damage in the human NK system. These were experiments done about 4 years ago . . . I think we did some experiments with mouse targets and human NK's and did not get nuclear damage, but I'd have to go back and look at those experiments. They wouldn't have been done using fragmentation as an assay, but using Triton solubility.

G. Granger: Duane, did you consider that in the human system, maybe there was fragmentation but the assay may not have picked it up. For example maybe the nucleosome sizes are different so that you might have to use greater centrifugal force to see the fragmentation.

D. Sears: Well, we would have had to use less, because at 15,000 g, you don't see anything thats stays in the supernatant. We're doing it by detergent lysis of the cells, so we're opening up the nucleus and everything else. This particular set of data was not by fragments found in the supernatants. We can do that, but you don't get as many counts, so we just open the whole cell up.

CELL SURFACE THIOLS, METHYLATION, AND COMPLEMENT-LIKE COMPONENTS ARE INVOLVED IN THE EARLY EVENTS OF CML WHEREAS PROTEASES PARTICIPATE IN THE LATER, Ca^{++}-DEPENDENT EVENTS

Doug Redelman and Dorothy Hudig

Department of Microbiology

University of Nevada-Reno, Reno, NV   89557

INTRODUCTION

The long term goals of our work are to define the chemical and metabolic functions required for cell-mediated lysis, to identify the molecules that participate in the lytic process, and ultimately, to characterize how the molecules mediate the required functions. We have used both murine cytotoxic T lymphocytes (CTL) and human natural killer (NK) cells as model systems. The data to be summarized here were obtained principally with the murine CTL system.

Determining reliable techniques to generate effector populations with high specific activity was an important early objective since these types of effector populations would be required for biochemical analyses. We found that the CTL generated in secondary mixed lymphocyte responses (II°MLR) were appropriate effectors since they had high CML activity and could be readily maintained for extended periods by culturing with exogenous T cell growth factor (TCGF). The effectors that we have routinely used in these studies probably contained approximately 50-80% CTL based upon their lytic activity and frequency of target cell binding. The importance of using effectors with high activity was emphasized when we examined the metabolic requirements to mediate lysis. For example, we found that agents such as azide or cyanide that interfere with oxidative phosphorylation did not block the lytic activity of these cells. The inhibitory effects of these agents for populations having lower cytolytic activity most likely reflected an indirect effect on cell motility rather than a direct effect on CTL-mediated lysis (CML) (1).

We have used these high activity CTL populations to identify several distinct types of CML inhibitors, including substrates and inhibitors of serine-dependent proteases, penetrating and non-penetrating thiol oxidants and thiol alkylating agents (2), inhibitors of methylation (3), and drugs that inhibit specific complement components (4). We have used both cation pulse procedures and binding studies to determine which phases of CML were affected by these different types of inhibitors (3,4). We have also begun the initial characterization of which CTL molecules are involved in lysis by using antibody to a non-penetrating thiol alkylating agent to immunoprecipitate ^{125}I labelled CTL surface molecules (5). The current status of these studies will be summarized here.

MATERIALS AND METHODS

CTL were generated in II$^{\circ}$ MLR cultures containing responder spleen cells from CBA mice immunized with allogeneic tumor cells and mitomycin-treated spleen stimulator cells from P815-bearing CD2F$_1$ mice. In some experiments, the effector cells were maintained in an actively proliferating state by culturing for 4-14 days with medium having TCGF activity. The TCGF-maintained cells continued to express the same degree of target cell specificity observed after the initial MLR culture (1,2).

Inhibitors were tested in conventional ^{51}Cr-release CML assays (2) and in modified (3,4) cation-pulse procedures (6) to determine the stages of lysis susceptible to inhibition. In these latter experiments, the cultured CTL and the ^{51}Cr-labeled targets were each washed with a Ca^{++}-free medium that contained the other inorganic components of RPMI-1640, glucose, EGTA, and 1% FBS. The effectors and targets were mixed in this Mg^{++}-containing medium and conjugates were formed by centrifugation at room temperature. The conjugates were then warmed to 37°, pulsed with Ca^{++} for 5-15 min, and incubated for 6-120 min with excess EDTA to allow isotope release to reach completion. In some cases, targets labeled with fluorescein diacetate (FDA) were used to determine the frequency of the effector cell which could form stable, visually enumerated conjugates. Inhibitors were added to the cation pulse assays at different times to determine which steps were affected. Effects on the early Mg^{++}-dependent CTL-target interaction were determined by comparing the inhibitory activity of agents added before or after the initial conjugate formation. Effects on the later Ca^{++}-dependent phase were determined by adding the inhibitors to preformed conjugates. Since there was no lytic activity in the absence of Ca^{++}, these conjugates could be incubated with the inhibitor at 37° for 5-20 min before Ca^{++} addition to provide adequate time for the inhibitor to enter the cells and/or to mediate its effect. Finally, effects on the terminal cation-independent phase were examined by adding the inhibitors concurrently with EDTA at the end of the Ca^{++} pulse. None of the inhibitors to be discussed had any inhibitory activity when added with the EDTA.

INHIBITORS OF METHYLATION AND THIOL ALKYLATING AGENTS

Inhibitors of methylation, i.e., a combination of 2'-deoxycoformycin (dCF) to block adenosine deaminase, adenosine (AR), and L-homocysteine thiolactone (L-Hcy), were most effective when they were added prior to the formation of conjugates. Inhibitors of methylation had considerably less effect on CML if added after centrifugation, even if the conjugates were incubated with the inhibitors for 20 min at 37° prior to adding the Ca^{++}. The quaternary ammonium salt of monobromobimane (qBBr, a non-penetrating thiol aklylating agent) displayed a similar pattern of inhibition. Thus, it appeared that methylation reactions and participation of the cell surface thiol groups were essential for one or more of the early Mg^{++}-dependent step(s) in CML. These processes became much less sensitive to inhibition, although not totally resistant, after effector-target conjugates were formed.

INHIBITION OF CML BY PROTEASE SUBSTRATES AND PROTEASE INHIBITORS

We have previously reported that both low and high molecular weight inhibitors or substrates of serine-dependent proteases can block both murine CML and human NK activity (2). Since high molecular weight irreversible protease inhibitors such as human plasma α_1-antichymotrypsin (α_1-X) do not affect CML unless they are present during the assay, it appears that the putative enzyme is either not active or is not available until CML is initiated by effector-target interaction. The substrates with the greatest inhibitory activity are the derivatives of tyrosine, such as acetyl-tyrosine ethyl ester (ATEE) or the more soluble tyrosine ethyl ester (TEE) or tyrosine methyl ester (TME). We found that these substrates of chymotrypsin-like enzymes had as much ability to inhibit CML when they were added at the same time as the Ca^{++} pulse as when they were added before centrifugation. Furthermore, we also found that ATEE or TEE, at concentrations in excess of those required to inhibit CML or NK, had virtually no effect on the formation of visually enumerated stable conjugates.

INHIBITON OF CML BY K-76 COONa, AN INHIBITOR OF COMPLEMENT

The protease inhibitor data suggested that the protease, which we propose to be required for CML, acts during the Ca^{++} phase. The chymotrypsin-like specificity of the protease resembles that of C5 convertase which is the only enzyme of the complement system with an aromatic amino acid cleavage specificity. A C5-like molecule and an appropriate enzyme to activate it would be sufficient to initiate the assembly of a C5b-C9-like membrane attack complex (MAC) and mediate CML. For this reason, we were particularly interested in determining the effects on CML of the fungal product K-76 COONa since it blocks complement mediated lysis by interacting with C5 and preventing its activation to C5b (7).

K-76 COONa, when included in the CML assay at concentrations equivalent to those which block complement mediated lysis (7), did inhibit cytolysis (4). However, although pretreatment of C5 with K-76 COONa inhibits its subsequent activity (7), we found that pretreatment of effector and/or target cells with K-76 COONa had no detectable effect on subsequent cytolytic function. Pretreatment was ineffective even at concentrations of K-76 COONa greatly in excess of those that inhibited CML when present in the assay. We then tested the effects of K-76 COONa when it was added at different times in a cation pulse procedure. Our expectation, based on the apparent parallels between C5 activation and the Ca^{++}-dependent phase of CML, was that K-76 COONa would resemble ATEE and inhibit effectively when it was added after conjugate formation. However, we found that K-76 COONa was much less active if it was added at any time after the initial effector-target interaction. In further contrast to the results with the protease substrates, we found that the drug prevented the formation of stable NK-target conjugates (8).

In summary, our data indicated that K-76 COONa probably acted at a very early point near the time of initial effector-target interaction. Since pretreatment of effectors failed, it argued that the K-76 COONa sensitive molecule was unavailable before the Mg^{++}-dependent events. Finally, the inability to block CML during the Ca^{++}-dependent phase argued against the drug acting on a C5-like molecule. K-76 COONa is also known to block Factor I (9), the enzyme responsible for hydrolyzing C3b to iC3b. Some of our other results have suggested that an effect on a Factor I-like molecule may be a more plausible explanation for the CML inhibition by the drug.

THE ESSENTIAL CELL SURFACE THIOL-BEARING MOLECULE

We were initially surprised that non-penetrating thiol reactive compounds would be able to inhibit CML because one would expect few external thiol groups on the surface of a cell that is exposed to an oxygen atmosphere. Since there should be relatively few cell surface thiol groups capable of reacting with qBBr, anti-qBBr immunoprecipitation of lysates from surface ^{125}I labeled, qBBr modified CTL should reveal a relatively small number of bands following PAGE and autoradiography. This expectation was realized when we examined lysates from qBBr-treated CTL (5). The principal bands were at approximately 180-200 kD and approximately 40-50 kD with a fainter band at approximately 90 kD. Our initial hypothesis was that the high molecular weight band was T200 since it has been implicated in CML. However, exhaustive immunoprecipitation with anti-T200 did not remove the band precipitated with anti-qBBr. Likewise, pre-precipitation with anti-qBBr did not prevent the subsequent immunoprecipitation of the characteristic band by anti-T200 antibody. It now seems more likely that the bands at approximately 90 and approximately 180 kD correspond to the two chains of Lymphocyte Function Antigen (LFA) (10,11). The intense band at 40-50 kD could correspond to a Class I MHC product since we noted that lysates from C57B1/6 cells, which are known to have an unpaired Cys residue in the H-2K^b molecule (12), produced higher relative amounts of this band than did lysates from CBA cells. Alternatively, this band may correspond to a chain from the recently described putative T cell receptor (13). The latter possibility is consistent with our preliminary inability to immunoprecipitate the 40-50 kD band with antibody to β 2-microglobulin, as one should be able to do if the band were a Class I MHC product.

CONCLUSIONS

Our studies of the inhibition of CML with protease substrates support the concept of complement-like molecules being involved in CML. However, our findings do place some constraints on how these molecules could be participating. For example, we were unable to block CML by pretreating effectors with inhibitors such as α_1-X that are irreversible inhibitors of serine dependent enzymes. Since these inhibitors do block CML when included in the assay, it implies that the enzyme is either inactive or unavailable before CTL-target contact. Furthermore, if there is a C5-like molecule involved in CML, then our data place some narrow restrictions on how it may participate. If it is sufficiently similar to C5 to be blocked by K-76 COONa, then it must be available only during the time immediately surrounding the initial CTL-target interaction since neither pretreatment nor treatment during the Ca^{++}-dependent phase with K-76 COONa was effective. This possibility does not seem the most likely since the protease inhibitor data suggest that the molecule should be available for activation during the Ca^{++} phase. There are several explanations for these apparent discrepancies, but two of the simpler ones are that there is either no C5-like molecule involved or, that if there is, it is sufficiently different from C5 to be insensitive to K-76 COONa inhibitory effects. If there is no C5-like molecule being activated during the Ca^{++}-dependent phase, then one must ask what the protease is actually doing. The final answer to this question will require the isolation of the protease and the identification of its natural substrate.

The data concerning the initial events in CML can be viewed as more internally consistent and these data support some interesting and provocative inferences about the possible mechanism of CML. Our findings, and the results from other investigators, are consistent with molecules resembling C3, Factor I and the complement receptor (CR_3) for iC3b all being involved in one or more of the early events of CML. One CR_3-like molecule, namely LFA, is known to be involved in the early binding events (10). Our data also suggest that LFA may bear the cell surface thiol groups that are necessary for CML. The thiols could form specific disulfide bonds that would transiently stabilize the interactions required for cell activation. These interactions could involve cross-linking between LFA and T cell receptor molecules to deliver an activation signal. The involvement of C3-like and Factor I-like molecules is inferred from the LFA data and from our results with K-76 COONa, which is known to inactivate Factor I (9). Thus, we would agree with the suggestions of others that molecules resembling complement receptors are involved in several types of cell-mediated cytotoxic and phagocytic reactions (14).

These molecules may participate in more types of reactions than those initiating cytolysis or phagocytosis. Antibody to LFA is known to inhibit T cell activation (10) just as it blocks CML. We have recently found that K-76 COONa also blocks T cell activation (4), as one would predict if Factor I-like and CR_3-like molecules were involved in T cell activation. Furthermore, in parallel with the effects on CML, we found that K-76 COONa inhibited early events in T cell activation. T cells cultured with lectins and K-76 COONa failed to develop TCGF receptors as detected by functional activity or by the anti-Tac monoclonal antibody (4). Therefore, we would suggest that a group of molecules resembling the CR_3, Factor I, and C3 is generally involved in delivering activation signals to T lymphocytes.

REFERENCES

1. Redelman, D. 1982. The mechanism of cell-mediated cyto-toxicity II. The apparent biochemical requirements for cytolysis are influenced by the source and frequency of murine cytotoxic T lymphocytes. Cell. Immunol. 74:172.

2. Redelman, D., and D. Hudig. 1980. The mechanism of cell-mediated cytotoxicity. I. Killing by murine cytotoxic T lymphocytes requires cell surface thiols and activated proteases. J. Immunol. 124:870.

3. Redelman, D., and D. Hudig. 1983. The mechanism of cell-mediated cytotoxicity. III. Protease-specific inhibitors preferentially block later events in CTL-mediated lysis than do inhibitors of methylation or thiol-reactive agents. Cell. Immunol. 81:9.

4. Redelman, D., and Hudig. 1984. The mechanism of cell-mediated cytotoxicity. IV. K-76 COONa, which inhibits the activity of Factor I and of C5, inhibits early events in cytotoxic T lymphocyte-mediated cytolysis and in T lymphocyte activation. Cell. Immunol., in press.

5. Redelman, D., and D. Hudig. 1983. T-200-like molecules are involved in cell-mediated lysis by rabbit, human, and mouse effector cells. In Intercellular Communication in Leukocyte Function. Parker, J. W., and R. L. O'Brien ed.'s, John Wiley and Sons, Ltd., Chichester, p. 171.

6. Goldstein, P., and E. T. Smith. 1977. Mechanism of T-cell-mediated cytolysis: The lethal hit stage. Contemp. Top. Immunobiol. 7:273.

7. Hong, K., T. Kinoshita, W. Miyazaki, T. Izawa, and K. Inoue. 1979. An anticomplementary agent, K-76 monocarboxylic acid: Its site and mechanism of inhibition of the complement activation cascade. J. Immunol. 122:2418.

8. Hudig, D., D. Redelman, L. Minning, and K. Carine. 1984. Inhibition of human lymphocyte natural cytotoxicity and antibody-dependent cell-mediated cytotoxicity by K-76 COONa, a reagent that blocks complement activity. J. Immunol., in press.

9. Hong, K., T. Kinoshita, H. Kitajima, and K. Inoue. 1979. Inhibitory effect of K-76 monocarboxylic acid, an anticomplementary agent, on the C3b inactivator system. J. Immunol. 127:104.

10. Springer, T. A., D. Davignon, M.-K. Ho, K. Kurzinger, E. Martz, and F. Sanchez-Madrid. 1982. LFA-1 and Lyt-2,3, molecules associated with T lymphocyte-mediated killing; and Mac-1, an LFA-1 homologue associated with complement receptor function. Immunol. Rev. 68:171.

11. Pierres, M., C. Goridis, and P. Goldstein. 1982. Inhibition of murine T cell-mediated cytolysis and T cell proliferation by a rat monoclonal antibody immunoprecipitating two lymphoid cell surface polypeptides of 94,000 and 180,000 molecular weight. Eur. J. Immunol. 12:60.

12. Coligan, J. E., T. J. Kindt, H. Uehara, J. Martinko, and S.
    G. Nathenson. 1981. Primary structure of a murine
    transplantation antigen. Nature. 291:35.

13. Hedrick, S. M., D. I. Cohen, E. A. Nielson, and M. M. Davis.
    1984. Isolation of cDNA clones encoding T cell-specific
    membrane-associated proteins. Nature. 308:149.

14. Springer, T. A., and J. C. Unkeless. 1984. Analysis of
    macrophage differentiation and function with monoclonal
    antibodies. Contemp. Top. Immunobiol. 13:1.

ANTIGEN/MITOGEN INDUCED CYTOLYTIC ACTIVITY AND IL-2 SECRETION IN MEMORY-LIKE CTL-HYBRIDOMAS

Y. Kaufmann*, M. Moscovitch*, R.J. Robb**,
S.A. Rosenberg*** and G. Berke*

*Department of Cell Biology, The Weizmann Institute of
Science, Rehovot 76100, Israel; **E.I. duPont deNemours
and Co., Glenolden Laboratory, Glenolden, PA 19036 and
***Surgery Branch, National Cancer Institute, Bethesda,
MD 20205, USA

SUMMARY

Memory-like monoclonal CTL hybridomas, derived from fusion of
the AKR thymoma BW5147 with secondary CTL generated in vivo or in
MLC cultures, have been used to study the mechanism whereby
antigen/mitogen induces anamnestic CTL responses. Specifically,
we have asked whether induction of cytolytic activity can be
promoted by an antigenic/mitogenic signal without involvement of
IL-2 receptors, IL-2, or other extrinsic factors. We have found
that antigen/lectin alone can trigger the cytolytic potential of
the hybridomas and induce IL-2 secretion. Pure IL-2 and conditioned medium were ineffective inducers of cytotoxicity.
Moreover, IL-2 receptors were not detected on the hybrid cells
before and after antigenic stimulation, demonstrating that expression of IL-2 receptors and induction of specific killing activity
are not genetically linked. Non-activated and activated cells
conjugated with target cells equally well, suggesting that induction of cytolytic activity involves a post target cell binding
step. Close linkage between cytotoxicity and IL-2 secretion has
been observed: induction of killing was consistently associated
with IL-2 secretion and stimulation of both activities could be
blocked by Cyclosporin A. IL-2 was secreted by the CTL hybrids as
early as 3 h following stimulation. We propose that the immediate
supply of IL-2 by such memory CTL enhances antigenic response of
other, IL-2-dependent T cells.

INTRODUCTION

Activation of precursors and memory CTL has been the subject of much investigation in recent years (reviewed in 1-3). A widely accepted hypothesis is that activation requires two "signals," namely, a specific antigen and interleukin 2 (IL-2; Ref. 4). Recent reports, however, suggest that at least in some cases an antigenic signal alone is sufficient to induce differentiation of CTL (5, 6). Other studies demonstrate that cytolytic activity can be triggered in CTL (7) and in some CTL-hybridomas (8), by purified IL-2 and by IL-2-containing conditioned medium, in the absence of an antigenic signal. Stimulation of cytotoxicity without an extrinsic supply of IL-2 has been explained by an autocrine mechanism in which some CTL secrete and utilize IL-2 in response to the stimulating antigen (5, 6, 9). Coexpression of IL-2 receptors and killing activity has been taken to indicate that IL-2 plays an essential role in the maturation of CTL (7). Both types of results imply involvement of external IL-2, through IL-2 receptors, in CTL differentiation. Because in previous studies IL-2-dependent CTL (either bulk MLC cultures or CTL lines and clones) have been employed, the results do not allow a clear distinction between the effect(s) of the factor on the acquisition of cytolytic activity by CTL and its contribution to survival of the cells in tissue culture. We have previously described monoclonal CTL-hybridomas which proliferate autonomously and can be activated by lectin or antigen (Ag) to kill target cells (TC) specifically and to secrete IL-2 (10, 11). Such memory-like CTL hybridomas, which do not depend for their growth on external factors and other cell subsets, provide an ideal tool for studying the involvement of external IL-2 and its receptors in the induction of cytolytic activity. We show here that 2 memory-like CTL-hybridomas with inducible killing activity lack IL-2 receptors and do not respond to conditioned medium, indicating that antigenic signal(s) <u>alone</u> can promote CTL maturation without involvement of external IL-2.

RESULTS AND DISCUSSION

A. <u>Antigen or lectin, but not conditioned medium stimulate cytolytic activity and IL-2 secretion by memory-like CTL hybridomas</u>

We have used two unrelated clones of CTL hybridomas, Md26.15 (M-hybridoma) and P47.21 (P-hybridoma) that had been derived from fusion of AKR thymoma cells (BW5147) and BALB/c anti-EL4 CTL following secondary stimulation in mixed lymphocyte culture, or in peritoneal exudate lymphocyte, respectively (10). Both hybridomas appear to be directed against H-2D[b] determinant(s). They grow independently of known exogenous stimuli and can be induced to secrete IL-2 by T cell mitogens or irradiated cells presenting H-2D^b antigens (11). Initially, the hybridomas were screened and selected for specific killing. Lysis of EL4 (H-2D^b) TC was detected in a 6-h cytolytic assay. Later on, it became apparent that the hybridomas were devoid of immediate (1-2 h) cytolytic activity and that their killing potential was stimulated by TC during the long cytolytic assay (11). In addition, following a 20-h pre-incubation with the TC or mitogenic lectins, cytolytic activity was enhanced and IL-2 was detected in supernatants. Repeated cloning of the hybridomas yielded cytolytic subclones which consistently secreted IL-2 upon stimulation (11), indicating that the two activities, cytolysis and IL-2 secretion, were mediated by a single cell.

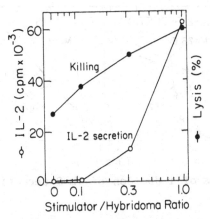

FIGURE 1. Stimulation of Md26.15 hybridoma with Ag-presenting cells.

Hybrid cells were preincubated for 5 h at 37° with irradiated (4000 rad) EL4 cells at the indicated ratios. Supernatants, diluted 1:4, were assayed for IL-2 with IL-2-dependent CTL line, CTLL-2 as described (11). Irradiated EL4 were added to preincubated hybrid cells to complete the stimulator/hybridoma ratio to 1. Killing activity was tested on freshly added ^{51}Cr-labeled EL4 TC at effector/TC ratio of 1 for 3.5 hr. Spontaneous release was 8%.

In this study we have asked what is the basis for stimulation of the hybridomas' cytolytic activity and whether IL-2 or other extrinsic factor(s) are involved in it. To test the effect of antigen-presenting cells, M-hybridomas were co-cultured for 5 hr with graded amounts of irradiated EL4, and their cytolytic activity was examined on ^{51}Cr-labeled EL4 TC. Figure 1 shows that the amount of stimulating antigen determined the level of responsiveness. Cells which had not been preincubated with Ag caused 25% lysis, a level reflecting the limited stimulation which occurred during the killing assay. Killing increased considerably as a result of pre-incubating the hybridomas with irradiated TC. IL-2 was detected in supernatants following 5 h of stimulation.

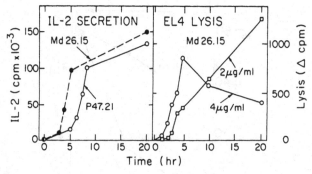

FIGURE 2. Kinetics of induction of IL-2 secretion and cytolytic activity.

IL-2 secretion. Md26.15 hybridoma, 5×10^5 cells/ml, was stimulated in 24-well Costar plates with irradiated EL4 cells at 5×10^5 cells/ml, P47.21 hybridoma, 5×10^5 cells/ml, was stimulated with 4 ug/ml Con A. Conditioned media were collected for IL-2 assay at the indicated times following onset of stimulation. The figure shows proliferation of CTLL-2 test cells (11) promoted by 12.5% and 50% conditioned media from M and P hybridomas, respectively.
EL4 lysis. Md26.15 hybridoma, 2.5×10^5 cells/ml, was stimulated with Con A (2 or 4 ug/ml) for the indicated times. The lytic activity was assessed, after removal of residual Con A, on EL4 TC at E:T of 1:1 in a 3.5 hr lytic assay. The results show Δ cpm between stimulated and non-stimulated hybrids.

The kinetics of stimulatory response of the hybridomas' killing and IL-2 secretion were investigated. The results were consistent with triggering of both processes by a common cell surface receptor. Thus, Figure 2 shows that IL-2 could be detected in conditioned medium of EL4-stimulated M-hybridomas and Con A-stimulated P-hybridomas by 3 and 5 h, respectively. Induction of killing was observed as early as 2 h following onset of stimulation. The decrease in cytolytic activity of M-hybridomas observed after 10 h of preincubation with 4 ug/ml Con A was probably due to autologous lectin-dependent cytotoxicity. Induction of specific cytotoxicity within 2 h suggests that activation is not dependent on effector cell multiplication. Anamnestic CTL response in vivo, but not primary CTL response, occurs in the presence of cyclophosphamide (an inhibitor of cell proliferation; 12). Therefore, the immediate induction of hybrid cells appears to reflect memory CTL response.

A possible interpretation for the concomitant induction of secretion and cytotoxicity might be that the antigen triggers secretion of IL-2 and/or other factor(s) which in turn bind(s) to the cells and promotes their killing potential. To test this possibility, M-hybridomas were preincubated for 20 h with pure IL-2 (13) or with conditioned medium derived from Con A stimulated rat splenocytes (CS). Cytolytic activity was tested afterwards in a short assay, to avoid considerable activation during the assay (Fig. 3). Neither pure IL-2 nor CS could replace Ag-presenting cells in stimulating specific killing activity; mixtures of conditioned medium with cell-presenting Ags did not show synergistic effects (not shown). Moreover, supernatants derived from activated hybridomas were also devoid of inducible activity. Similar results were obtained with the P-hybridomas (11). The finding that CS, known to contain several lymphokines and T cell differentiation factors (14-16), had no effect on the cytolytic potential of the hybridomas showed that such extrinsic factors were probably not involved in its activation.

To further clarify the role of IL-2 we asked whether hybridomas express high affinity cell-surface receptors capable of binding free IL-2 (17). Thus, P- and M-hybridomas were examined for binding of radiolabeled pure IL-2, as previously described (17). Hybrid cells prior to and after antigenic stimulation were unable to bind a significant number of IL-2 molecules. Furthermore, treatment of the cells under conditions which removed bound IL-2 (18) did not expose receptor activity (Table 1). Stimulation of cytolytic activity of immature cells not responding to external IL-2 and devoid of functional IL-2 receptors, demonstrated that induction of cytolytic potential may occur not via IL-2 receptors, and that expression of specific killing is not necessarily associated with IL-2 dependency, as previously suggested (19). We

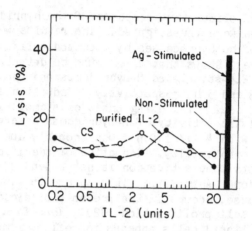

FIGURE 3. Pure IL-2 and IL-2-containing conditioned medium do not stimulate cytolytic activity of the CTL-hybridoma.

Md26.15 hybrid cells were incubated for 20 hr with an equivalent number of irradiated EL4 (Ag-stimulated, ▅), or without pretreatment (▭), or with IL-2, purified (>99%) from stimulated Jurkat cells (13), or with conditioned medium from stimulated rat splenocytes (CS). One unit of IL-2 is defined as 20 times the amount of the factor needed to promote 50% of the maximal (^{3}H) Thy uptake by 5×10^3 CTLL-2 test cells. Following preincubation hybrid cells were washed, stimulators were removed (11) and killing of EL4 TC was tested for 3.5 hr at E/T of 1. Spontaneous release was 15%.

conclude that activation of cytolytic potential of such memory-like CTL hybridomas is induced by Ag-presenting cells alone (or T cell mitogen), and that it is <u>not</u> mediated via external IL-2 or other factor(s) secreted by activated cells. The suggestion of genetic linkage between specific killing and expression of IL-2 receptors is based on analyses of IL-2 dependent long-term CTL clones and CTL hybridomas derived from them (19). Association between these two functions in that case could merely reflect selection for IL-2 dependency under long-term culture conditions (5, 6).

Table I. Test for IL-2 receptors on stimulated and non-stimulated hybrid cells

Tested cells	Stimulator	Free IL-2	IL-2 receptors*	
			Nontreated cells	pH4-treated cells
		pmole	No. of receptors per cell	
CTL line	None	95	3790	N.T.
P47.21	None	320	5	0
		143	10	6
		95	8	4
	EL4	205	2	0
		137	2	5
		91	4	5
Md26.15	None	320	0	11
		143	11	8
		95	0	10
	EL4	205	0	5
		137	12	5
		91	0	0

*Radiolabeled purified IL-2 was prepared from stimulated Jurkat cells (13). IL-2 binding was measured as described (17). Briefly, hybrid cells, either stimulated for 3 days with 1 equivalent irradiated EL4 or not stimulated, or IL-2 dependent CTL were incubated for 20 min at $37^{\circ}C$ with various concentrations of the radiolabeled factor. pH 4 wash was done to remove IL-2 bound to the receptors (18); the cells were treated for 30 sec at pH 4, washed in RPMI/BSA and then put into the binding assay. Viability of all cells was higher than 90%.

B. Induction of IL-2 secretion and cytolytic activity are associated

A linkage between the induction of cytolytic activity and IL-2 secretion in memory CTL may enhance the efficiency of a secondary T cell response. The finding that the two activities of the CTL hybridomas are induced in response to the same Ag-presenting cells (11) suggests that their triggering is associated. To further examine this linkage, we applied agents known to interfere with the induction of one activity and examined their effect on the second. Anti-LFA-1 monoclonal antibody (mAb), which had been previously reported to block CTL killing activity (20, 21), was first examined. P-hybridomas were stimulated by Con A and M-hybridomas by irradiated EL4 cells in the presence of anti-LFA-1 mAb (H35-89.9; Ref. 21). IL-2 secretion and hybrid cell proliferation were tested after 20 h and 40 h, respectively. To test the effect of anti-LFA-1 on the stimulation of killing potential and on expression of cytolytic activity, the mAb was included in the killing reactions promoted by non-activated and pre-activated hybridomas, respectively. Thus, when the hybrid cells were activated prior to the killing assay, lysis reflected a CTL-mediated killing reaction. However, if the hybridomas were tested in the killing assay without pre-stimulation, lysis reflected two processes: maturation of the hybrid cells induced by TC during the assay and TC lysis. While IL-2 secretion and cytotoxicity were inhibited by anti-LFA-1 with similar efficiency, proliferation was unaffected (Fig. 4). Because cytotoxicity of pre-activated cells was blocked by anti-LFA-1, it was impossible to conclude whether anti LFA-1 inhibited the stimulation phase of non-activated cells.

Distinguishing between stimulation of killing potential and the expression of cytolytic activity became possible with Cyclosporin A (CsA). CsA is a fungus metabolite previously reported to block T cell proliferation, IL-2 secretion and expression of IL-2 receptors in bulk MLC cultures (22, 23), and to inhibit Ag-dependent proliferation of T helper and cytotoxic clones (24). Like anti-LFA-1, CsA abolished the Ag-induced secretion of IL-2 without affecting proliferation of the hybridomas (Fig. 5). However, unlike anti-LFA-1, CsA caused only moderate inhibition of killing by pre-activated hybridomas, suggesting that the killing reaction itself is relatively resistant to this drug. This result is consistent with a previous report showing that cytotoxicity of bulk MLC culture is not affected by CsA (25). In contrast, TC lysis by non-activated hybridomas, which had to be stimulated by TC during the killing assay, was as sensitive to the inhibitory effect of CsA as IL-2 secretion, suggesting that stimulation of killing potential is associated with induction of IL-2 secretion. The finding that CsA has little effect on killing suggests that the receptor-Ag interactions necessary to induce IL-2 secretion and CTL maturation and those required to mediate TC lysis may be different.

542

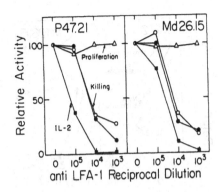

FIGURE 4. Anti-LFA-1 blocks Ag/mitogen induction of IL-2 secretion and cytolytic activity, but not autonomous proliferation of CTL-hybridomas.

Anti-LFA-1, produced by hybridoma H35-89.9 (Pierres et al., 21) and concentrated from ascites, was used.

Proliferation. Hybrid cells were incubated (2×10^3 cells/well) for 40 hr in the presence of anti-LFA-1 and harvested after a 4-hr terminal pulse with (^{3}H)thymidine. In the absence of anti-LFA-1 thymidine uptake by M and P hybridomas was 280 and 440×10^3 cpm, respectively.

IL-2 secretion. P and M hybrid cells at 2.5×10^5/ml were incubated in 2 ml Costar wells with Con A (2 ug/ml), or an equivalent number of irradiated EL4, respectively, in the presence of anti-LFA-1 for 20 hr. Conditioned media at several dilutions were assayed for IL-2 (11). (^{3}H)thymidine uptake by the test cells induced with 50% supernatant of Con A-activated P-hybridoma and 25% supernatant of EL4-activated M-hybridoma were 69.5 and 91.0 cpm x 10^3, respectively. Anti LFA-1 did not affect the response of CTLL-2 test cells to IL-2.

Killing. Specific lysis of EL4 TC by non-stimulated (open circles) or pre-stimulated (closed circles) hybridomas in the presence of anti-LFA-1 was examined at an E:T of 1.5:1 in a 5 hr assay. Lysis induced in absence of mAb by pre-activated and non-activated P-hybridomas was 47.2% and 25.2% and by M-hybridomas 33.2% and 19.5%, respectively.

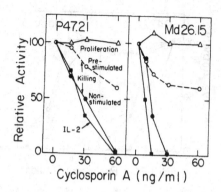

FIGURE 5. Induction of cytolytic activity and IL-2 secretion is abrogated by CsA while specific TC lysis by pre-activated hybridomas is marginally affected.

Proliferation. Hybrid cells (3.3×10^3/well with 3.3×10^3 irradiated EL4 cells) were incubated with CsA for 20 h and harvested after a 4 h terminal pulse with ^{3}H-thymidine. In the absence of CsA thymidine uptake by P and M hybridomas was 104.5 and 94.1×10^3 cpm. Irradiated EL4 incorporated 5×10^3 cpm.

IL-2 secretion. Hybrid cells were stimulated for 20 hr with irradiated EL4, as in Fig. 4. (^{3}H)thymidine uptake by the test cells induced with 50% supernatant of P and M hybridomas was 41.0 and 112.9 cpmx10^3, respectively. CsA had no effect on the response of CTLL-2 to IL-2.

Killing. The hybrid cells were either non-stimulated (closed circles) or prestimulated (open circles) for 20 hr with irradiated EL4 cells. Stimulator cells were removed (11), and lysis of EL4 TC was examined in the presence of CsA at an E:T of 1:1, in a 6 hr assay. The lysis induced in the absence of CsA by pre-activated and non-activated P-hybridoma was 38.3% and 23.8% and by M-hybridoma, 46.2% and 27.0%, respectively.

C. Characteristics of activated vs. non-activated hybridomas

We have previously reported that these CTL hybridomas do not express cell surface Lyt-2 molecules and suggested that expression of Lyt-2 is not essential for specific killing activity (26).

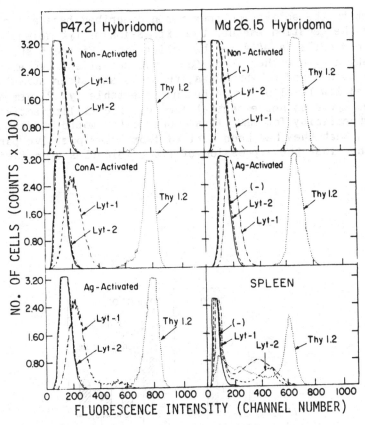

FIGURE 6. FACS analysis of the expression of surface antigens on stimulated and non-stimulated hybridomas.

Hybrid cells were stimulated with either Con A (2 ug/ml) for 20 hr or with irradiated EL4 cells for 4 days. Con A was removed by alpha-MM, and all stimulated hybridomas were purified on density gradients (11) and stained with fluorescein conjugated mAbs (Becton-Dickinson); anti Thy 1.2, anti Lyt-1 and anti Lyt-2 produced by clones 30-H 12, 53.7.3 and 53.6.7, respectively. Normal C57BL/6 splenocytes were used as positive controls. For each cell population a negative control of unstained cells (-) is shown.

Relevant to the activation phenomenon described here and elsewhere
(11) is the question whether the expression of Lyt molecules on
the hybrid cells is affected by activation. Figure 6 shows that
stimulation with either TC or Con A did not affect Lyt expression,
namely, both P and M hybridomas, prior to and after stimulation,
expressed low level of Lyt 1 but no detectable Lyt-2, demonstrating that Lyt-2 is not essential for specific killing activity.
Their specificity for MHC class I product(s) would suggest,
however, that they had been derived from Lyt-2 positive parental
cells that lost the expression of Lyt-2 molecules upon fusion.

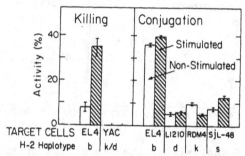

FIGURE 7. Non-stimulated M-hybridomas conjugate specifically
with TC.

Md26.15 hybrid cells were stimulated with Con A (2 ug/ml) for
20 hr. Con A was removed by alpha-MM (11).
Conjugation assay. 0.5×10^6 non-stimulated or stimulated hybrid
cells were mixed with 0.5×10^6 fluorescently (FDA) labeled TC in
0.5 ml culture medium. Conjugation was affected by a 15 min
incubation at 24°C followed by centrifugation, 200 g, 10 min at
24°. The pellets were resuspended 15 times in pasteur pipette and
percent conjugated TC was scored under a UV microscope.
Killing assay. Nonstimulated or stimulated hybridomas were tested
for killing of ^{51}Cr labeled EL4 at effector to TC ratio of 3/1,
for 3 hr.

To examine the basis for activation, we asked whether potentiation of the effector function following stimulation was expressed at a pre- or post-binding step of cytolytic reaction. We used the CTL-TC conjugation assay (27) to monitor the frequency of TC binding M-hybridoma cells, before and after mitogenic stimulation. Fluorescently labeled TC were examined for conjugation with hybridomas at a ratio of 1:1. Specificity was determined using both specific (EL4) and nonspecific (L1210, RDM4, and SJL.48) TC. No significant difference in the frequency of TC-binding hybridoma cells was detected prior to and after stimulation, as 40% of EL4 TC were engaged in conjugation with either activated or non-activated hybridomas (Fig. 7). The ability of hybridomas to conjugate with specific TC prior to stimulation suggests that an effector cell activity required for a post-binding step is triggered by the stimulant. Based on this finding, we propose that potentiation of cytolytic activity of precursor cells by Ag/lectin is involved in a metabolic activation of CTL which is required for onset of the lethal hit. The ability of non-activated hybrid cells to bind specifically TC and the rapid onset (2-3 h) of stimulation suggest that they reflect an advanced stage in CTL maturation.

Acknowledgments: We thank M. Pierres and P. Golstein for providing the H35-89.9 anti LFA-1 mAB. The work was supported by the United States-Israel Binational Science Foundation, Grant No. 2642/81.

REFERENCES

1. MacDonald, H.R. 1982. Differentiation of cytolytic T lymphocytes. Immunol. Today 3:183.

2. Larsson, E.L., Gullberg, M., Beretta, A., and Coutinho, A. 1982. Requirement for the involvement of clonally distributed receptors in the activation of cytotoxic T lymphocytes. Immunol. Rev. 68:67.

3. Nabholz, M. and MacDonald, H.R. 1983. Cytolytic T lymphocytes. Ann. Rev. Immunol. 1:273.

4. Möller, G. (ed.) 1980. T cell stimulating growth factors. Immunol. Rev. 51:1-357.

5. Von Boehmer, H. and Turton, K. 1983. Autonomously proliferating K/D-restricted cytolytic T cell clones. Eur.J. Immunol. 13:176.

6. Andrus, L., Granelli-Piperno, A., and Reich, E. 1984. Cytotoxic T cells both produce and respond to interleukin 2. J. Exp. Med. 59, 647.

7. Lefrancois, L., Klein, J.R., Patkau, V. and Bevan, M.J. 1984. Antigen-independent activation of memory cytotoxic T cells by interleukin 2. J. Immunol. 132:1845.

8. Conzelman, A., Corthesy, P., Cianfriglia, M., Silva, A., and Nabholz, M. 1982. Hybrids between rat lymphoma and mouse T cells with inducible cytolytic activity. Nature (Lond.) 298, 170.

9. Widmer, M.B. and Bach, F.H. 1981. Antigen-driven helper cell-independent cloned cytolytic T lymphocytes. Nature (Lond.) 294:750.

10. Kaufmann, Y., Berke, G. and Eshhar, Z. 1981. Cytotoxic T lymphocyte hybridomas that mediate specific tumor-cell lysis in vitro. Proc. Natl. Acad. Sci. USA 78:2502.

11. Kaufmann, Y. and Berke, G. 1983. Monoclonal cytotoxic T lymphocyte-hybridomas capable of specific killing activity, antigenic responsiveness and inducible interleukin(s) secretion. J. Immunol 131:50.

12. Walker, C.M., Rawls, W.RE., and Rosenthal, K.L. 1984. Generation of memory cell-mediated immune response after secondary infection of mice with pichinde virus. J. Immunol. 132:469.

13. Robb, R.J., Kutny, R.M., and Chowdhry, V. 1983. Purification and partial sequence analysis of human T cell growth factor. Proc. Natl. Acad. Sci. USA 80:5990.

14. Raulet, D.H. and Bevan, M.J. 1982. A differentiation factor required for the expression of cytotoxic T cell function. Nature (Lond.) 296:754.

15. Wagner, H., Hardt, C., Rouse, B.T., Rollinghoff, M., Scherich, P. and Pfizenmaier, K. 1982. Dissociation of the proliferative and differential signals controlling murine cytotoxic T lymphocyte responses. J. Exp. Med. 155:1876.

16. Finke, H.J., Scott, J., Gillis, S., and Hilfiker,M.L. 1983. Generation of alloreactive cytotoxic T lymphocytes. Evidence for a differentiation factor distinct from IL-2. J. Immunol. 130:763.

17. Robb, R.J., Munck, A. and Smith, K.A. 1981. T cell growth factor receptors. Quantitation, specificity and biological relevance. J. Exp. Med. 165:1455.

18. Robb, R.J. and Lin, Y. 1983. T cell growth factor: purification, interaction with the cellular receptor and in vitro synthesis. In: Thymic Hormones and Lymphokines, Goldstein, A.L., ed., Plenum Press, New York, in press.

19. Conzelman, A., Silva, A., Cianfriglia, M., Tougne, C., Sekaly, R.P. and Nabholz, M. 1982. Correlated expression of TCGF dependence, sensitivity to Vicia villosa lectin, and cytolytic activity in hybrids between cytolytic T cells and T lymphomas. J. Exp. Med. 156:1335.

20. Davignon, D., Martz, E., Reynolds, T., Kurzinger, K. and Springer, T.A. 1981. Lymphocyte function-associated antigen one (LFA-1): A surface antigen distinct from Lyt-2/3 that participates in T lymphocyte-mediated killing. Proc. Natl. Acad. Sci. USA 78:4535.

21. Pierres, M., Goridis, C. and Golstein, P. 1982. Inhibition of murine T cell-mediated cytolysis and T cell proliferation by a rat monoclonal antibody immunoprecipitating two lymphoid cell surface polypeptides of 94,000 and 180,000 molecular weight. Eur. J. Immunol. 12:60.

22. Bunjes, D., Hardt, C., Rollinghoff, H. and Wagner, H. 1981. Cyclosporin A mediates immunosuppression of primary cytotoxic T cell responses by impairing the release of Interleukin 1 and Interleukin 2. Eur. J. Immunol. 11:657.

23. Palacios, R. 1981. Cyclosporin A inhibits the proliferative response and the generation of helper, suppressor and cytotoxic T cell functions in the autologous mixed lymphocyte reaction. Cell. Immunol. 61:453.

24. Orosz, C.C., Fidelus, R.K., Roopenian, D.C., Widmer, M.B., Ferguson, R.M. and Bach, F.H. 1982. Analysis of cloned T cell function, I. Dissection of cloned T cell proliferative responses using Cyclosporin A. J. Immunol. 129:1865.

25. Wang, B., Heacock, E., Collins, K., Hutchinson, I., Tilney, N. and Mannick, J. 1981. Suppressive effects of Cyclosporin A on the induction of alloreactivity in vitro and in vivo. J. Immunol. 127:89.

26. Kaufmann, Y., Golstein, P., Pierres, M., Springer, T.A. and Eshhar, Z. 1982. LFA-1 but not Lyt-2 is associated with killing activity of cytotoxic T lymphocyte hybridomas. Nature (Lond.) 300:357.

27. Berke, G., Gabison, D. and Feldman, M. 1975. The frequency of effector cells in populations containing cytotoxic T lymphocytes. Eur. J. Immunol. 5:813.

DISCUSSION

B. Bonavida: Do the CTL hybridomas secrete CTL differentiation factors?

Y. Kaufmann: I didn't test this. However, one hybridoma, when stimulated with a lectin, produced both IL2 and colony stimulating factor.

C. Ware: Just out of curiosity, does the hybridoma express the L3T4 antigen analogous to the human T4 antigen?

Y. Kaufmann: We have never tested this.

QUANTITATIVE MODELS FOR THE KINETICS OF CELL-MEDIATED

CYTOTOXICITY AT THE SINGLE CELL LEVEL

Alan S. Perelson and
Catherine A. Macken*

Theoretical Division
Los Alamos National Laboratory
Los Alamos, New Mexico 87545

INTRODUCTION

Is there a role for quantitative theory in helping us understand cell mediated cytotoxicity? In many areas of science, but
particularly physics and chemistry, theory has played a fundamental, and in some cases an essential, role in advancing knowledge. In physics a primary activity of theorists is to envision
and then explore in a quantitative manner alternative constructions
for the universe. A theorist might ask how the orbits of the eight
closest planets surrounding the sun would change if there were a
ninth planet, or how bubble chamber tracks might look if there were
a new elementary particle, or how a clock would run if it were in a
space ship traveling at 99% the speed of light, or what the dif-
fraction pattern of nucleic acid would be if the molecule were a
double helix. By engaging in flights of fantasy and examining in a
quantitative manner the consequences of alternative designs of the
universe, great progress has been made in the physical sciences.
Given such successes, one is tempted to believe that there is a
role for similar theoretical activities in cell biology and immunology. Here we demonstrate how a theoretical approach can be used
to gain insights into T cell mediated cytotoxicity.

First we discuss a model for the kinetics of lethal hitting
developed by Perelson and Bell (1). The model is used to answer

---

*Permanent address: Centre for Computing and Biometrics,
Lincoln College, Canterbury, New Zealand

the following questions: What would be the observed kinetics of lethal hitting in conjugates containing a single lymphocyte and multiple target cells a) if all target cells were simultaneously at risk of being hit and b) if only a single target were at risk of being hit at any given time? Comparing the model with data we conclude that all target cells are not simultaneously at risk. Next, we discuss a model for the rate at which a lethally hit target cell disintegrates, based upon the possibility that disintegration involves a number of sequential biochemical events (2,3). We then combine our models of lethal hitting and target cell disintegration to obtain a multistage model that can account for the kinetics of target cell lysis (4).

Comparing the multistage model to data on the kinetics of cytolysis in conjugates containing multiple CTL, we find that the rate of target cell disintegration increases with the number of CTL bound per target cell (5). This finding suggests that the rate of target cell disintegration is influenced by events that occur after a target cell has been lethally hit once.

A MODEL OF LETHAL HITTING

Let us construct for a well-defined situation alternative views of how a CTL might act in generating lethal hits. In order to distinguish between the alternatives it is necessary to consider LT_n conjugates in which a CTL is bound to n target cells, with n = 2, 3 or 4. For such conjugates one can ask whether or not all n target cells are hit at once. Since truly simultaneous events are rare in nature and difficult to detect, it is better to ask whether or not all n target cells are simultaneously at risk of being hit. Simultaneous risk of all bound target cells is what one would expect if a soluble mediator were secreted into the medium. Because of "biological variability" one might expect differences in susceptibilities of target cells to soluble mediators, and hence all target cells might not be scored as being lethally hit at the same time in an experiment such as the one performed by Zagury et al. (6). In this experiment preformed LT_n conjugates were incubated at 37°C in the presence of Ca^{++}. After t time units had elapsed, EDTA was added to the medium to prevent further lethal hitting, and the state of the target cells determined at 3 hr. Target cells that were lethally hit before EDTA addition presumably were lysed at 3 hr. In LT_2 and LT_3 conjugates some, but not all, target cells were lysed, and hence Zagury et al. (6) concluded that target cells were hit sequentially rather than simultaneously. But Zagury et al. (6) failed to consider the effects of biological variability and other sources of random variation. However we believe that, rather fortuitously, his conclusion is correct.

In order to analyze the effects of variability let us assume that in a collection of LT_1 conjugates not all target cells are hit at the same time but rather that there is a distribution of hitting times. In experiment, one tends to find that lethal hitting takes anywhere from 2 min to approxiately 20 min (7-9). We summarize this distribution of hitting times by saying that if one examines a single LT_1 conjugate there is a probability, $p(t)$, that the target cell is hit by time t. If hits are delivered at random, then one expects $p(t)$ to be given by an exponential distribution, i.e.,

$$p(t) = 1 - e^{-\lambda t} \; , \tag{1}$$

where λ is the mean rate at which a CTL can hit a target cell. The exact form of $p(t)$ is not important, only the fact that there is some variation in the time by which target cells are hit.

Now consider an LT_n conjugate with $n \geq 2$. Let us assume that there is nothing different about target cells in LT_n conjugates as compared with target cells in LT_1 conjugates. That is, if there is a distribution in times at which target cells would be hit in LT_1 conjugates, then let us assume that the same distribution applies to a target cell in an LT_n conjugate, but with some modification, as described below, due to the sequenatial or simultaneous nature of the T cell attack.

There are at least two alternative ways in which we can envision a CTL attacking n bound target cells: (1) all target cells can be simultaneously at risk of being attacked, or (2) only one target cell at a time might be at risk. In large conjugates other possibilities exist but will not be discussed here. If all n target cells are at risk of being hit and if $p(t)$ is the probability that a target cell is hit by time t, then $P_n(m,t)$, the probability that m out of n target cells are hit by time t is given by the binomial distribution, i.e.,

$$P_n(m,t) = \binom{n}{m}[p(t)]^m[1 - p(t)]^{n-m} \; . \tag{2}$$

If the CTL generates hits at random at rate λ, then the rate at which a single target cell is hit is λ/n, and Eq. (2) becomes

$$P_n(m,t) = \binom{n}{m}[1 - e^{-\lambda/n}]^m[e^{-\lambda/n}]^{n-m} \; . \tag{3}$$

On the other hand, if only one cell at a time is at risk of being hit and hits are generated at random with rate λ, then the probability of the CTL having sequentially hit m out of the n target cells is given by a (modified) Poisson distribution,

$$P_n(m,t) = e^{-\lambda t}\, \frac{(\lambda t)^m}{m!} \quad , \qquad 0 \leq m \leq n - 1 , \qquad\qquad (4a)$$

and

$$P_n(n,t) = 1 - \sum_{m=0}^{n-1} \frac{e^{-\lambda t}(\lambda t)^m}{m!} \quad . \qquad\qquad\qquad (4b)$$

A more complete derivation of Eqs. (2) - (4) can be found in references (1) and (10). If only a single target cell at a time is at risk, but if hits are generated with a non-exponential distribution, i.e., p(t) is not of the form of Eq. (1), then Eq. (4) would need to be replaced by a more involved expression that is beyond the scope of this paper.

Up to this point our discussion of the two alternative scenarios of hitting has been rather abstract. An example might help distinguish what we mean by all n target cells being at risk versus a single target cell being at risk. For the purposes of this example let us assume that a CTL generates hits at the membrane interface between itself and a target cell. We call such an interface a membrane attack area. In an LT_n conjugate there are n membrane attack areas. If on warming a conjugate to 37°C all n membrane attack areas become active, then all n target cells are simultaneously at risk. Alternatively, if only a single attack area becomes active, then only one target cell is at risk. After one target cell is hit, the cell must then activate a different membrane attack area.

Lethal Hitting Appears to Occur Sequentially

Table 1 compares the predictions of the sumultaneous risk and sequential risk models with the data of Zagury et al. (6). The rate of hitting, λ, was estimated from data on the percentage of conjugates with at least one target cell hit. Then using that value of λ, the percentage of conjugates with at least two or at least three hit target cells was predicted [see Perelson and Bell (1) for details]. From Table 1 it is very clear that the simultaneous risk model does not fit the data. The predictions always underestimate the observed value. The sequential hit model gives a sufficiently good fit that it can be used as the basis of a model for the kinetics of target cell lysis.

Notice in Table 1 that both the simultaneous and sequential risk models predict that not all target cells are hit at the same time. Thus Zagury's observation that in individual LT_3 conjugates some but not all target cells were hit by time t provides insufficient information to conclude that hitting is sequential. For example, if Zagury had observed that 13% of LT_3 conjugates have 2 target cells hit and only 1% of LT_3 conjugates have 3 target cells hit by 5 min, he might have concluded that hitting was sequential. Yet as shown in Table 1, this is precisely what one would expect from a simultaneous risk model if there were some dispersion in the time at which each target cell was hit. It is only in conjunction with a quantitative model that an experiment such as Zagury's can be used to rigorously test the hypothesis that hitting is sequential.

TABLE 1

COMPARISON OF PREDICTIONS UNDER THE SEQUENTIAL (I) AND

SIMULTANEOUS (II) RISK MODELS WITH OBSERVATIONS

ON LETHAL HITTING IN LT_n CONJUGATES

	Percentage of Conjugates Exhibiting Lysis at 3 hr of at Least								
	Two Target Cells						Three Target Cells		
	LT_2			LT_3			LT_3		
Time of EDTA Addition (min)	Observed[c]	Predicted[a] I	II	Observed	Predicted[b] I	II	Observed	Predicted[b] I	II
3	26	26	15	ND[d]	8	6	ND	1	0.3
5	42	49	32	30	19	14	4	5	1
10	ND	84	65	ND	48	37	ND	22	7
15	92	96	84	80	69	58	45	43	17

[a] Using least squares estimate of $\lambda = 0.33$ min^{-1} from (1)
[b] Using least squares estimate of $\lambda = 0.16$ min^{-1} from (1)
[c] Measured by Zagury et al. (6)
[d] Not determined.

If our conclusion from the analysis of Zagury's data is correct and target cells within LT_n conjugates are hit sequentially, one needs to explain how a CTL focuses its attention on only one target cell, hits that cell, and then focuses on another cell that has not yet been hit. Zagury et al. (6) report that in LT_3 conjugates one target cell appears to be more firmly attached to the CTL than the other two. The tightly attached cell may be the one under attack. Sanderson (11,12) has shown that upon being lethally hit, target cells undergo zeiosis, spectacular blebbing of the membrane that gives the impression that the cell is boiling. By time-lapse cinematography Sanderson has shown the CTL remains in contact with a target cell up to the time of zeiosis; the target cell detaches at variable times after zeiosis begins; and in those cases where a target cell detaches without zeiosis occurring, the target cell did not die. We thus propose that after a lethal hit has been delivered, zeiosis breaks chemical bonds between surface structures on the CTL involved in cytolysis and target cell structures, and allows these surface structures (e.g., receptors) to redistribute on the CTL surface and bind a different target cell in the same conjugate. If a critical number of such bonds are necessary to trigger a lethal hit, then whichever of the remaining target cells accumulates enough bonds between itself and the CTL will be the next to be hit. The work by Dennert et al. (this volume) and others (14) indicates that the CTL orients its microtubule organizing center (MTOC) in the direction of the target cell under attack. In LT_n conjugates the MTOC is oriented toward a single target cell (Dennert, personal communication) and presumably reorients toward a new target cell once the target cell under attack has been hit. This reorientation might be triggered by a critical number of receptors diffusing away from the area of contact with the hit target cell and binding to an unhit one.

TARGET CELL DISINTEGRATION

Once lethally hit, we assume a target cell begins disintegrating. The length of time it takes a target cell to disintegrate is highly variable. To explain this variability Berke (2) suggested that target cell disintegration involves "an accumulative series of lethal events." Because the exact timing and number of lethal events leading to disintegration are unknown, we assume that at least some critical number, c, of events must occur, with each event taking a random length of time. If the critical events occur at a mean rate, μ, then according to the Poisson distribution the probability of at least c events occurring in d time units is

Pr(target disintegrates by d time units after being hit)

$$= 1 - \sum_{k=0}^{c-1} (\mu d)^k e^{-\mu d}/k! \quad . \tag{5}$$

If two events are required for disintegration, then the right side of Eq. (5) reduces to

$$1 - e^{-\mu d}(1 + \mu d) \quad .$$

LYSIS AS A TWO-STAGE PROCESS

Lysis consists of lethal hitting followed by target cell disintegration. Thus, to model the overall kinetics of the lytic process we must take into account the kinetics of both the lethal hitting and the disintegration stages of the process. Based upon the success of the sequential risk model in fitting the data of Zagury et al. (6), we shall assume that lethal hitting occurs sequentially. Macken and Perelson (4) combine Eqs. (4) and (5) to obtain an expression for the probability that, by time t, k target cells lyse in an LT_n conjugate. Fitting the resulting expression to data, we have found that the kinetics of target cell disintegration is described well by a model involving two, or possibly three, critical events. In Fig. 1 we compare the predictions of this two-stage model with data published by Zagury et al. (6).

To further test the model, we, in collaboration with B. Bonavida's group at UCLA, undertook a series of experiments involving multiple CTL bound to a single target cell (5). Reasoning that if each of the n CTL in an L_nT conjugate could deliver a lethal hit, then the CTL which hit first would be the one that programmed the target cell for lysis. Once hit, the target cell should then disintegrate with kinetics governed by Eq. (5). As shown in Fig. 2 the two-stage model gave excellent agreement with data, and again we found that disintegration involved at least two or three critical events. Further, we discovered that the mean time for a hit target cell to disintegrate, c/μ, decreased with the number of CTL bound per target cell until the number of CTL reached three (see Table 2). This result was rather surprising because it indicated that the rate of target cell disintegration depended upon the number of CTL in the conjugate. If disintegration were a killer cell independent event, then the rate of disintegration would not depend upon the number of CTL present. This finding thus suggests that the CTL affects the target cell after it has been lethally damaged. Sanderson (11) previously reached a similar conclusion. One possible explanation for our finding is that a single lethal hit does enough damage to eventually kill a target cell but that multiple CTL can inflict greater damage and thus hasten the target cell's ultimate destruction.

TABLE 2

No. CTL bound per target cell	Mean time for target cell disintegration (min)
1	52
2	39
3	27
4	28

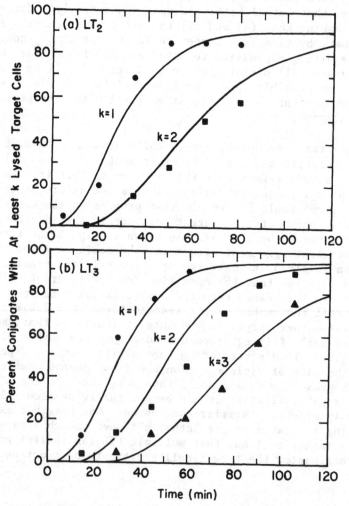

Fig. 1. The kinetics of target cell lysis in LT_2 and LT_3 conjugates. Data was taken from Ref. (6). The solid line is the best fitting theoretical curve obtained by non-linear regression. See (4) for details. Reproduced from (4) with permission.

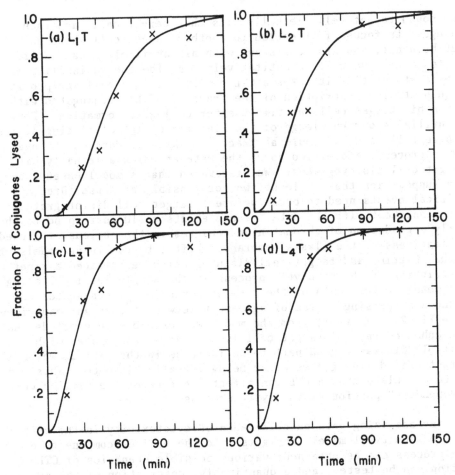

Fig. 2. The kinetics of target cell lysis in multiple lymphocyte-
target cell conjugates. The data points (x) indicate the
fraction of conjugates containing lysed target cells.
Ten separate experiments utilizing the single cell assay
of Grimm and Bonavida (13) were averaged to obtain the
indicated data points. The solid line is the best fitting
theoretical curve obtained by nonlinear regression. See
(5) for details. Reproduced from (5) with permission.

CONCLUSIONS

We have developed a quantitative model of T cell mediated
cytotoxicity at the single cell level. From the model a number of
insights have been gained. First, by examining alternative scenarios
of the lethal hitting process in conjugates containing multiple
target cells, we were able to rigorously rule out the possibility
that a CTL simultaneously attacks all bound target cells. Second,
we found that a scenario in which the CTL focuses its attention on

one bound target cell, lethally hits that target cell, and then changes its focus of attention to another target cell which has not yet been hit, appears consistent with all available data. Third, we found that we could quantitatively describe the variability in the length of time it takes a CTL to hit a target cell and provide a quantitative description of the fraction of LT_n conjugates with $m \leq n$ hit target cells at time t after conjugate formation. Fourth, by utilizing our knowledge of the kinetics of lethal hitting at the single cell level we could abstract from kinetic data on the overall lytic process information about the rate at which a lethally hit target cell disintegrates. We discovered that a model based upon the supposition that at least two, or possibly at least three, critical events need to occur before a target cell disintegrates was consistent with the data. These events could correspond to the early degradation of chromatin and changes in the nucleus, followed by leakiness of the plasma membrane. Fifth, by combining models of lethal hitting and target cell disintegration we obtained a kinetic description of the cytolytic process at the single level. Testing the model against data on the rate of lysis in LT conjugates we found a surprising degree of agreement between theory and experiment (see Fig.2). Further, from the model we were able to conclude that the enhanced rate of target cell lysis seen in conjugates with multiple CTL was due in part to an increase in the rate at which a target cell disintegrates after being lethally hit once. This led us to postulate that a CTL can affect the rate of the "killer cell independent" portion of the lytic process.

By analyzing data on cell mediated cytotoxicity in the context of a mathematical model, insights into the various components of the process can be obtained, various possible scenarios of CTL action can be tested, and a quantitative description of the overall process and its constituent parts can be obtained. Although our modeling and analysis has been confined to CTL·mediated lysis, a similar approach should find value in the analysis of NK mediated lysis.

ACKNOWLEDGMENT

We thank Carol England for cheerfully typing the camera-ready manuscript.

This work was performed under the auspices of the U.S. Department of Energy. A.S.P. is the recipient of an N.I.H. Research Career Development Award 5 K04 AI00450-05.

REFERENCES

1. Perelson, A. S., and G. I. Bell. 1982. Delivery of lethal
    hits by cytotoxic T lymphocytes in multicellular conjugates
    occurs sequentially but at random times. J. Immunol.
    129:2796.
2. Berke, G. 1980. Interaction of cytotoxic T lymphocytes and
    target cells. Prog. Allergy 27:69.
3. Russel, J. H. 1983. Internal disintegration model of
    cytotoxic lymphocyte-induced target damage. Immunol. Rev.
    72:97.
4. Macken, C. A., and A. S. Perelson. 1984. A multistage model
    for the action of cytotoxic T lymphocytes in multicellular
    conjugates. J. Immunol. 132:1614.
5. Perelson, A. S., C. A. Macken, E. A. Grimm, L. S. Roos, and B.
    Bonavida. 1984. Mechanism of cell-mediated cytotoxicity at
    the single cell level. VIII. Kinetics of lysis of target
    cells bound by more than one cytotoxic T lymphocyte.
    J. Immunol. 132:2190.
6. Zagury, D., J. Bernard, P. Jeannesson, N. Thiernesse, and
    J.-C. Cerottini. 1979. Studies on the mechanism of T
    cell-mediated lysis at the single effector cell level. I.
    Kinetic analysis of lethal hits and target cell lysis in
    multicellular conjugates. J. Immunol. 123:1604.
7. Martz, E. 1975. Early steps in specific tumor cell lysis by
    sensitized mouse T-lymphocytes. I. Resolution and
    characterization. J. Immunol. 115:261.
8. Martz, E. 1977. Mechanism of specific tumor-cell lysis by
    alloimmune T lymphocytes: resolution and characterization of
    discrete steps in the cellular interaction. Contemp. Top.
    Immunobiol. 7:301.
9. Martz, E., W. L. Parker, M. K. Gately, and C. D. Tsoukas.
    1982. The role of calcium in the lethal hit of T
    lymphocyte-mediated cytolysis. Adv. Exp. Med. Biol. 146:121.
10. Perelson, A. S., and C. A. Macken. 1984. Kinetics of cell
    mediated cytotoxicity: stochastic and deterministic models.
    Math. Biosci. In press.
11. Sanderson, C. J. 1981. The mechanism of T-cell mediated
    cytotoxicity. VIII. Zeiosis corresponds to irreversible phase
    (programming for lysis) in steps leading to lysis. Immunol.
    42:201.
12. Sanderson, C. J. 1982. Morphological aspects of lymphocyte
    mediated cytotoxicity. Adv. Exp. Med. Biol. 146:3.
13. Bonavida, B., T. P. Bradley, and E. A. Grimm. 1983. The
    single-cell assay in cell-mediated cytotoxicity. Immunol.
    Today 4:196.
14. Geiger, B., D. Rosen, and G. Berke. 1982. Spatial relation-
    ships of microtubule-organizing centers and the contact area
    of cytotoxic T lymphocytes and target cells. J. Cell Biol.
    95:137.

AUTHOR INDEX

Acha-Orbea, H, 99
Adams, D.O., 65, 74
Agpar, J.R., 387
Ameisen, J.C., 23
Anderson, C.G., 83
Anderson, D.C., 311
Auriault, C., 23

Berke, G., 473, 535
Bhakdi, S., 3
Blanca, I., 203
Bluestone, J., 121
Blumenthal, R. 121
Bonavida, B., 179, 193, 415
Brooks, C.G., 221
Burakoff, S.J., 311

Capron, A., 23
Capron, M, 23
Carson, D.A., 365
Cerottini, J.C., 343
Chervenak, R., 493
Christiaansen, J.E., 509
Cohen, J.J., 493

Deem, R.L., 239
Dennert, G., 83
Dick, M.D., 401
Duke, R.C., 493

Eisen, H.N., 429
Elsbach, P., 35
Evans, C.H., 281

Frederickse, P., 121

Gately, M.K., 401
Granger, D.L., 53
Grimm, E.A., 161
Gromkowski, S.H., 291

Hanna, M.G., Jr., 281
Hengartner, H., 99
Henkart, M., 121
Henkart, P., 121
Herberman, R.B., 203
Hibbs, J.B., Jr, 53
Hiserodt, J.C., 138
Howe, R.C., 453
Hudig, D., 271, 527

Johnson, W.J., 75
Jondal, M., 257
Joseph, M., 23

Kao, L., 35
Katz, J., 415
Kaufmann, Y., 535
Konigsberg, P.J., 99
Koprowski, H., 75
Krensky, A.M., 311
Kullman, C., 257
Kupfer, A, 83
Kusnierz, J.P., 23

Lehninger, A.L., 53
Lindgren, J.A., 257
Lotz, M., 365

MacDonald, H.R., 343
Macchi, B., 401

563

INDEX

Printed in the United States
by Baker & Taylor Publisher Services